ESSENTIALS OF HEALTH CARE FINANCE

Second Edition

William O. Cleverley, Ph.D.
Ohio State University

AN ASPEN PUBLICATION®
Aspen Publishers, Inc.

1986

Rockville, Maryland
Royal Tunbridge Wells

Library of Congress Cataloging in Publication Data

Cleverley, William O.
Essentials of health care finance.

"An Aspen publication."
Rev. ed. of: Essentials of hospital finance. 1978.
Includes bibliographies and index.
1. Hospitals—Finance. 2. Hospitals—Accounting. 3. Health facilities—Finance. 4. Health
facilities—Accounting. I. Cleverley, William O. Essentials of hospital finance. II. Title.
[DNLM: 1. Costs and Cost Analysis. 2. Financial Management. 3. Health Services—
economics. W 74 C635e]
RA971.3.C528   1986   362.1′068′1   86-14053
ISBN: 0-87189-374-6

Editorial Services: Carolyn Ormes

Library of Congress Catalog Card Number: 86-14053
ISBN: 0-87189-374-6

Printed in the United States of America

2 3 4 5

To my parents
James and Evelyn Cleverley

Table of Contents

Preface

This book is a major adaptation of an earlier book that I wrote, entitled *Essentials of Hospital Finance*. That book was very favorably received by both practitioners and students and appeared to fill a market void for an easy-to-understand elementary text on hospital finance. The book was published in 1978 and, like most things in life, has aged and become less useful. A large number of individuals convinced me that I should rewrite and expand the earlier text.

Among the reasons for rewriting was the major change in the payment environment facing most hospitals and other health care organizations. The initiation of the prospective payment system (PPS) by Medicare in 1983 was, of course, the single most important change, but it was not the only change. Many health care providers found that their basis for payment was changing in other market areas. Hospitals found themselves negotiating for discounts with health maintenance organizations and preferred provider organizations. Cost reimbursement was quickly becoming a very small, perhaps even a nonexistent, element of their total business.

So much of the financial management literature had evolved around a cost payment theme, and most of it was of little or no value. In many cases, the structure provided for financial decision making in a cost-reimbursed world was 180 degrees from the financial structure of today's health care firm. For example, capital financing decisions of the past were almost totally concerned with tax-exempt revenue bonds. Cost of financing was not especially critical because third party payers paid their proportion of total debt service cost. Emphasis was placed on the timing of debt principal payments in relation to reimbursed depreciation rather than on the absolute interest rate on the financing. Today, the mode of analysis is clearly different, and decisions reached based upon old algorithms of financial analysis could have catastrophic consequences.

Another reason for revision was related to the absence of problems in the original book. Many practitioners and students have told me that they learn finance best from working out real-life problems. The original book provided case examples in the narrative but did not include any assignment material for the reader to work on after reading a chapter. From my own teaching experiences, I realized that the need for such material was a very valid concern. Most of us learn quantitative disciplines by working out problems that relate to a particular area. Thus, the present book includes assignment material and solutions in each chapter. The solutions are included to enable those readers who are not involved in a formalized course of study an opportunity to test their knowledge and understanding of the material.

The original book was geared specifically to a hospital audience. Since 1978, however, it has become increasingly clear that we are not involved in the management of hospitals, but rather of health care firms. Most hospitals have already taken steps to diversify into new and expanding health care markets, such as long-term care and ambulatory care. This trend will clearly continue, and probably accelerate, in the future. The emphasis of the present book is on finance for health care firms in general, and it uses illustrations from different health care sectors to develop major points.

Finally, readers have suggested that the book be expanded to provide additional coverage on other topics. The initiation of PPS and the growing competition among hospitals have underscored the need for expanded coverage. For example, the original text provided minimal coverage on costing. Product costing and standard costing were not topics that health care executives thought very much about. Usually, products and services provided by hospitals and other health care firms were not sold on a fixed price basis, and they were not sold in competitive markets. This situation has clearly changed. The present text thus devotes four chapters to the general areas of costing and management control.

Similarly, strategic financial planning was not discussed in the earlier text because few firms engaged in any real long-range financial planning. There was not any major compelling reason to do so when financing could be arranged to meet almost all needs. However, strategic financial planning is clearly critical in today's environment, and a chapter is devoted to this topic in the revised text. Other additional topics have been included in existing chapters; for example, equity capital formation has been made a subtopic of the chapter on capital formation.

The ultimate objective of this book is to improve the understanding and use of financial information by decision makers in the health care industry. Informed and intelligent use of financial information is critical to the continued financial viability of all business firms. To this end, the comments and suggestions of readers and users of this volume are invited.

Acknowledgments

I am indebted to many individuals for their ideas and assistance in the development of this book. Without their help and guidance, its preparation and completion would clearly not have been possible.

I am especially thankful for the help of my students. They read the manuscript and pointed out many ways in which the material could be restructured to give greater emphasis to key points. They also worked out the problems to ensure that they are as error-free as possible. I would like especially to thank Anne Olsen in this regard. Anne spent considerable time reviewing the problems and their solutions and provided very valuable input.

Sara Toomey, Lee Bolzenius, and Kim Hayes provided skillful typing of material that was not always easy to produce or read.

I also want to thank the people at Aspen Publishers, Inc. This is the fourth book that I have done with them, and I am always impressed with their professionalism.

Finally, I want to acknowledge the support and love of my family. My wife Linda has always encouraged me in everything that I do. My three children—Michelle, Meredith, and Jamie—have been understanding when writing was difficult and my disposition was less than desirable.

Chapter 1

Financial Information and the Decision-Making Process

This book is intended to improve decision makers' understanding and use of financial information in the health care industry. It is not an advanced treatise in accounting or finance but an elementary discussion of how financial information in general, and health care industry financial information in particular, are interpreted and used. It is written for individuals who are not experienced health care financial executives. Its aim is to make the language of health care finance readable and relevant for general decision makers in the health care industry.

Three interdependent factors have created the need for this book:

1. rapid expansion of the health care industry
2. health care decision maker's general lack of business and financial background
3. financial and cost criteria's increasing importance in health care decisions

The health care industry's expansion is a trend visible even to individuals outside the health care system. The hospital industry, the major component of the health care industry, consumes about 4.5 percent of the Gross National Product; other types of health care systems, though smaller than the hospital industry, are expanding at even faster rates. Table 1–1 lists the types of major health care institutions and indexes their relative size.

The rapid growth of health care facilities providing direct medical services has substantially increased the number of decision makers who need to be familiar with financial information; even greater expansion in the number of decision makers indirectly involved in health care has compounded the need. Most of these decision makers work with health care regulations. Effective decision making in their jobs depends on an accurate interpretation of

1

Table 1-1 Health Care Expenditures 1974 –1984 (billions)

	1984	1974	% Change
Total health expenditures	384.3	116.3	230.4
Percentage of GNP	10.5	8.1	29.6
Health services and supplies:	368.2	108.9	238.1
Personal health care:	339.7	101.5	234.7
Hospital care	156.3	45.0	247.3
Physicians' services	76.1	21.2	259.0
Dentists' services	24.6	7.4	232.4
Other professional services	8.8	2.2	300.0
Drug and medical supplies	25.8	11.0	134.5
Eyeglasses and appliances	6.9	2.8	146.4
Nursing home care	31.4	8.5	269.4
Other health services	9.8	3.3	197.0
Expenses for prepayment and administration	16.1	4.7	242.6
Government public health	12.4	2.7	359.3
Research and construction	16.1	7.5	114.7

Source: Health Care Financing Administration, Office of Financial and Actuarial Analysis, Division of National Cost Estimates.

financial information. Many health care decision makers involved directly in health care delivery—doctors, nurses, dieticians, pharmacists, radiation technologists, physical therapists, inhalation therapists—are medically or scientifically trained but lack education and experience in business and finance. Their specialized education, in most cases, did not include such courses as accounting. However, advancement and promotion within health care organizations increasingly entails assumption of administrative duties, requiring almost instant knowledgeable reading of financial information. Communication with the organization's financial executives is not always helpful. As a result, nonfinancial executives often end up ignoring financial information.

Governing boards, significant users of financial information, are expanding in size in many health care facilities, in some cases to accommodate demands for more consumer representation. This trend can be healthy for both the community and the facilities. However, many board members, even those with backgrounds in business, are being overwhelmed by financial reports and statements. There are important distinctions between the financial statements of business organizations (with which some board members are familiar) and those of health care facilities that governing board members must recognize to carry out their governing mission satisfactorily.

Decision makers involved in regulation have also multiplied. These decision makers work primarily with quantitative information provided by the facilities they regulate; much of this information is financial, especially that from rate regulatory commissions. Many of these important and influential decision makers have some background in accounting and finance, but it may not be sufficient for their assigned tasks. In most situations, the agency staff serve only as a source of input for decisions that are made by a governing board. These boards usually represent a public constituency and may have little or no understanding of or experience with financial data. It is highly important for these individuals to have some minimum level of financial awareness if effective regulatory decisions are to be made.

The increasing importance of financial and cost criteria in health care decision making is the third factor creating a need for more knowledge of financial information. For many years, accountants and financial people have been caricatured as individuals with narrow vision, incapable of seeing the forest for the trees. In many respects, this may have been an accurate portrayal. However, few individuals in the health care industry today would deny the importance of financial concerns, especially cost. Careful attention to these concerns requires *knowledgeable* consumption of financial information by a variety of decision makers. It is not an overstatement to say that inattention to financial criteria can lead to excessive costs and eventually to insolvency.

INFORMATION AND DECISION MAKING

The major function of information in general, and financial information in particular, is to oil the decision-making process. Decision making is basically the selection of a course of action from a defined list of possible or feasible actions. In many cases, the actual course of action followed may be essentially no action—decision makers may decide to make no change from their present policies. It should be recognized, however, that both action and no action represent policy decisions.

Figure 1–1 shows how information is related to the decision-making process and gives an example to illustrate the sequence. Generating information is the key to decision making. The quality and effectiveness of decision making depends on accurate, timely, relevant information. It is important to note that the difference between data and information is more than semantic: data become information *only* when they are useful and appropriate to the decision. Many financial data never become information because they are not viewed as relevant or are unavailable in an intelligible form.

Figure 1–1 Information in the Decision-Making Process

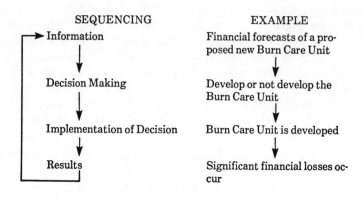

For the illustrative purposes of the burn care unit example in Figure 1–1, only two possible courses of action are assumed: to build or not build a burn care unit. In most situations, there may be a continuum of alternative courses of action. For example, a burn care unit might be varied by bed size or facilities included in the unit. In this case, prior decision making seems to have reduced the feasible set of alternatives to a more manageable and limited number for analysis.

Once a course of action has been selected in the decision-making phase, it must be accomplished. Implementing a decision may be extremely complex. In the burn care unit example, carrying out the decision to build the unit would require enormous management effort to ensure that the projected results are actually obtained. Periodic measurement of results in a feedback loop, as in Figure 1–1, is a method commonly used to make sure that decisions are actually implemented according to plan.

As previously stated, results that are forecast are not always guaranteed. Controllable factors, such as failure to adhere to prescribed plans, and uncontrollable circumstances, such as a change in reimbursement, may obstruct planned results.

Decision making is usually surrounded by uncertainty. No anticipated result of a decision is guaranteed. Events may occur that have been analyzed but not anticipated. A results matrix concisely portrays the possible results of various courses of action, given the occurrence of possible events. Table 1–2 provides a results matrix for the sample burn care unit; it shows that approximately 50 percent utilization will enable this unit to operate in the black and not drain resources from other areas. If forecasting shows that utilization below 50 percent is unlikely, decision makers may very well elect to build.

A good information system should enable decision makers to choose those courses of action that have the highest expectation of results. Based on the results matrix of Table 1–2, a good information system should specifically

- list possible courses of action
- list possible events that might occur, affecting the expected results
- indicate the probability of those events occurring
- accurately estimate the results, given an action/event combination (e.g., profit in Table 1–2)

One thing an information system does not do is evaluate the desirability of results. Decision makers must evaluate results in terms of their organizations' or their own preferences. For example, construction of a burn care unit may be expected to lose $200,000 a year, but it could save a significant number of lives. Weighing these results, or criteria, is purely a decision maker's responsibility—not an easy task, but one that can be improved with accurate and relevant information.

USES AND USERS OF FINANCIAL INFORMATION

As a subset of information in general, financial information is important in the decision-making process. In some areas of decision making, financial information is especially relevant. For our purposes, we identify five uses of financial information that may be important in decision making:

1. evaluating the *financial condition* of an entity
2. evaluating *stewardship* within an entity
3. assessing the *efficiency* of operations
4. assessing the *effectiveness* of operations
5. determining the *compliance* of operations with directives

Table 1–2 Results Matrix for the Burn Care Example

	Event		
Alternative Actions	*25% Utilization*	*50% Utilization*	*75% Utilization*
Build unit	$400,000 Loss	$10,000 Profit	$200,000 Profit
Do not build unit	0	0	0

Financial Condition

Evaluating an entity's financial condition is probably the most common use of financial information. Usually, an organization's financial condition is equated with its viability or capacity to continue pursuing its stated goals at a consistent level of activity. Viability is a far more restrictive term than solvency; some health care organizations may be solvent but not viable. For example, a hospital may have its level of funds restricted so that it must reduce its scope of activity but still remain solvent. A reduction in approved rates by a designated regulatory or rate setting agency may be the vehicle for this change in viability.

Assessing the financial condition of business enterprises is essential to our economy's smooth and efficient operation. Most business decisions in our economy are directly or indirectly based on perceptions of financial condition. This includes the largely nonprofit health care industry. Though attention is usually directed at organizations as whole units, assessment of the financial condition of organizational divisions is equally important. In the burn unit example, information on the future financial condition of the unit is valuable. If continued losses from this operation are projected, impairment of the financial condition of other divisions in the organization could be in the offing.

Assessing financial condition also includes consideration of short-run versus long-run effects. The relevant time frame may change, depending on the decision under consideration. For example, suppliers are typically interested only in an organization's short-run financial condition because that is the period in which they must expect payment. However, investment bankers, as long-term creditors, are interested in the organization's financial condition over a much longer time period.

Stewardship

Historically, evaluating stewardship was the most important use of accounting and financial information systems. These systems were originally designed to prevent the loss of assets or resources through employees' malfeasance. This use is still very important. In fact, the relatively infrequent occurrence of employee fraud and embezzlement may be due in part to the deterrence of well-designed accounting systems.

Efficiency

Efficiency in health care operations is becoming an increasingly important objective for many decision makers. Efficiency is simply the ratio of outputs to inputs—not the quality of outputs (good or not good) but the lowest possible cost of production. Adequate assessment of efficiency implies the availability of standards against which actual costs may be compared. In many health care organizations, these standards may be formally introduced into the budgetary process. Thus a given nursing unit may have an efficiency standard of 4.3 nursing hours per patient day of care delivered. This standard may then be used as a benchmark to evaluate the relative efficiency of the unit. For example, actual employment of 6.0 nursing hours per patient day may cause management to assess staffing patterns.

Effectiveness

Assessment of the effectiveness of operations is concerned with the attainment of objectives through production of outputs, not the relationship of outputs to cost. Measuring effectiveness is much more difficult than measuring efficiency because most organizations' objectives or goals are typically not stated quantitatively. Because measurement of effectiveness is difficult, there is a tendency to place less emphasis on effectiveness and more on efficiency. This may result in the delivery of unneeded services at an efficient cost. For example, development of outpatient surgical centers may reduce costs per surgical procedure and thus create an efficient means of delivery. However, the necessity of those surgical procedures may still be questionable.

Compliance

Finally, financial information may be used to determine whether compliance with directives has taken place. The best example of an organization's internal directives is its budget, an agreement between two management levels regarding use of resources for a defined time period. External parties may also impose directives, many of them financial in nature, for the organization's adherence. For example, rate-setting or regulatory agencies may set limits on rates determined within an organization. Financial reporting by the organization is required to ensure compliance.

Table 1–3 presents a matrix of users and uses of financial information in the health care industry. It identifies areas or uses that may interest particular decision-making groups. It does not consider relative importance.

Table 1–3 Users and Uses of Financial Information

Users	Uses				
	Financial Condition	Stewardship	Efficiency	Effectiveness	Compliance
External:					
Health system agencies	X		X	X	X
Unions	X		X		
Rate-setting organizations	X		X	X	X
Creditors	X		X	X	
Third party payers			X		X
Suppliers	X				
Public	X		X	X	
Internal:					
Governing board	X	X	X	X	X
Top management	X	X	X	X	X
Departmental management			X		X

Not every use of financial information is important in every decision. For example, in approving a health care organization's rates, a governing board may be interested in only two uses of financial information: (1) assessment of financial condition and (2) assessment of operational efficiency. Other uses may be irrelevant. The board wants to ensure that services are being provided efficiently and that the rates being established are sufficient to guarantee a stable or improved financial condition. As Table 1–3 illustrates, most health care decision-making groups use financial information to assess financial condition and efficiency.

FINANCIAL ORGANIZATION

It is important to understand the management organizational structure of businesses in general and health care organizations in particular. The Figure 1–2 chart outlines the management structure of a typical hospital. It illustrates the delegation of authority from the board of trustees through the president and downward to the various vice presidents and department heads.

Our primary attention is directed to the finance functions. The Financial Executives Institute (FEI) has categorized financial management functions as either controllership or treasurership. While few health care organizations have specifically identified treasurers and controllers at this time, the

Figure 1–2 Financial Organization Chart

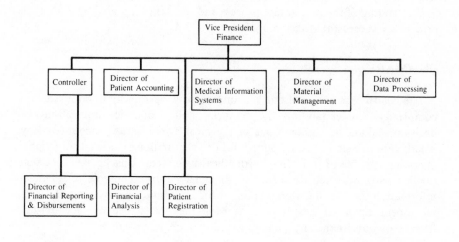

separation of duties is important to the understanding of financial management. The following describes functions in the two FEI categories:

1. Controllership

    - planning for control
    - reporting and interpreting
    - evaluating and consulting
    - tax administration
    - government reporting
    - protection of assets
    - economic appraisal

2. Treasurership

    - provision of capital
    - investor relations
    - short-term financing
    - banking and custody
    - credits and collections
    - investments
    - insurance

The effectiveness of financial management in any business is the product of many factors, such as environmental conditions, capabilities of personnel, and information quality. A major portion of the total financial management task is the provision of accurate, timely, and relevant information. Much of this activity is carried out through the accounting process. An adequate understanding of the accounting process and the data generated by it are thus critical to successful decision making.

SUMMARY

The health care sector of our economy is growing rapidly in both size and complexity. Understanding the financial and economic implications of decision making has become one of the most critical areas encountered by health care decision makers. Successful decision making can lead to a viable operation capable of providing needed health services. Unsuccessful decision making can and often does lead to financial failure. The role of financial information in the decision making process cannot be overstated. It is incumbent upon all health care decision makers to become accounting-literate in our financially changing health care environment.

ASSIGNMENTS

1. Only in recent years have hospitals begun to develop meaningful systems of cost accounting. Why did they not begin such development sooner?
2. Your hospital has been approached by a major employer in your market area to negotiate a preferred provider arrangement (PPA). The employer is seeking a 25 percent discount from your current charges. Describe a structure that you might use to summarize the financial implications of this decision. Describe the factors that would be critical in this decision.
3. What type of financial information should be routinely provided to board members?

SOLUTIONS AND ANSWERS

1. Prior to 1983, most hospitals were paid actual costs for delivering hospital services. With the introduction of Medicare's prospective payment system in 1983, hospitals now receive prices by diagnostic related groupings (DRGs) that are fixed in advance. Cost control, and therefore cost accounting, are critical in a fixed price environment.
2. This problem could be set up in a results matrix (see Table 1–2). The two actions to be charted are to accept or to reject the PPA opportunity. Possible events would center on the magnitude of volume changes, for example, to lose 1,000 patient days or gain 500 patient days. A key concern in estimating the financial impact would be the hospital's incremental revenue and incremental cost positions. In short, how large would the revenue reduction and cost reduction be if significant volume were lost? Actual gains or losses of business would be functions of the hospital's market position.
3. Board members do not need to see detailed financial statements on a routine basis. They need to see financial information that relates to their established plans to ensure that the plans are being met. If significant deviations have occurred, more details may be necessary to take corrective action or to modify established plans.

Chapter 2

Financial Environment of Health Care Organizations

Almost any measure of size would indicate that the health care industry is big business. Its proportion of the Gross National Product has been steadily increasing for several decades and now represents 10.5 percent of GNP. Paralleling this growth, the pressures for cost control within the system have increased tremendously. Health care organizations that are not able to deal effectively with these pressures face an uncertain future. In short, as the expected demand for health services continues to rise over the next several decades as our population ages, successful health care organizations must become increasingly cost-efficient.

FINANCIAL VIABILITY

Health care organizations (HCOs) are basic providers of health services, but they are also businesses. The environment of an HCO viewed from a financial perspective could be schematically represented as follows:

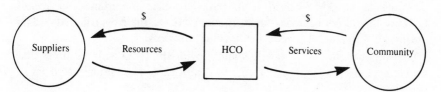

In the long run, the HCO must receive dollar payments from the community in an amount at least equal to the dollar payments it makes to its suppliers. In very simple terms, this is the essence of financial viability.

The community in the above schematic is the provider of funds to the HCO. The flow of funds is either directly or indirectly related to the delivery of services by the HCO. For our purposes, the community may be categorized as follows:

1. Patients
   a. Self-pay
   b. Third party

      • Blue Cross and Blue Shield
      • commercial insurance
      • Medicaid
      • Medicare
      • self-insured employer
      • other

2. Nonpatients
   a. grants
   b. contributions
   c. tax support
   d. miscellaneous

In most HCOs, the great proportion of funds is derived from patients who directly receive services. The largest percentage of these payments usually comes from third party sources, such as Blue Cross, Medicare, and Medicaid. In addition, some nonpatient sources of funds are derived from government sources in the form of grants for research purposes or direct payments in subsidized HCOs, such as county facilities. Some HCOs also receive significant sums of money from individuals, foundations, or corporations in the form of contributions. While these sums may be small relative to the total amounts of money received from patients, their importance in overall viability should not be understated. In many HCOs, these contributed dollars mean the difference between net income and loss.

The suppliers in the above schematic provide the HCO with resources that are necessary in the delivery of quality health care. The major categories of suppliers are:

• employees
• equipment suppliers
• service contractors
• vendors of consumable supplies
• lenders

Payments for employees are usually the largest single category of expenditures. For example, in many hospitals, payments for employees represent about 60 percent of total expenditures. Table 2–1 is an actual income statement for a hospital, showing percentages of revenues and expenses. Payments for physicians' services also represent important financial requirements. In addition, lenders such as commercial banks or investment bankers, supply dollars in the form of loans and receive from the HCO a promise to repay the loans with interest according to a defined repayment schedule. This financial requirement has grown steadily as HCOs have become more dependent upon debt financing.

SOURCES OF OPERATING REVENUE

Table 2–2 provides a historical breakdown of the relative size of the health care industry and its individual industrial segments. The largest segment is the hospital industry, which absorbs about 40 percent of all health care expenditure dollars. This percentage has been declining over the last few years and is expected to decline further as other industry segments grow faster. The physician segment absorbs approximately 19 percent of total health care expenditures; this represents a modest increase over the last decade when expressed as a percentage of total health care expenditures. Nursing homes represent the third largest health care segment, constituting about 8 percent of all health care expenditures. Many individuals believe future growth will be the fastest in this segment as the population ages.

Table 2–3 depicts the sources of operating funds for the three largest health care segments: hospitals, physicians, and nursing homes. Dramatic differences in financing among these three segments can be easily seen.

The hospital industry derives more than 50 percent of its total funding from public sources, largely Medicare and Medicaid. Of the two, Medicare is by far the larger, representing about 27 percent of all hospital revenue. This gives the federal government enormous control over hospitals and their financial positions. Few hospitals can choose to ignore the Medicare program because of its sheer size. Another 38 percent of total hospital funding results from private insurance (largely Blue Cross), commercial insurance carriers, and self-insured employers. Direct payments by patients to hospitals represent approximately 7.5 percent of total revenue. The implications of this distribution for hospitals is the creation of an oligopsonistic marketplace. The buying power for hospital services is concentrated in relatively few third party purchasers; namely the federal government, the state government, Blue Cross, a few commercial insurance carriers, and some large self-insured employers.

Table 2–1 Statement of Revenue and Expenses, Memorial Hospital, Year Ended June 30, 1986

	1986	Percentage
Operating revenue:		
Gross patient service revenue	$25,960,705	100.0
Allowances	1,484,550	5.7
Provision for uncollectible accounts	806,667	3.1
	2,291,217	8.8
Net patient service revenue	23,669,488	91.2
Other operating revenue	567,271	2.2
	24,236,759	93.4
Operating expenses:		
Salaries and wages	11,729,643	45.2
Employee benefits	1,767,041	6.8
Supplies and purchased services	8,122,005	31.2
Depreciation and amortization	1,263,284	4.9
Interest	1,345,140	5.2
	24,227,113	93.3
Excess (deficiency) of operating revenue over expenses	9,646	.1
Nonoperating revenue:		
Investment income on board-designated assets	226,576	.9
Unrestricted gifts and bequests	102,588	.4
Other nonoperating revenue	131,747	.5
Gain (loss) on sale of board-designated investments	(5,325)	–.–
Net rental income after depreciation, interest, and other expenses	12,230	–.–
	467,816	1.8
Excess of revenue over expenses before cumulative effect of change in accounting method	477,462	1.9
Cumulative effect on prior years of change in accounting method—Note F[a]	(199,841)	(.8)
Excess of revenue over expenses	$ 277,621	1.1

[a]See notes to financial statements

The physician marketplace is somewhat different from the marketplace for hospital services. A much larger percentage of physician funding is derived from direct payments by patients—approximately 28 percent. And, compared with hospital funding, a slightly larger percentage of physician funding

Table 2–2 National Health Care Expenditures

	Selected Years					
	1984	*1983*	*1982*	*1981*	*1980*	*1974*
	(billions)					
Total health expenditures	$384.3	$355.4	$322.3	$285.8	$248.0	116.3
	(percentage)					
Gross National Product	10.50	10.80	10.50	9.70	9.40	8.10
Health services and supplies:	95.81	95.69	95.59	95.42	95.20	93.64
Personal health care	88.39	88.15	88.33	88.77	88.35	87.27
Hospital care	40.67	41.42	41.86	41.25	40.85	38.69
Physicians' services	19.80	19.41	19.17	19.17	18.87	18.23
Dentists' services	6.40	6.13	6.05	6.05	6.21	6.36
Other professional services	2.28	2.25	2.20	2.24	2.26	1.89
Drug and medical supplies	6.71	6.67	6.76	7.17	7.46	9.46
Eyeglasses and appliances	1.80	1.74	1.71	1.96	2.06	2.41
Nursing home care	8.17	8.10	8.22	8.36	8.23	7.31
Other health services	2.55	2.39	2.36	2.45	2.38	2.84
Expenses for prepayment & administration	4.19	4.39	4.16	3.71	3.71	4.04
Government public health	3.23	3.15	3.10	3.01	3.10	2.32
Research and construction	4.19	4.31	4.41	4.62	4.80	6.45

Source: Health Care Financing Administration, Office of Financial and Actuarial Analysis, Division of National Cost Estimates.

results from private insurance sources, largely Blue Shield and commercial insurance carriers. Physicians derive approximately 44 percent of their total funds from this source, compared with 38 percent in the hospital segment. Public programs, while still significant, are the smallest source of physician funding, representing less than 28 percent of total funds. This situation results because more physician services, such as routine physical exams and many deductible and copayment services, are excluded from Medicare payment.

The nursing home segment realizes almost no funding from private insurance sources. Its source of funding is split almost equally between public programs and direct payments by or on behalf of patients. The major public program for nursing homes is Medicaid, not Medicare. Medicare payments to nursing homes are largely restricted to skilled nursing care, while the majority of Medicaid payments to nursing homes are for intermediate-level care.

Table 2–3 Sources of Health Services Funding, 1983

	Hospitals		Nursing Homes		Physicians	
	Dollars (billions)	Percent	Dollars (billions)	Percent	Dollars (billions)	Percent
Total expenditures	147.2	100.00	28.8	100.00	69.0	100.00
Private expenditures:	68.8	46.74	14.9	51.74	49.7	72.03
Direct payments	11.1	7.54	14.4	50.00	19.6	28.41
Insurance	56.2	38.18	0.3	1.04	30.1	43.62
Other	1.5	1.02	0.2	0.69	0.0	0.00
Public expenditures:	78.4	53.26	14.0	48.61	19.3	27.97
Medicare	40.4	27.45	0.5	1.74	13.4	19.42
Medicaid	13.6	9.24	12.4	43.06	2.9	4.20
Other medical care	0.7	0.48	0.5	1.74	0.2	.29
Veterans	6.3	4.28	0.5	1.74	0.1	.14
Department of Defense	5.3	3.60	0.0	0.00	2.1	3.04
Workers compensation	2.6	1.77	0.0	0.00	0.2	.29
State and local hospital	7.9	5.37	0.0	0.00	0.0	0.00
Other personal care	1.7	1.15	0.0	0.00	0.3	.43

Source: Health Care Financing Administration, Office of Financial and Actuarial Analysis, Division of National Cost Estimates.

HOSPITAL PAYMENTS SYSTEMS

One of the most important financial differences between hospitals and other businesses is the way in which its customers or patients make payment for the services they receive. Most businesses have only one basic type of payment: billed charges. Each customer is presented with a bill that represents the product of the quantity of goods or services received and their appropriate prices. Some selective discounting of the price may take place to move slow inventory during slack periods or to encourage large volume orders. The basic payment system, however, remains the same: a fixed price per unit of service that is set by the business, not the customer.

In contrast, the typical hospital may have four or more different payment systems in effect at any given time. Each of these payment systems has a different effect upon the hospital's financial position and might lead to different conclusions with respect to business strategy. It is thus extremely important to understand the financial implications of the various payment systems used by hospitals. The four major payment systems to be discussed here are:

1. historical cost reimbursement
2. specific services (charge payment)

3. negotiated bids
4. diagnosis related group

Historical Cost Reimbursement

Until recently, historical cost reimbursement was the predominant form of payment for most hospitals. In addition to Medicare, most state Medicaid plans and a large number of Blue Cross plans paid hospitals on the basis of "reasonable" historical costs. Today, the major payers are abandoning historical cost reimbursement and substituting other payment systems. However, historical cost reimbursement still exists and in some hospitals may represent a significant proportion of total revenue.

Two key elements in historical cost reimbursement are reasonable cost and apportionment. Reasonable cost is simply a qualification introduced by the payer to limit its total payment. Examples of costs often defined as unreasonable and therefore not reimbursable are costs for charity care, patient telephones, and nursing education. Apportionment refers to the manner in which costs are assigned or allocated to a specific payer such as Medicaid. For example, assume a hospital has total reasonable costs of $10 million that represents the costs of servicing all patients. If Medicaid is a historical cost reimbursement payer, an allocation or apportionment of that $10 million is necessary to determine Medicaid's share of the total cost. Quite often, the apportionment is related to charges. For example, if charges for services to Medicaid patients were $3 million and total charges to all patients were $15 million, then $3/15$ or 20 percent of the $10 million cost would be apportioned to Medicaid.

Several important financial principles of cost reimbursement should be emphasized. First, cost reimbursement can insulate management somewhat from the financial results of poor financial planning. New clinical programs that do not achieve targeted volume or exceed projected costs may still be viable because of extensive cost reimbursement. This assumes the payer does not regard the costs as unreasonable. Second, cost reimbursement can often be increased through careful planning, just as taxes can often be reduced through tax planning. The key objective is to maximize the amount of cost apportioned to cost payers subject to any tests for reasonableness.

Specific Services

Usually, a portion of a hospital's patients make payment based upon charges for the specific services provided, such as nursing, surgery, pharmacy, or laboratory. These charges may be regulated by external parties, such as state rate-setting commissions, or they may be completely unregulated and left to the discretion of hospital management. Commercial insurance carriers, self-insured employers, and self-pay patients are usually the largest sources of specific services payment.

Specific services payment has several important implications for financial management. First, specific services revenue may represent the major source of profit to the hospital. In this case, pricing or rate setting becomes an important hospital policy (rate setting is addressed later in this chapter). Second, the hospital's rate structure should be based on projected volume and cost factors. Any unexpected deviation from the hospital's plan merits prompt attention.

Negotiated Bids

Negotiated bids represent a new type of payment for many hospitals. This type of payment results from a specific contractual arrangement between the hospital and a payer. A special contract with a health maintenance organization or a local employer are common examples of a negotiated bid arrangement. In some states, Medicaid might also be considered a source of negotiated-bid revenue. For example, in 1983, California hospitals bid for Medicaid contracts on the basis of rate per patient day. Hospitals that submitted low bids (e.g., a low rate per patient day) would often receive contracts to provide hospital services to Medicaid patients in a given area.

In a negotiated-bid payment environment, financial planning and control are critical—even more critical than in a specific services payment situation. The fee arrangement is usually contractually fixed for a period of time, usually a year. Unexpected increases in costs will not usually be a basis for contract renegotiation. Cost accounting and analysis are also important. It is imperative that management knows what it costs to provide a unit of service required in the contract. For example, if the negotiated bid is to provide all hospital services to subscribers of a health maintenance organization for a fixed fee per subscriber, the hospital must know both the volume and the cost of the required services. Ideally, the cost accounting system should define the incremental costs likely to be incurred in a given contract so that they can be compared to the incremental revenue likely to result from the contract.

Diagnosis Related Groups

Payment by diagnosis related group (DRG) became universal for hospitals in 1983 when Medicare initiated payment on this basis. Because of the sheer size of the Medicare program in most hospitals, hospital management was quickly forced to become familiar with the DRG payment system. In the Medicare DRG payment system, specific prices are established for 467 specific diagnostic categories. These prices are updated each year by Medicare to reflect inflationary changes.

From the hospital's perspective, the prices established by Medicare are fixed and not appealable. The hospital may decide not to continue providing a given DRG service because it loses money, but it cannot get Medicare to change prices in specific DRGs.

The financial implications of DRG payment are fairly clear. First, cost control becomes critical to long-term financial viability. Hospitals must produce a given DRG at a reasonable cost. There are four primary ways that cost for a DRG can be reduced:

1. Reduce the prices paid for resources.
2. Reduce the length of stay.
3. Reduce the intensity of service provided.
4. Improve production efficiency.

It is important to note that two of the four methods for DRG cost reduction involve medical staff decision making, namely reducing length of stay and reducing service intensity. It is thus necessary that hospital management focus more intensely on product lines. Ultimately, hospitals need to analyze the relative profitability of given DRGs comprising particular clinical services, such as psychiatry or surgery. Clearly, cost accounting by DRG is essential to any intelligent analysis of relative DRG profitability. Hospital cost accounting systems are usually structured around departments, such as dietary, laboratory, and physical therapy. However, DRGs require services from a number of departments, and therefore costs must be assigned from these departments to individual DRGs. This is no small problem, and accurate cost information is essential.

RATE SETTING

Stages in the Rate-Setting Process

Rate setting is an extremely complex and important management activity. The success or failure of the organization may ultimately depend on the quality of management decision making in this area. Assuming that reasonably accurate projections of both output and expense are available, there are at least three stages in the rate-setting process:

1. determining required net income
2. determining patient payment composition
3. determining bad debt and charity deductions

In most situations, net income is essential to the viability of the organization. The real issue is how much net income is acceptable. In this short discussion, it is not possible to answer this question in detail. However, in general, the rates must be established at levels that will meet budgeted financial requirements, that is:

Budgeted financial requirements = Total operating revenue

where:

Total operating revenue = Gross patient service revenue − Allowances and uncollectibles + Other operating revenue

The required amount of income can now be defined as:

Required net income = Budgeted financial requirements − Budgeted operating expenses

It should be noted that the above calculations ignore the existence of nonoperating revenue. It sizable and stable sums of nonoperating revenue are available, they may be used to subsidize operations. This is clearly an important policy determination and should be made by the board after a careful consideration of projected financial plans.

Budgeted financial requirements are cash requirements or expenditures that an entity must meet during the budget period. These requirements usually comprise four elements:

1. budgeted expenses, excluding depreciation
2. requirements for debt principal payment
3. requirements for increases in working capital
4. requirements for capital expenditures

Budgeted expenses at the departmental level should include both direct and indirect or allocated expenses. Depreciation charges are excluded because depreciation is an expense, not an expenditure; it does not require an actual cash outlay.

Debt principal payments include only the principal portion of debt service due. In some cases, additional reserve requirements may be established, and these may require additional funding. Interest expense is already included in budgeted expenses and should not be included in this category.

Working capital requirements include such things as necessary build-ups in inventory, accounts receivable, and precautionary cash balances. Planned financing of increases in working capital is a legitimate financial requirement.

Capital expenditure requirements may be of two types. First, actual capital expenditures may be made for approved projects. Those projects not financed with indebtedness require a cash investment. Second, prudent fiscal management requires that funds be set aside and invested to meet reasonable requirements for future capital expenditures. This amount should be related to the replacement cost depreciation of existing fixed assets. An HCO should fund some proportion of its replacement cost depreciation.

Determination of the patient payment composition is the next important stage in effective rate setting. It must be remembered that not all patients will actually pay the rates established. Many third party payers—especially Blue Cross, Medicare, and Medicaid—do not pay billed charges. Therefore, the rate structure should incorporate the effect of these contractual allowances in the establishment of rates.

Finally, an estimation of write-offs for bad debts must be made. Just as most third party payers do not pay billed charges, some self-pay patients may not pay all of their bills. Significant amounts of bad debts or charity care are especially common in hospitals with large outpatient operations and in hospitals that service medically indigent patients.

A Rate-Setting Model

It is possible to develop a very simple but realistic rate setting model based on the above discussion. In algebraic form, revenue should be determined as follows:

$$\text{Revenue} = \frac{\text{Budgeted expenses} + \text{Desired net income} - \text{Noncharge paying patient payments}}{\text{Proportion of charge paying patients}}$$

The following example may help illustrate this formula. Let us assume that a hospital has 20 patients in the following payment categories:

DRG payment patients	10
Cost payment patients	4
Charity care patients	1
Charge payment patients	5
	20

Further, assume that the hospital has budgeted operating expenses of $22,000, or $1,100 per patient, and the DRG payment rate is $1,000 per patient. If the hospital needs to earn a $3,000 net income, it must set its rates as follows:

$$\text{Revenue} = \frac{\$22,000 + 3,000 - 10,000 - 4,400}{.25}$$

$$= \$42,400 \text{ or } \$2,120 \text{ per patient}$$

The following income statement would result if the above expectations were realized:

Gross patient revenue:

DRG patients (10 × $2,120)	$21,200
Cost patients (4 × $2,120)	8,480
Charity patients (1 × $2,120)	2,120
Charge patients (5 × $2,120)	10,600
Total	$42,400

Allowances and uncollectibles:

DRG patients [10 × (2,120 − $1,000)]	$11,200
Cost patients [4 × ($2,120 − $1,100)]	4,080
Charity patients [1 × ($2,120 − 0)]	2,120
Charge patients [5 × ($2,120 − $2,120)]	0
Total	$17,400
Net patient revenue	$25,000
Operating expenses	$22,000
Net operating income	$ 3,000

A number of conclusions can be drawn from this example. First, rates may often be significantly above actual expenses. The hospital in this example had a rate structure that was almost 100 percent above its expenses, but it realized just $3,000 or 7 percent of its gross patient revenue as income. Health care executives and board members should not be surprised by this occurrence. Secondly, payer subsidies clearly exist. In this example, charge paying patients paid almost twice the rate of cost patients ($1,100) and more than twice the rate of DRG patients ($1,000). Third, the impact of charity care is directly related to the marginal cost of providing that care. In our example, removing the one charity care patient with no resulting reduction in expense would change required rates only marginally:

$$\text{Revenue} = \frac{\$22,000 + 3,000 - 10,000 - 4,632}{5/19}$$

$$= \$39,398 \text{ or } \$2,073.60 \text{ per patient}$$

However, removing $1,100 of cost (the average cost of treating one patient) would lead to a sizable reduction in rates:

$$\text{Revenue} = \frac{\$20,900 + 3,000 - 10,000 - 4,400}{5/19}$$

$$= \$36,100 \text{ or } \$1,900 \text{ per patient}$$

Finally, it should be noted that reductions in operating expenses can lead to sizable reductions in required rates if the percentage of cost patients is relatively low. In our example, a 10 percent reduction in operating expense ($2,200) would yield a 17 percent reduction in rate per patient:

$$\text{Revenue} = \frac{\$19,800 + 3,000 - 10,000 - 3,960}{.25}$$

$$= \$35,360 \text{ or } \$1,768 \text{ per patient}$$

Cost reduction has in fact become a primary objective for many hospitals as their percentage of cost payment business declines.

THE MEDICARE PROSPECTIVE PAYMENT SYSTEM FOR HOSPITALS

It is somewhat risky to describe in detail the mechanics of Medicare's prospective payment system (PPS), given the fact that the system is still evolving. However, the enormous impact that this payment system has on the entire health care system dictates that some attempt be made here to examine its operation and implications. Still, readers are cautioned that the information provided here may not be accurate at the time of reading.

PPS was officially launched by Medicare on October 1, 1983. All hospitals participating in the Medicare program are required to participate in PPS, except:

- psychiatric hospitals
- rehabilitation hospitals
- children's hospitals
- long-term care hospitals
- distinct psychiatric and rehabilitation units
- hospitals outside the 50 states
- hospitals in states with an approved waiver

PPS provides payment for all hospital nonphysician services provided to hospital inpatients. This payment also covers services provided by outside suppliers, such as laboratory or radiology units. Medicare makes one comprehensive payment to the hospital, which is then responsible for paying outside suppliers or nonphysician services.

The basis of PPS payment is the diagnosis related grouping (DRG) system developed by Yale University. The DRG system takes all possible diagnoses from the ICD-9-CM system and classifies them into 23 major diagnostic categories based on organ systems. These 23 categories are further broken down into 467 distinct medically meaningful groupings or DRGs (Appendix 2–A contains a list of the 467 DRGs). Medicare contends that the resources required to treat a given DRG entity should be similar for all patients within a DRG category.

Total payments to a hospital under Medicare can be split into two components: (1) the prospective portion and (2) the reasonable cost portion. The prospective portion in turn encompasses three factors: (1) DRG payments, (2) indirect medical education payments, and (3) outlier payments (see Figure 2–1).

DRG payments result from the multiplication of the hospital dollar rate and the specific case weight of an actual DRG. For example, assume that a hospital with a dollar rate of $3,000 treated DRG #1 (craniotomy age > 17 except for trauma), which has a case weight of 3.3548. The actual DRG payment would be $3,000 × 3.3548 = $10,064.40.

Figure 2–1 Breakdown of Medicare Payments to a Hospital

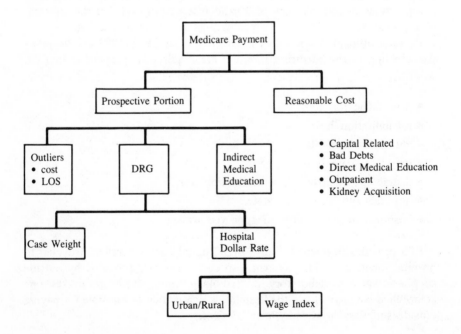

The hospital's dollar rate is a unique value assigned to a hospital. It is a function of (1) urban/rural status and (2) the wage index of its location. In the transition years of PPS, a hospital's dollar rate was also affected by its 1982 base year cost and its geographic region. However, these two factors have now been eliminated.

The indirect medical education allowance is a percentage added to the DRG payment, based on the number of full-time equivalent (FTE) interns/residents and beds the hospital has. At the time of this writing, the percentage was calculated as follows:

$$11.59\% \times 10 \times \frac{\text{FTE interns and residents}}{\text{Beds}}$$

Thus, a hospital with 400 beds and 50 FTE interns and residents would receive a separate add-on percentage of 14.4875. Applying this rate to our DRG #1 example would mean an additional payment of $1,458.08 (.144875 × $10,064.40). The rationale for this separate add-on is the recognition that teaching hospitals often utilize more tests and procedures. Some of this extra cost is due to teaching activities; some of it may also be due to care for severely ill patients.

Outlier payments, the last element in the prospective portion, are authorized in those cases in which either the patient's length of stay is unusually long or the patient's actual costs are considerably above the approved DRG rate. Outlier payments for length-of-stay (LOS) deviations are permitted when the actual LOS exceeds the Medicare mean by 20 days or 1.94 standard deviations, whichever is less. In the case of DRG #1, if the 20-day criterion were used, a patient would need to stay in the hospital beyond 39 days (19.4 + 20) before any additional payment would be made. After the 39th day, a per diem rate equal to 60 percent of the average cost would be paid.

Thus, in our example, a patient with a 50-day LOS for DRG #1 would produce the following outlier payment to the hospital:

$$(50-39) \times \frac{\$10,064.40 \times .60}{19.4} = \$3423.97$$

The multiplication by 60 percent reflects the fact that only a portion of the hospital's cost is variable. Medicare assumes that the variable costs of outlier patients are 60 percent; alternatively, it assumes that the fixed costs are 40 percent.

Calculations for cost outliers are quite complex and beyond the scope of this book. As in the case of LOS outliers, only the cost beyond the cut-off point is reimbursed, and then only at 60 percent. For example, a cost outlier with a $60,000 total cost and a cut-off cost value of $20,000 would generate only $24,000 additional reimbursement (.60 × $40,000).

There is still a portion of the total Medicare payment that is related to reasonable cost (see Figure 2–1). Costs that are still paid for on this basis include:

- direct medical education costs
- kidney acquisition costs
- bad debts for copayments and deductibles
- outpatient costs
- capital-related costs

Capital related costs—largely depreciation, interest, leases, rentals, and returns on equity payments to investor-owned hospitals—are expected eventually to be included in the prospective payment portion. At this writing, however, they were still paid for on a reasonable cost basis.

To complete this quick review of the Medicare PPS, a number of additional key terms and concepts should be explained:

- *Sole community hospitals* (SCHs). Hospitals that are designated as SCHs are still in PPS, but they may opt for special treatment. They may have 75 percent of their dollar rate based upon their specific costs in the base year and only 25 percent related to national rates.
- *Referral centers.* A hospital in a rural area that is designated as a referral center substitutes urban rates for its rural rate. Since urban rates are higher, this is a significant advantage.
- *Peer review organizations* (PROs). PROs are designated by Medicare to review the validity of an actual DRG assignment, the quality of the care provided, and the appropriateness of the admission and discharge. All hospitals must contract with a PRO to receive Medicare payments.
- *DRG Recalibration.* At least every four years, the DRG classification and weighting factors must be changed. These changes reflect changes in technology, treatment patterns, and other factors affecting resource utilization.
- *Principal diagnosis.* The principal diagnosis is the diagnosis of the condition that was responsible for the patient's admission. This factor is integral to the actual DRG assignment.
- *Physician attestation.* Medicare regulations require that the attending physician attest in writing to the principal diagnosis, the secondary

diagnosis, and the names of the procedures performed before the fiscal intermediary assigns a DRG code and initiates payment.

- *DRG gaming.* DRG gaming is a term that describes attempts by hospitals to get patients assigned to DRG categories with higher case mix weights. The hospital attempts to do this through the assignment of the principal and secondary diagnoses, which must be attested to by the attending physician.

SUMMARY

Compared with most businesses, health care organizations are financially complex. Not only do they provide a large number of specific services, but their individual services often have different effective price structures. One customer may choose to pay on the basis of cost while another may pay full charges. This variation in payment patterns creates problems in the establishment of prices for products and services. Indeed, the revenue function of a typical health care entity is usually much more complex than that of a comparably sized non-health care business.

Health care entities also depend quite heavily upon a very limited number of key clients for most of their operating funding. Their largest client is often the federal government or the state government. Doing business with the government involves a significant amount of reporting to ensure compliance and adherence to government regulations. Moreover, since the federal government is such a large purchaser of services, a thorough understanding of the nature and implications of the Medicare payment system's rules and regulations is a must for effective management of a health care organization.

Yet, though health care organizations may be complex from a financial perspective, they are still businesses. Their financial viability requires the receipt of funds in amounts sufficient to meet their financial requirements.

ASSIGNMENTS

1. What is the prospective amount that would be paid to ABC Medical Center for treating DRG #39 (Lens Procedure)? Assume that the hospital has an effective dollar rate per case weight of one equal to $3,500. Assume further that the case is not an outlier. Finally, assume that the hospital is a teaching hospital with 100 FTE residents and 400 beds.

2. From the following data, determine the amount of revenue that needs to be generated to meet hospital financial requirements:

Volume:

Medicare cases	1000
Cost payment cases	400
Charity care and bad debt cases	100
Charge paying cases	500
Total cases	2000

Financial data:

Budgeted expenses	$6,000,000
Debt principal payment	200,000
Working capital increase	250,000
Capital expenditures	400,000

Present payment structure:

- Medicare pays only $2,800 per case, or a total of $2,800,000.
- All other cost payers pay their share of existing expenses.

3. Why is the accumulation of funded reserves for capital replacement more critical for nonprofit health care entities than for investor-owned health care facilities?

4. Rural hospitals receive less payment for specific DRGs than urban hospitals. What might be the rationale to justify these differences?

5. Depreciation expense is recognized as a reimbursable cost by a number of payers who pay prospective rates for operating costs. Would you prefer accelerated depreciation (sum of the year's digits) or price-level depreciation for a five-year-life asset with a $150,000 cost? Assume that inflation is projected to be six percent per year.

6. Nonprofit organizations should not make profits; instead, either their rates should be reduced or their services expanded. Evaluate the choices.

7. Using the data from Problem 2 above, calculate the impact of a ten percent reduction in operating expenses, that is, down to $5,400,000, upon the required revenue and rate structure. Discuss the implications of your findings.

SOLUTIONS AND ANSWERS

1. Payment would be calculated as follows:
    DRG payment:

    Case weight $\times$ Dollar rate = DRG payment

    $.5010 \times \$3,500.00 = \$1,753.50$

    Indirect medical education payment:

    Indirect medical education proportion $\times$ DRG payment
        = Indirect medical education payment

    $$\left[.1159 \times 10 \times \frac{100}{400}\right] \times \$1,753.50 = \$508.08$$

    Total payment:

    $\$1,753.50 + 508.08 = \$2,261.58$

2. The relevant calculation is as follows:

$$\text{Revenue} = \frac{\text{Budgeted expenses} + \text{Desired net income} - \text{Noncharge paying patient payments}}{\text{Proportion of charge paying patients}}$$

$$\text{Revenue} = \frac{\$6,000,000 + \$850,000 - \$4,000,000}{.25}$$

$$= \$11,400,000 \text{ or } \$5,700 \text{ per case}$$

Desired net income = $850,000 = $200,000 + $250,000 + $400,000

Noncharge paying patient payments = Medicare payments + Cost payer payments

$$= \$2,800,000 + \frac{400}{2,000} \times \$6,000,000$$

$$= \$4,000,000$$

$$\text{Proportion of charge paying patients} = \frac{500}{2,000} = .25$$

3. A nonprofit entity does not have the same opportunities for capital formation that an investor-owned organization does. Specifically, the nonprofit entity cannot sell new shares or ownership interests. It is, by and large, constrained in its ability to replace its assets and expand into new markets, to its accumulated funded reserves, and to new debt. In some special situations, nonprofit organizations may receive contributions but these amounts are usually not significant.

4. The major rationale for urban/rural hospital payment differences relates to severity-of-illness differences. Many individuals believe that urban hospitals are more likely to treat more severely ill patients. Rural hospitals contend that much of the variation is due to differences in the efficiency and effectiveness of care. At this time, it is not clear precisely what the causes of urban/rural hospital cost differences are, but such differences do exist.

5. The relevant comparative data might be as follows:

	Price Level Depreciation*	Sum of the Years Digits Depreciation
Year 1	$ 31,800	$ 50,000
Year 2	33,708	40,000
Year 3	35,730	30,000
Year 4	37,874	20,000
Year 5	40,147	10,000
	$179,259	$150,000

*Depreciation in year t $= \frac{150,000}{5}(1.06)^t$. This term reflects compounding of straight line depreciation at 6 percent per year.

In most cases, price-level-adjusted depreciation would be better. However, for short-lived assets, accelerated depreciation may provide greater levels of reimbursement in earlier years to offset lower returns in later years. The lower the rate of asset inflation, the more desirable accelerated depreciation becomes.

6. Profit is essential to most business organizations because accounting expenses do not equal cash requirements. Additional funds or profit must be available to meet the financial requirements of debt principal payments, increases in working capital, and capital expenditures.

7. The relevant calculation would be as follows:

$$\text{Revenue} = \frac{\$5,400,000 + \$850,000 - \$3,880,000}{.25}$$

$$= 9,480,000 \text{ or } \$4,740 \text{ per case}$$

A 10 percent reduction in operating expenses permitted a 17 percent reduction in rates ($5,700 to $4,740 per case). Cost control is critical in health care entities, especially in those with relatively low levels of cost payers. A reduction in rates is especially important when competing for major contracts in which price is a predominant determinant.

List of Major Diagnostic Categories (MDCs), Diagnosis Related Groups (DRGs), Relative Weighting Factors, and Mean Length of Stay (LOS) Used in the Prospective Payment System

MDC 1: Diseases and Disorders of the Nervous System

DRG	Title	Weights	Mean LOS
1	Craniotomy Age >17 Except For Trauma	3.3548	19.4
2	Craniotomy For Trauma Age >17	3.2829	15.8
3	Craniotomy Age <18	2.9489	12.7
4	Spinal Procedures	2.2452	16.0
5	Extracranial Vascular Procedures	1.6780	9.8
6	Carpal Tunnel Release	.3993	2.6
7	Periph + Cranial Nerve + Other Nerv Syst Proc Age >69 +/or C.C.	1.0279	5.3
8	Periph + Cranial Nerve + Other Nerv Syst Proc Age <70 w/o C.C.	.7239	4.1
9	Spinal Disorders + Injuries	1.3958	9.1
10	Nervous System Neoplasms Age >69 and/or C.C.	1.3087	9.6
11	Nervous System Neoplasms Age <70 w/o C.C.	1.2545	8.5
12	Degenerative Nervous System Disorders	1.1136	9.4

DRG	Title	Weights	Mean LOS
13	Multiple Sclerosis + Cerebellar Ataxia	1.0150	8.9
14	Specific Cerebrovascular Disorders Except TIA	1.3527	9.9
15	Transient Ischemic Attacks	.6673	5.6
16	Nonspecific Cerebrovascular Disorders With C.C.	.8592	7.4
17	Nonspecific Cerebrovascular Disorders w/o C.C.	.8392	7.2
18	Cranial + Peripheral Nerve Disorders Age >69 and/or C.C.	.7915	6.6
19	Cranial + Peripheral Nerve Disorders Age <70 w/o C.C.	.6975	5.7
20	Nervous System Infection Except Viral Meningitis	1.3141	7.6
21	Viral Meningitis	.6301	4.5
22	Hypertensive Encepholopathy	.7869	6.4
23	Nontraumatic Stupor + Coma	1.1568	5.9
24	Seizure + Headache >69 and/or C.C.	.7279	5.6
25	Seizure + Headache Age 18-69 w/o C.C.	.6392	4.9
26	Seizure + Headache Age 0-17	.4349	3.3
27	Traumatic Stupor + Coma. Coma >1 Hr	1.1368	4.1
28	Traumatic Stupor + Coma. Coma <1 Hr Age >69 and/or C.C.	1.0701	5.9
29	Traumatic Stupor + Coma <1 Hr Age 18-69 w/o C.C.	.7175	3.8
30	Traumatic Stupor + Coma <1 Hr Age 0-17	.3576	2.0
31	Concussion Age >69 and/or C.C.	.6051	4.6
32	Concussion Age 18-69 w/o C.C.	.4519	3.3
33	Concussion Age 0-17	.2483	1.6
34	Other Disorders of Nervous System Age >69 and/or C.C.	.9927	7.1
35	Other Disorders of Nervous System Age <70 w/o C.C.	.8460	6.2

MDC 2: Diseases and Disorders of the Eye

DRG	Title	Weights	Mean LOS
36	Retinal Procedures	.7093	5.0
37	Orbital Procedures	.5630	3.4
38	Primary Iris Procedures	.4325	3.0
39	Lens Procedures	.5010	2.8
40	Extraocular Procedures Except Orbit Age >17	.3977	2.4
41	Extraocular Procedures Except Orbit Age 0-17	.3695	1.6
42	Intraocular Procedures Except Retina, Iris + Lens	.5906	3.8
43	Hyphema	.3828	4.2
44	Acute Major Eye Infections	.6298	6.5
45	Neurological Eye Disorders	.5641	4.3
46	Other Disorders of the Eye Age >17 With C.C.	.5964	4.1
47	Other Disorders of the Eye Age >17 w/o C.C.	.5064	3.0
48	Other Disorders of the Eye Age 0-17	.4060	2.9

		Mean
DRG	**Title**	**Weights**	**LOS**

MDC 3: Diseases and Disorders of the Ear, Nose, and Throat

DRG	Title	Weights	Mean LOS
49	Major Head + Neck Procedures	2.5270	13.6
50	Sialoadenectomy	.7160	4.6
51	Salivary Gland Procedures Except Sialoadenectomy	.6702	4.2
52	Cleft Lip + Palate Repair	.6488	3.8
53	Sinus + Mastoid Procedures Age >17	.5895	3.5
54	Sinus + Mastoid Procedures Age 0-17	.6961	3.2
55	Miscellaneous Ear, Nose + Throat Procedures	.4153	2.5
56	Rhinoplasty	.4144	2.8
57	T + A Proc Except Tonsillectomy +/or Adenoidectomy Age >17	.5251	2.7
58	T + A Proc Except Tonsillectomy +/or Adenoidectomy Age 0-17	.3130	1.5
59	Tonsillectomy and/or Adenoidectomy Only Age >17	.3147	2.0
60	Tonsillectomy and/or Adenoidectomy Only Age 0-17	.2643	1.5
61	Myringotomy Age >17	.4273	2.1
62	Myringotomy Age 0-17	.3121	1.3
63	Other Ear, Nose + Throat O.R. Procedures	1.1090	5.8
64	Ear. Nose + Throat Malignancy	1.0812	5.7
65	Dyseguilibrium	.4857	4.6
66	Epistaxis	.4116	3.7
67	Epiglottitis	.6762	4.3
68	Otitis Mecia + URI Age >69 and/or C.C.	.6289	6.0
69	Otitis Mecia + URI Age 18-65 w/o C.C.	.5417	4.8
70	Otitis Mecia + URI Age 0-17	.3697	3.1
71	Laryngotracheitis	.3589	2.9
72	Nasal, Trauma + Deformity	.4857	3.8
73	Other Ear, Nose + Throat Diagnoses Age >17	.5217	3.5
74	Other Ear, Nose + Throat Diagnoses Age 0-17	.3463	2.1

MDC 4: Diseases and Disorders of the Respiratory System

DRG	Title	Weights	Mean LOS
75	Major Chest Procedures	2.6044	14.4
76	O.R. Proc on the Resp System Except Major Chest With C.C.	1.8734	10.6
77	O.R. Proc on the Resp System Except Major Chest w/o C.C.	1.8178	9.5
78	Pulmonary Embolism	1.4095	10.4
79	Respiratory Infections + Inflammations Age >69 and/or C.C.	1.7982	11.2
80	Respiratory Infections + Inflammations Age 18-69 w/o C.C.	1.7445	10.9
81	Respiratory Infections + Inflammations Age 0-17	.8743	6.1
82	Respiratory Neoplasms	1.1400	7.4

DRG	Title	Weights	Mean LOS
83	Major Chest Trauma Age >69 and/or C.C.	.9809	8.1
84	Major Chest Trauma Age <70 w/o C.C.	.7738	5.3
85	Pleural Effusion Age >69 and/or C.C.	1.1461	8.4
86	Pleural Effusion Age <70 w/o C.C.	1.1217	7.6
87	Pulmonary Edema + Respiratory Failure	1.5529	7.7
88	Chronic Obstructive Pulmonary Disease	1.0412	7.5
89	Simple Pneumonia + Pleurisy Age >69 and/or C.C.	1.1029	8.5
90	Simple Pneumonia + Pleurisy Age 18-69 w/o C.C.	.9849	7.6
91	Simple Pneumonia + Pleurisy Age 0-17	.5131	4.6
92	Interstitial Lung Disease Age >69 and/or C.C.	1.0370	7.8
93	Interstitial Lung Disease Age <70 w/o C.C.	.9724	6.9
94	Pneumothorax Age >69 and/or C.C.	1.4374	9.2
95	Pneumothorax Age <70 w/o C.C.	1.1252	7.7
96	Bronchitis + Asthma Age >69 and/or C.C.	.7996	6.9
97	Bronchitis + Asthma Age 18-69 w/o C.C.	.7256	6.2
98	Bronchitis + Asthma Age 0-17	.4275	3.7
99	Respiratory Signs + Symptoms Age >69 and/or C.C.	.8035	5.5
100	Respiratory Signs + Symptoms Age <70 w/o C.C.	.7730	5.1
101	Other Respiratory Diagnoses Age >69 and/or C.C.	.9035	6.8
102	Other Respiratory Diagnoses Age <70	.9024	6.1

MDC 5: Diseases and Disorders of the Circulatory System

DRG	Title	Weights	Mean LOS
103	Heart Transplant	.0000	.0
104	Cardiac Valve Procedure With Pump + With Cardiac Cath	6.8527	20.9
105	Cardiac Valve Procedure With Pump + w/o Cardiac Cath	5.2308	16.2
106	Coronary Bypass With Cardiac Cath	5.2624	20.4
107	Coronary Bypass w/o Cardiac Cath	3.9891	13.5
108	Cardiothor Proc. Except Valve + Coronary Bypass, With Pump	4.3756	13.3
109	Cardiothoracic Procedures w/o Pump	3.6963	12.1
110	Major Reconstructive Vascular Procedures Age >69 and/or C.C.	2.9328	14.3
111	Major Reconstructive Vascular Procedures Age <70 w/o C.C.	2.5851	13.2
112	Vascular Procedures Except Major Reconstruction	2.3500	11.2
113	Amputation for Circ System Disorders Exept Upper Limb + Toe	2.6800	21.6
114	Upper Limb + Toe Amputation for Circ System Disorders	2.1067	16.6
115	Permanent Cardiac Pacemaker Implant With AMI or CHF	3.9150	15.8

DRG	Title	Weights	Mean LOS
116	Permanent Cardiac Pacemaker Implant w/o AMI or CHF	2.8665	9.3
117	Cardiac Pacemaker Replace + Revis Exc Pulse Gen Repl Only	1.8210	6.4
118	Cardiac Pacemaker Pulse Generator Replacement Only	1.7809	4.2
119	Vein Ligation + Stripping	1.0610	7.2
120	Other O.R. Procedures on the Circulatory System	2.5204	15.0
121	Circulatory Disorders With AMI + C.V. Comp. Disch. Alive	1.8648	11.9
122	Circulatory Disorders With AMI w/o C.V. Comp. Disch. Alive	1.3651	9.8
123	Circulatory Disorders with AMI, Expired	1.1360	3.1
124	Circulatory Disorders Exc AMI, With Card Cath + Complex Diag	2.2200	8.4
125	Circulatory Disorders Exc AMI, With Card Cath w/o Complex Diag	1.6455	5.0
126	Acute + Subacute Endocarditis	2.6645	18.4
127	Heart Failure + Shock	1.0408	7.8
128	Deep Vein Thrombophlebitis	.8639	9.6
129	Cardiac Arrest	1.5506	4.6
130	Peripheral Vascular Disorders Age >69 and/or C.C.	.9645	7.1
131	Peripheral Vascular Disorders Age <70 w/o C.C.	.9491	6.4
132	Atherosclerosis Age >69 and/or C.C.	.9182	6.7
133	Atherosclerosis Age <70 w/o C.C.	.8599	5.2
134	Hypertension	.7049	6.1
135	Cardiac Congenital + Valvular Disorders Age >69 and/or C.C.	.9922	6.1
136	Cardiac Congenital + Valvular Disorders Age 18-69 w/o C.C.	.9674	4.9
137	Cardiac Congenital + Valvular Disorders Age 0-17	.6381	3.3
138	Cardiac Arrhythmia + Conduction Disorders Age >69 and/or C.C.	.9297	5.7
139	Cardiac Arrhythmia + Conduction Disorders Age <70 w/o C.C.	.8303	4.8
140	Angina Pectoris	.7548	5.5
141	Syncope + Collapse Age >69 and/or C.C.	.6475	5.0
142	Syncope + Collapse Age <70 w/o C.C.	.5680	4.3
143	Chest Pain	.6814	4.4
144	Other Circulatory Diagnoses With C.C.	1.1267	7.0
145	Other Circulatory Diagnoses w/o C.C.	1.0020	6.4

MDC 6: Diseases and Disorders of the Digestive System

DRG	Title	Weights	Mean LOS
146	Rectal Resection Age >69 and/or C.C.	2.7082	19.1
147	Rectal Resection Age <70 w/o C.C.	2.5087	17.9

DRG	Title	Weights	Mean LOS
148	Major Small + Large Bowel Procedures Age >69 and/or C.C.	2.5493	17.0
149	Major Small + Large Bowel Procedures Age <70 w/o C.C.	2.2154	15.2
150	Peritoneal Adhesiolysis Age >69 and/or C.C.	2.3746	15.3
151	Peritoneal Adhesiolysis Age <70 w/o C.C.	2.0274	13.4
152	Minor Small + Large Bowel Procedures Age >69 and/or C.C.	1.4851	10.6
153	Minor Small + Large Bowel Procedures Age <70 w/o C.C.	1.2599	9.3
154	Stomach, Esophageal + Duodenal Procedures Age >69 and/or C.C.	2.6901	14.8
155	Stomach, Esophageal + Duodenal Procedures Age 18-69 w/o C.C.	2.3336	13.0
156	Stomach, Esophageal + Duodenal Procedures Age 0-17	.8470	6.0
157	Anal Procedures Age >69 and/or C.C.	.7985	6.0
158	Anal Procedures Age <70 w/o C.C.	.6408	5.2
159	Hernia Procedures Except Inguinal + Femoral Age >69 and/or C.C.	.9297	7.1
160	Hernia Procedures Except Inguinal + Femoral Age 18-69 w/o. C.C.	.7676	6.0
161	Inguinal + Femoral Hernia Procedures Age >69 and/or C.C.	.7068	5.7
162	Inguinal + Femoral Hernia Procedures Age 18-69 w/o C.C.	.5854	4.8
163	Hernia Procedures Age 0-17	.4358	2.1
164	Appendectomy With Complicated Princ. Diag Age >69 and/or C.C.	1.8320	11.9
165	Appendectomy With Complicated Princ. Diag Age <70 w/o C.C.	1.6154	11.3
166	Appendectomy w/o Complicated Princ. Diag Age >69 and/or C.C.	1.4328	9.4
167	Appendectomy w/o Complicated Princ. Diag Age <70 w/o C.C.	1.0818	7.4
168	Procedures on the Mouth Age >69 and/or C.C.	.8631	4.3
169	Procedures on the Mouth Age <70 w/o C.C.	.8992	4.2
170	Other Digestive System Procedures Age >69 and/or C.C.	2.6602	14.6
171	Other Digestive System Procedures Age <70 w/o C.C.	2.3976	13.3
172	Digestive Malignancy Age >69 and/or C.C.	1.2268	8.2
173	Digestive Malignancy Age <70 w/o C.C.	1.0517	6.7
174	G.I. Hemorrhage Age >69 and/or C.C.	.9281	6.7
175	G.I. Hemorrhage Age <70 w/o C.C.	.8236	5.8
176	Complicated Peptic Ulcer	1.2438	8.1
177	Uncomplicated Peptic Ulcer >69 and/or C.C.	.7422	6.6
178	Uncomplicated Peptic Ulcer <70 w/o C.C.	.6141	5.5

DRG	Title	Weights	Mean LOS
179	Inflammatory Bowel Disease	1.0153	8.0
180	G.I. Obstruction Age >69 and/or C.C.	.8197	6.2
181	G.I. Obstruction Age <70 w/o C.C.	.7845	5.9
182	Esophagitis, Gastroent. + Misc. Digest. Dis Age >69 +/or C.C.	.6185	5.4
183	Esophagitis, Gastroent. + Misc. Digest. Dis Age 18-69 w/o C.C.	.5652	4.8
184	Esophagitis, Gastroenteritis + Misc. Digest. Disorders Age 0-17	.3822	3.3
185	Dental + Oral Dis. Exc Extractions + Restorations, Age >17	.6681	4.2
186	Dental + Oral Dis. Exc Extractions + Restorations, Age 0-17	.4155	2.9
187	Dental Extractions + Restorations	.3990	2.7
188	Other Digestive System Diagnoses Age >69 and/or C.C.	.7444	5.1
189	Other Digestive System Diagnoses Age 18-69 w/o C.C.	.6576	4.5
190	Other Digestive System Diagnoses Age 0-17	.3379	2.1

MDC 7: Diseases and Disorders of the Heptobiliary System and Pancreas

DRG	Title	Weights	Mean LOS
191	Major Pancreas, Liver + Shunt Procedures	4.1791	20.8
192	Minor Pancreas, Lever + Shunt Procedures	3.9197	20.1
193	Biliary Track Proc Exc Tot Cholecystectomy Age >69 +/or C.C.	2.4513	17.3
194	Biliary Track Proc Exc Tot Cholecystectomy Age <70 w/o C.C.	1.9881	13.9
195	Total Cholecystectomy With C.D.E. Age >69 and/or C.C.	2.1690	16.0
196	Total Cholecystectomy With C.D.E. Age <70 w/o C.C.	2.0594	15.8
197	Total Cholecystectomy w/o C.D.E. Age >69 and/or C.C.	1.4868	11.5
198	Total Cholecystectomy w/o C.D.E. Age <70 w/o C.C.	1.2752	10.1
199	Hepatobiliary Diagnostic Procedure for Malignancy	2.4574	17.9
200	Hepatobiliary Diagnostic Procedure for Non-Malignancy	2.5818	15.1
201	Other Hepatobiliary or Pancreas O.R. Procedures	2.7291	16.9
202	Cirrhosis + Alcoholic Hepatitis	1.1965	9.3
203	Malignancy of Hepatobiliary System or Pancreas	1.0937	8.0
204	Disorders of Pancreas Except Malignancy	.9682	7.5
205	Disorders of Liver Exc Malig. Cirr. Alc Hepa Age >69 and/or C.C.	1.0822	7.9
206	Disorders of Liver Exc Malig. Cirr. Alc Hepa Age <70 w/o C.C.	.9247	6.8
207	Disorders of the Biliary Track Age >69 and/or C.C.	.8492	6.6
208	Disorders of the Biliary Track Age <70 w/o C.C.	.7315	5.5

DRG	Title	Weights	Mean LOS

MDC 8: Diseases and Disorders of the Musculoskeletal System and Connective Tissue

DRG	Title	Weights	Mean LOS
209	Major Joint Procedures	2.2912	17.1
210	Hip + Femur Procedures Except Major Joint Age >69 and/or C.C.	2.0833	17.8
211	Hip + Femur Procedures Except Major Joint Age 18-69 w/o C.C.	1.9530	15.9
212	Hip + Femur Procedures Except Major Joint Age 0-17	1.7132	11.1
213	Amputations for Musculoskeletal System + Conn. Tissue Disorders	2.1315	14.3
214	Back + Neck Procedures Age >69 and/or C.C.	1.8427	15.6
215	Back + Neck Procedures Age <70 w/o C.C.	1.4920	13.0
216	Biopsies of Musculoskeletal System + Connective Tissue	1.5596	11.3
217	Wnd Debrid + Skn Grft Exc Hand, for Muscuskeletal + Conn. Tiss. Dis	2.2824	13.1
218	Lower Extrem + Humer Proc Exc Hip, Foot, Femur Age >69 +/or C.C.	1.4250	10.9
219	Lower Extrem + Humer Proc Exc Hip, Foot, Femur Age 18-69 w/o C.C.	1.0790	8.3
220	Lower Extrem + Humer Proc Exc Hip, Foot, Femur Age 0-17	.9339	5.3
221	Knee Procedures Age >69 and/or C.C.	1.2727	8.3
222	Knee Procedures Age <70 w/o C.C.	.9897	6.4
223	Upper Extremity Proc Exc Humerus + Hand Age >69 and/or C.C.	1.0723	6.9
224	Upper Extremity Proc Exc Humerus + Hand Age <70 w/o C.C.	.8952	5.6
225	Foot Procedures	.6476	4.8
226	Soft Tissue Procedures Age >69 and/or C.C.	.7984	5.1
227	Soft Tissue Procedures Age <70 w/o C.C.	.6337	4.2
228	Ganglion (Hand) Procedures	.3626	2.2
229	Hand Procedures Except Ganglion	.5998	3.4
230	Local Excision + Removal of Int Fix Devices of Hip + Femur	1.3594	8.9
231	Local Excision + Removal of Int Fix Devices Except Hip + Femur	.9519	5.3
232	Arthroscopy	.6063	3.6
233	Other Musculoskelet Sys + Conn Tiss O.R. Proc Age >69 +/or C.C.	1.7737	13.1
234	Other Musculoskelet Sys + Conn Tiss O.R. Proc Age <70 w/o C.C.	1.2454	8.2
235	Fractures of Femur	1.7586	13.6
236	Fractures of Hip + Pelvis	1.3855	11.9

DRG	Title	Weights	Mean LOS
237	Sprains, Strains, + Dislocations of Hip, Pelvis + Thigh	.7929	6.4
238	Osteomyelitis	1.5511	12.3
239	Pathological Fractures + Musculoskeletal + Conn. Tiss. Malignancy	1.0979	9.2
240	Connective Tissue Disorders Age >69 and/or C.C.	.9709	8.6
241	Connective Tissue Disorders Age <70 w/o C.C.	.9048	8.0
242	Septic Arthritis	1.5880	11.2
243	Medical Back Problems	.7551	7.5
244	Bone Diseases & Septic Arthropathy Age >69 and/or C.C.	.7792	7.5
245	Bone Diseases & Septic Arthropathy Age <70 w/o C.C.	.7177	6.3
246	Non-Specific Arthropathies	.7147	6.8
247	Signs + Symptoms of Musculoskeletal System + Conn Tissue	.6559	5.8
248	Tendonitis, Myositis + Bursitis	.6136	5.4
249	Aftercare, Musculoskeletal System + Connective Tissue	1.0203	7.6
250	Fx. Sprns, Strns + Disl of Forearm, Hand, Foot Age >69 +/or C.C.	.7428	6.0
251	Fx. Sprns, Strns + Disl of Forearm, Hand, Foot Age 18-69 w/o C.C.	.5964	4.2
252	Fx. Sprns, Strns + Disl of Forearm, Hand, Foot Age 0-17	.3533	1.8
253	Fx. Sprns, Strns + Disl of Uparm, Lowleg Ex Foot Age >69 +/or C.C.	.7466	6.6
254	Fx. Sprns, Strns + Disl of Uparm, Lowleg Ex Foot Age 18-69 w/o C.C.	.6258	5.3
255	Fx. Sprns, Strns + Disl of Uparm, Lowleg Ex Foot Age 0-17	.4687	2.9
256	Other Diagnoses of Musculoskeletal System + Connective Tissue	.8706	6.5

MDC 9: Diseases and Disorders of the Skin, Subcutaneous Tissue and Breast

DRG	Title	Weights	Mean LOS
257	Total Mastectomy for Malignancy Age >69 and/or C.C.	1.1085	9.3
258	Total Mastectomy for Malignancy Age <70 w/o C.C.	1.0729	8.9
259	Subtotal Mastectomy for Malignancy Age >69 and/or C.C.	1.0141	7.4
260	Subtotal Mastectomy for Malignancy Age <70	.9325	6.4
261	Breast Proc for Non-Malig Except Biopsy + Loc Exc	.7329	4.8
262	Breast Biopsy + Local Excision for Non-Malignancy	.4617	3.0
263	Skin Grafts for Skin Ulcer or Cellulitis Age >69 and/or C.C.	2.4737	21.3
264	Skin Grafts for Skin Ulcer or Cellulitis Age <70 w/o C.C.	2.2031	18.2

DRG	Title	Weights	Mean LOS
265	Skin Grafts Except for Skin Ulcer or Cellulitis With C.C.	1.4959	8.6
266	Skin Grafts Except for Skin Ulcer or Cellulitis w/o C.C.	.9485	5.9
267	Perianal + Pilonical Procedures	.6113	5.0
268	Skin. Subcutaneous Tissue + Breast Plastic Procedures	.5388	3.0
269	Other Skin, Subcut Tiss + Breast O.R. Proc Age >69 +/or C.C.	.9947	5.7
270	Other Skin, Subcut Tiss + Breast O.R. Proc Age <70 w/o C.C.	.8123	4.5
271	Skin Ulcers	1.3802	12.1
272	Major Skin Disorders Age >69 and/or C.C.	.8620	7.8
273	Major Skin Disorders Age <70 w/o C.C.	.8286	7.3
274	Malignant Breast Disorders Age >69 and/or C.C.	1.0108	7.5
275	Malignant Breast Disorders Age <70 w/o C.C.	.9014	6.4
276	Non-Malignant Breast Disorders	.6066	4.2
277	Cellulitis Age >69 and/or C.C.	.8663	8.3
278	Cellulitis Age 18-69 w/o C.C.	.8096	7.2
279	Cellulitis Age 0-17	.4789	4.2
280	Trauma to the Skin, Subcut Tiss + Breast Age >69 +/or C.C.	.6201	5.4
281	Trauma to the Skin, Subcut Tiss + Breast Age 18-69 w/o C.C.	.5377	4.2
282	Trauma to the Skin, Subcut Tiss + Breast Age 0-17	.3460	2.2
283	Minor Skin Disorders Age >69 and/or C.C.	.6394	5.3
284	Minor Skin disorders Age <70 w/o C.C.	.5971	4.4

MDC 10: Endocrine, Nutritional, and Metabolic Diseases and Disorders

285	Amputations for Endocrine, Nutritional + Metabolic Disorders	2.8658	24.0
286	Adrenal + Pituitary Procedures	2.8952	16.1
287	Skin Grafts + Wound Debride for Endoc, Nutrit + Metab Disorders	2.8143	22.8
288	O.R. Procedures for Obesity	1.5695	10.0
289	Parathyroid Procedures	1.3736	8.3
290	Thyroid Procedures	.8549	6.0
291	Thyroglossal Procedures	.4909	2.9
292	Other Endocrine, Nutrit + Metab O.R. Proc Age >69 +/or C.C.	2.0307	10.8
293	Other Endocrine, Nutrit + Metab O.R. Proc Age <70 w/o C.C.	1.4951	8.0
294	Diabetes Age ≥36	.8087	7.7
295	Diabetes Age 0-35	.7457	5.6

DRG	Title	Weights	Mean LOS
296	Nutritional + Misc. Metabolic Disorders Age >69 and/or C.C.	.8979	7.3
297	Nutritional + Misc. Metabolic Disorders Age 18-69 w/o C.C.	.7923	6.0
298	Nutritional + Misc. Metabolic Disorders Age 0-17	.7538	5.4
299	Inborn Errors of Metabolism	.9407	6.8
300	Endocrine Disorders Age >69 and/or C.C.	.9731	7.8
301	Endocrine Disorders Age <70 w/o C.C.	.8143	6.4

MDC 11: Diseases and Disorders of the Kidney and Urinary Tract

DRG	Title	Weights	Mean LOS
302	Kidney Transplant	6.6322	24.1
303	Kidney, Ureter + Major Bladder Procedure for Neoplasm	2.5397	16.2
304	Kidney, Ureter + Maj Bldr Proc for Non-Malig Age >69 +/or C.C.	1.7952	12.8
305	Kidney, Ureter + Maj Bldr Proc for Non-Malig Age <70 w/o C.C.	1.7043	11.9
306	Prostatectomy Age >69 and/or C.C.	1.1399	8.6
307	Prostatectomy Age <70 w/o C.C.	.9513	7.2
308	Minor Bladder Procedures Age >69 and/or C.C.	1.0441	7.1
309	Minor Bladder Procedures Age <70 w/o C.C.	.9290	5.7
310	Transurethral Procedures Age >69 and/or C.C.	.7071	4.9
311	Transurethral Procedures Age <70 w/o C.C.	.5871	4.1
312	Urethral Procedures, Age >69 and/or C.C.	.7424	5.2
313	Urethral Procedures, Age 18-69 w/o C.C.	.6897	5.1
314	Urethral Procedures, Age 0-17	.4368	2.3
315	Other Kidney + Urinary Tract O.R. Procedures	2.4884	9.8
316	Renal Failure w/o Dialysis	1.3314	6.7
317	Renal Failure with Dialysis	.2385	1.2
318	Kidney + Urinary Tract Neoplasms Age >69 and/or C.C.	.9142	5.5
319	Kidney + Urinary Tract Neoplasms Age <70 w/o C.C.	.7942	4.2
320	Kidney + Urinary Tract Infections Age >69 and/or C.C.	.8123	7.0
321	Kidney + Urinary Tract Infections Age 18-69 w/o C.C.	.6803	5.6
322	Kidney + Urinary Tract Infections Age 0-17	.4553	3.7
323	Urinary Stones Age >69 and/or C.C.	.7131	4.9
324	Urinary Stones Age <70 w/o C.C.	.5472	3.9
325	Kidney + Urinary Tract Signs + Symptoms Age >69 and/or C.C.	.7247	5.4
326	Kidney + Urinary Tract Signs + Symptoms Age 18-69 w/o C.C.	.5875	4.3
327	Kidney + Urinary Tract Signs + Symptoms Age 0-17	.5027	3.1
328	Urethral Stricture Age >69 and/or C.C.	.6508	4.8

DRG	Title	Weights	Mean LOS
329	Urethral Stricture Age 18-69 w/o C.C.	.5326	3.9
330	Urethral Stricture Age 0-17	.2817	1.6
331	Other Kidney + Urinary Tract Diagnoses Age >69 and/or C.C.	.8919	6.3
332	Other Kidney + Urinary Tract Diagnoses Age 18-69 w/o C.C.	.7763	5.0
333	Other Kidney + Urinary Tract Diagnoses Age 0-17	.5146	3.2

MDC 12: Diseases and Disorders of the Male Reproductive System

DRG	Title	Weights	Mean LOS
334	Major Male Pelvic Procedures With C.C.	1.5612	12.7
335	Major Male Pelvic Procedures w/o C.C.	1.3590	11.8
336	Transurethral Prostatectomy Age >69 and/or C.C.	1.0079	8.4
337	Transurethral Prostatectomy Age <70 w/o C.C.	.8491	7.2
338	Testes Procedures, for Malignancy	.9069	6.3
339	Testes Procedures, Non-Malignant Age >17	.6093	4.5
340	Testes Procedures, Non-Malignant Age 0-17	.4381	2.4
341	Penis Procedures	.9983	6.0
342	Circumcision Age >17	.4228	2.8
343	Circumcision Age 0-17	.3828	1.7
344	Other Male Reproductive System O.R. Procedures for Malignancy	1.1204	7.4
345	Other Male Reproductive System O.R. Proc Except for Malig	.8334	5.6
346	Malignancy, Male Reproductive System, Age >69 and/or C.C.	.9395	6.9
347	Malignancy, Male Reproductive System, Age <70 w/o C.C.	.8304	5.7
348	Benign Prostatic Hypertrophy Age >69 and/or C.C.	.8864	6.2
349	Benign Prostatic Hypertrophy Age <70 w/o C.C.	.6998	4.9
350	Inflammation of the Male Reproductive System	.6096	5.2
351	Sterilization. Male	.2655	1.3
352	Other Male Reproductive System Diagnoses	.6385	4.4

MDC 13: Diseases and Disorders of the Female Reproductive System

DRG	Title	Weights	Mean LOS
353	Pelvic Evisceration, Radical Hysterectomy + Vulvectomy	1.9376	12.4
354	Non-Radical Hysterectomy Age >69 and/or C.C.	1.1108	9.6
355	Non-Radical Hysterectomy Age <70 w/o C.C.	1.0156	8.8
356	Female Reproductive System Reconstructive Procedures	.8460	8.1
357	Uterus + Adenexa Procedures, for Malignancy	1.9188	13.9
358	Uterus + Adenexa Proc for Non-Malignancy Except Tubal Interrupt	1.0890	8.0
359	Tubal Interruption for Non-Malignancy	.4279	2.3
360	Vagina, Cervix + Vulva Procedures	.5985	4.2

DRG	Title	Weights	Mean LOS
361	Laparoscopy + Endoscopy (Female) Except Tubal Interruption	.4864	2.6
362	Laparoscopic Tubal Interruption	.3126	1.4
363	D + C, Conization + Radio–Implant, for Malignancy	.6516	4.3
364	D + C, Conization Except for Malignancy	.4028	2.6
365	Other Female Reproductive System O.R. Procedures	1.7965	12.7
366	Malignancy, Female Reproductive System Age >69 and/or C.C.	.8444	5.2
367	Malignancy, Female Reproductive System Age <70 w/o C.C.	.5786	3.5
368	Infections, Female Reproductive System	.7944	6.7
369	Menstrual + Other Female Reproductive System Disorders	.6959	5.1

MDC 14: Pregnancy, Childbirth, and the Puerperium

DRG	Title	Weights	Mean LOS
370	Cesarean Section with C.C.	.9912	7.6
371	Cesarean Section w/o C.C.	.7535	6.1
372	Vaginal Delivery with Complicating Diagnoses	.5534	3.8
373	Vaginal Delivery w/o Complicating Diagnoses	.4063	3.2
374	Vaginal Delivery with Sterilization and/or D + C	.5492	3.6
375	Vaginal Delivery with O.R. Proc Except Steril and/or D + C	.6889	4.4
376	Postpartum Diagnoses w/o O.R. Procedure	.4158	2.9
377	Postpartum Diagnoses with O.R. Procedure	.4761	2.2
378	Ectopic Pregnancy	.8094	5.5
379	Threatened Abortion	.3169	2.2
380	Abortion w/o D + C	.2705	1.5
381	Abortion with D + C	.3602	1.4
382	False Labor	.1842	1.2
383	Other Antepartum Diagnoses with Medical Complications	.4317	3.4
384	Other Antepartum Diagnoses w/o Medical Complications	.3245	2.2

MDC 15: Newborns and Other Neonates with Conditions Originating in the Perinatal Period

DRG	Title	Weights	Mean LOS
385	Neonates, Died or Transferred	.6883	1.8
386	Extreme Immaturity, Neonate	3.6863	17.9
387	Prematurity with Major Problems	1.8459	13.3
388	Prematurity w/o Major Problems	1.1693	8.6
389	Full Term Neonate with Major Problems	.5482	4.7
390	Neonates with Other Significant Problems	.3523	3.4
391	Normal Newborns	.2241	3.1

DRG	Title	Weights	Mean LOS

MDC 16: Diseases and Disorders of the Blood and Blood-Forming Organs and Immunity Disorders

DRG	Title	Weights	Mean LOS
392	Splenectomy Age >17	2.7746	16.4
393	Splenectomy Age 0-17	1.5366	9.1
394	Other O.R. Procedures of the Blood + Blood Forming Organs	1.1146	6.1
395	Red Blood Cell Disorders Age >17	.7839	6.1
396	Red Blood Cell Disorders Age 0-17	.6295	4.1
397	Coagulation Disorders	.9863	6.7
398	Reticuloendothelial + Immunity Disorders Age >69 and/or C.C.	.8900	6.1
399	Reticuloendothelial + Immunity Disorders Age <70 w/o C.C.	.8459	5.6

MDC 17: Myeloproliferative Diseases and Disorders, Poorly Differentiated Malignancy and other Neoplasms NEC

DRG	Title	Weights	Mean LOS
400	Lymphoma or Leukemia with Major O.R. Procedure	2.8272	16.9
401	Lymphoma or Leukemia with Minor O.R. Proc Age >69 and/or C.C.	1.2409	8.9
402	Lymphoma or Leukemia with Minor O.R. Procedure Age <70 w/o C.C.	1.1316	7.1
403	Lymphoma or Leukemia Age >69 and/or C.C.	1.1715	7.1
404	Lymphoma or Leukemia Age 18-69 w/o C.C.	1.1787	6.4
405	Lymphoma or Leukemia Age 0-17	1.0517	4.9
406	Myeloprolif Disord or Poorly Diff Neoplasm W Maj O.R. Proc. + C.C.	2.2671	15.0
407	Myeloprolif Disord or Poorly Diff Neopl W Maj O.R. Proc w/o C.C.	2.1366	13.3
408	Myeloprolif Disord or Poorly Diff Neopl With Minor O.R. Proc.	1.1389	7.1
409	Radiotherapy	.8134	5.7
410	Chemotherapy	.3527	2.6
411	History of Malignancy w/o Endoscopy	.7221	4.7
412	History of Malignancy With Endoscopy	.3400	2.0
413	Othr Myeloprolif Disord or Poorly Diff Neopl Dx Age >69 +/or C.C.	1.0975	7.3
414	Othr Myeloprolif Disord or Poorly Diff Neopl Dx Age <70 w/o C.C.	1.0359	6.4

MDC 18: Infectious and Parasitic Diseases (Systemic or Unspecified Sites)

DRG	Title	Weights	Mean LOS
415	O.R. Procedure for Infectious + Parasitic Diseases	3.0027	15.1
416	Septecemia Age >17	1.5504	9.2
417	Septecemia Age 0-17	.7152	5.2
418	Postoperative + Post-Traumatic Infections	.9968	8.4
419	Fever of Unknown Origin Age >69 and/or C.C.	.8628	6.9
420	Fever of Unknown Origin Age 18-69 w/o C.C.	.8022	6.2
421	Viral Illness Age >17	.6045	5.4
422	Viral Illness + Fever of Unknown Origin Age 0-17	.4360	3.2
423	Other Infectious + Parasitic Diseases Diagnoses	1.2107	8.8

MDC 19: Mental Diseases and Disorders

DRG	Title	Weights	Mean LOS
424	O.R. Procedures With Principal Diagnosis of Mental Illness	2.1938	14.2
425	Acute Adjust React + Disturbances of Psychosocial Dysfunction	.6812	5.8
426	Depressive Neuroses	.9495	9.4
427	Neuroses Except Depressive	.7678	6.9
428	Disorders of Personality + Impulse Control	.9741	8.3
429	Organic Disturbances + Mental Retardation	.9523	8.8
430	Psychoses	1.0934	10.8
431	Childhood Mental Disorders	2.2519	15.4
432	Other Diagnoses of Mental Disorders	1.0525	7.2

MDC 20: Substance Use and Substance Induced Organic Mental Disorders

DRG	Title	Weights	Mean LOS
433	Substance Use + Subst Induced Organic Mental Disorders, Left APA	.4457	2.5
434	Drug Dependence	1.0404	9.1
435	Drug Use Except Dependence	1.0738	8.0
436	Alcohol Dependence	.8853	8.1
437	Alcohol Use Except Dependence	.6183	3.5
438	Alcohol + Substance Induced Organic Mental Syndrome	.8420	6.9

MDC 21: Injury, Poisoning, and Toxic Effects of Drugs

DRG	Title	Weights	Mean LOS
439	Skin Grafts for Injuries	1.8219	8.9
440	Wound Debridements for Injuries	1.4807	7.2
441	Hand Procedures for Injuries	.7180	3.0
442	Other O.R. Procedures for Injuries Age >69 and/or C.C.	1.9026	9.1
443	Other O.R. Procedures for Injuries Age < 70 w/o C.C.	1.5211	6.6

DRG	Title	Weights	Mean LOS
444	Multiple Trauma Age >69 and/or C.C.	.8830	6.7
445	Multiple Trauma Age 18-69 w/o C.C.	.7530	5.2
446	Multiple Trauma Age 0-17	.4846	2.4
447	Allergic Reactions >17	.4785	3.7
448	Allergic Reactions 0-17	.3505	2.9
449	Toxic Effects of Drugs Age >69 and/or C.C.	.7331	5.6
450	Toxic Effects of Drugs Age 18-69 w/o C.C.	.5957	3.9
451	Toxic Effects of Drugs Age 0-17	.2912	2.1
452	Complications of Treatment Age >69 and/or C.C.	.8492	5.5
453	Complications of Treatment Age <70 w/o C.C.	.9020	5.1
454	Other Injuries, Poisonings + Toxic Eff Diag Age >69 and/or C.C.	.8224	5.3
455	Other Injuries, Poisonings + Toxic Eff Diag Age <70 w/o C.C.	.6185	3.5

MDC 22: Burns

456	Burns, Transferred to Another Acute Care Facility	2.0902	11.6
457	Extensive Burns	6.8631	12.6
458	Non-Extensive Burns with Skin Grafts	2.8572	18.3
459	Non-Extensive Burns with Wound Debridement + Other O.R. Proc	2.7568	12.7
460	Non-Extensive Burns w/o O.R. Procedure	1.4225	9.0

MDC 23: Factors Influencing Health Status and Other Contacts with Health Services

461	O.R. Proc With Diagnoses of Other Contact With Health Services	1.6507	8.0
462	Rehabilitation	1.8268	13.5
463	Signs + Symptoms With C.C.	.7702	6.3
464	Signs + Symptoms w/o C.C.	.7322	6.0
465	Aftercare With History of Malignancy as Secondary Dx	.2071	1.5
466	Aftercare w/o History of Malignancy as Secondary Dx	.6377	3.7
467	Other Factors Influencing Health Status	.9799	6.1
468	Unrelated O.R. Procedure	2.1037	11.2
469	PDX Invalid as Discharge Diagnosis	.0000	.0
470	Ungroupable	.0000	.0

Abbreviations

OR	—Operating Room Procedure
CC	—Complication and/or Comorbidity
URI	—Upper Respiratory Infection
FUO	—Fever of Unknown Origin

NEC   —Not Elsewhere Classifiable
AMI   —Acute Myocardial Infarction
CHF   —Congestive Heart Failure
D&C   —Dilation and Curettage

Source: Federal Register. Vol. 48, No. 171, September 1, 1983.

Chapter 3

General Principles of Accounting

Information does not happen by itself; it must be generated by an individual or a formally designed system. Financial information is no exception. The accounting system generates most financial information to provide quantitative data, primarily financial in nature, that are useful in making economic decisions about economic entities.

FINANCIAL VERSUS MANAGERIAL ACCOUNTING

Financial accounting is the branch of accounting that provides general purpose financial statements or reports to aid a large number of decision-making groups, internal and external to the organization, in a variety of decisions. The primary outputs of financial accounting are four financial statements that will be discussed in chapter 4 (see Exhibits 4-1, 4-2, 4-3, 4-4, and 4-5).

1. balance sheet
2. statement of revenues and expenses
3. statement of changes in financial position
4. statement of changes in fund balance

The field of financial accounting is restricted in many ways regarding how certain events or business transactions may be accounted for. The term *generally accepted accounting principles* is often used to describe the body of rules and requirements that shape the preparation of the four primary financial statements. For example, an organization's financial statements that have been audited by an independent certified public accountant (CPA) would bear the following language:

In our opinion, the aforementioned financial statement present fairly the financial position of the XYZ Company at December 31, 1986, and the results of its operations and changes in its financial position for the year ended, in conformity with generally accepted accounting principles applied on a basis consistent with that of the preceding year.

Financial accounting is not limited to preparation of the four statements. An increasing number of additional financial reports are being required, especially for external users for specific decision-making purposes. This is particularly important in the health care industry. For example, hospitals submit cost reports to a number of third party payers, such as Blue Cross, Medicare, and Medicaid. They also submit financial reports to a large number of regulatory agencies, such as planning agencies, rate review agencies, service associations, and many others. In addition, CPAs often prepare financial projections that are used by investors in capital financing. These statements, though not usually audited by independent CPAs are, for the most part, prepared in accordance with the same generally accepted accounting principles that govern the preparation of the four basic financial statements.

Managerial accounting is primarily concerned with the preparation of financial information for specific purposes, usually for internal users. Since this information is used within the organization, there is less need for a body of principles restricting its preparation. Presumably, the user and the preparer can meet to discuss questions of interpretation. Uniformity and comparability of information, which are desired goals for financial accountants, are clearly less important to management accountants.

PRINCIPLES OF ACCOUNTING

Here we are concerned with both sets of accounting information—financial and managerial. Although managerial accounting has no formally adopted set of principles, it relies strongly on financial accounting principles. Understanding the principles and basics of financial accounting is therefore critical to understanding both financial and managerial accounting information.

The case example in our discussion of the principles of financial accounting is a newly formed, nonprofit community hospital, which we shall refer to as "Alpha Hospital."

Accounting Entity

Obviously, in any accounting there must be an entity for which the financial statements are being prepared. Specifying the entity upon which the accounting will focus defines the information that is pertinent. Drawing these boundaries is the underlying concept behind the accounting entity principle.

Alpha Hospital is the entity for which we will account and prepare financial statements. We are not interested in the individuals who may have incorporated Alpha or other hospitals in the community, but solely in Alpha Hospital's financial transactions.

Defining the entity is not as clear-cut as one might expect. Significant problems arise, especially when the legal entity is different from the accounting entity. For example, if one doctor owns a clinic through a sole proprietorship arrangement, the accounting entity may be the clinic operation, whereas the legal entity includes the doctor and the doctor's personal resources as well. A hospital may be part of a university or government agency, or it might be owned by a large corporation organized on a profit or nonprofit basis. Indeed, many hospitals have now become subsidiaries of a holding company as a result of corporate restructuring. Careful attention must be paid to the definition of the accounting entity in these situations. If the entity is not properly defined, evaluation of its financial information may be useless at best, and misleading at worst.

The common practice of municipalities directly paying the fringe benefits of municipal employees employed in the hospital illustrates this situation. Such expenses may never show up in the hospital's accounts, resulting in an understatement of the expenses associated with running the hospital. In many cases, this may produce a bias in the rate-setting process.

Money Measurement

Accounting in general, but financial accounting in particular, is concerned with measuring economic resources and obligations and their changing levels for the accounting entity under consideration. The accountant's yardstick for measuring is not metered to size, color, weight, or other attributes; it is limited exclusively to money. However, there are significant problems in money measurement, which will be discussed shortly.

Economic resources are defined as scarce means, limited in supply, but essential to economic activity. They include supplies, buildings, equipment, money, claims to receive money, and ownership interests in other enterprises. The terms *economic resources* and *assets* may be interchanged for most practical purposes. Economic obligations are responsibilities to transfer economic resources or provide services to other entities in the future, usually in return for economic resources received from other entities in the past through the purchase of assets, the receipt of services, or the acceptance of loans. For most practical purposes, the terms *economic obligations* and *liabilities* may be used interchangeably.

In most normal situations, assets exceed liabilities in money-measured value. Liabilities represent the claim of one entity on another's assets; any excess, or remaining residual interest, may be claimed by the owner. In fact, for entities with ownership interest, this residual interest is called "owner's equity."

In most nonprofit entities, including health care organizations, there is no residual ownership claim. Any assets remaining in a liquidated not-for-profit entity, after all liabilities have been dissolved, legally become the property of the state. Residual interest is referred to as "fund balance" for most health care organizations.

In the Alpha Hospital example, assume that the community donated $1 million in cash to the hospital at its formation, hypothetically assumed to be December 31, 1986. At that time, a listing of its assets, liabilities, and fund balance would be prepared in a balance sheet and read as below:

Alpha Hospital Balance Sheet
December 31, 1986

Assets	Liabilities and Fund Balance
Cash $1,000,000	Fund balance $1,000,000

Duality

One of the fundamental premises of accounting is a very simple arithmetic requirement: the value of assets must always equal the combined value of liabilities and residual interest, which we have called fund balance. This basic accounting equation, the *duality principle*, may be stated as follows:

$$\text{Assets} = \text{Liabilities} + \text{Fund balance}$$

This requirement means that a balance sheet will always balance—the value of the assets will always equal the value of claims, whether liabilities or fund balance, on those assets.

Changes are always occurring in organizations that affect the value of assets, liabilities, and fund balance. These changes are called transactions and represent the items that interest accountants. Examples of transactions are borrowing money, purchasing supplies, and constructing buildings. The important thing to remember is that each transaction must be carefully analyzed under the duality principle to keep the basic accounting equation in balance.

To better understand how important this principle is, let us analyze several transactions in our Alpha Hospital example:

- *Transaction No. 1.* On January 2, 1987, Alpha Hospital buys a piece of equipment for $100,000. The purchase is financed with a $100,000 note from the bank.
- *Transaction No. 2.* On January 3, 1987, Alpha Hospital buys a building for $2,000,000, using $500,000 cash and issuing $1,500,000 worth of 20-year bonds.
- *Transaction No. 3.* On January 4, 1987, Alpha Hospital purchases $200,000 worth of supplies from a supply firm on a credit basis.

If balance sheets were prepared after each of these three transactions, they would appear as follows:

- *Transaction No. 1*

Alpha Hospital Balance Sheet
January 2, 1987

Assets		Liabilities and Fund Balance	
Cash	$1,000,000	Notes payable	$ 100,000
Equipment	100,000	Fund balance	1,000,000
Total	$1,100,000	Total	$1,100,000

Assets: Increase $100,000 (equipment increases by $100,000)
Liabilities: Increase $100,000 (notes payable increase by $100,000)

- *Transaction No. 2*

Alpha Hospital Balance Sheet
January 3, 1987

Assets		Liabilities and Fund Balance	
Cash	$ 500,000	Notes payable	$ 100,000
Equipment	100,000	Bonds payable	1,500,000
Building	2,000,000	Fund balance	1,000,000
Total	$2,600,000	Total	$2,600,000

Assets: Increase $1,500,000 (cash decreases by $500,000 and building increases by $2,000,000)
Liabilities: Increase $1,500,000 (bonds payable increase by $1,500,000)

● *Transaction No. 3*

Alpha Hospital Balance Sheet
January 4, 1987

Assets		Liabilities and Fund Balance	
Cash	$ 500,000	Accounts payable	$ 200,000
Supplies	200,000	Notes payable	100,000
Equipment	100,000	Bonds payable	1,500,000
Building	2,000,000	Fund balance	1,000,000
Total	$2,800,000	Total	$2,800,000

Assets: Increase $200,000 (supplies increase by $200,000)
Liabilities: Increase $200,000 (accounts payable increase by $200,000)

In each of these three transactions, the change in asset value is matched by an identical change in liability value. Thus, the basic accounting equation remains in balance.

It should be noted that, as the number of transactions increases, the number of individual asset and liability items also increases. In most organizations, there is a very large number of these individual items, which are referred to as accounts. The listing of these accounts is often called a chart of accounts; it is a useful device for categorizing transactions related to a given health care organization. There is already significant uniformity among hospitals and other health care facilities in the chart of accounts used, however, there is also pressure, especially from external users of financial information, to move toward even more uniformity.

Cost Valuation

Many readers of financial statements make the mistake of assuming that reported balance sheet values represent the real worth of individual assets or liabilities. Asset and liability values reported in a balance sheet are based on their historical or acquisition cost. In most situations, asset values do not equal the amount of money that could be realized if the assets were sold. However, in many cases the reported value of a liability in a balance sheet is a good approximation of the amount of money that would be required to extinguish the indebtedness.

Examining the alternatives to historical cost valuation helps clarify why the cost basis of valuation is used. The two primary alternatives to historical cost valuation of assets and liabilities are market value and replacement cost valuation.

Valuation of individual assets at their market value sounds simple enough and appeals to many users of financial statements. Creditors are often especially interested in what values assets would bring if liquidated. Current market values give decision makers an approximation of liquidation values.

The market value method's lack of objectivity is, however, a serious problem. In most normal situations, established markets dealing in second-hand merchandise do not exist. Decision makers must rely on individual appraisals. Given the current state of the art of appraisal, two appraisers are likely to produce different estimates of market value for an identical asset. Accountants' insistence on objectivity in measurement thus eliminates market valuation of assets as a viable alternative.

Replacement cost valuation of assets measures assets by the money value required to replace them. This concept of valuation is extremely useful for many decision-making purposes. For example, management decisions to continue delivery of certain services should be affected by the replacement cost of resources, not their historical or acquisition cost—which is considered to be a sunk cost, irrelevant to future decisions. Planning agencies or other regulatory agencies should also consider incorporating estimates of replacement cost into their decisions to avoid bias. Considering only historical cost may improperly make old facilities appear more efficient than new or proposed facilities and projects.

While replacement cost may be a useful concept of valuation, however, it too suffers from lack of objectivity in measurement. Replacement cost valuation depends upon *how* an item is replaced. For example, given the rate of technological change in the general economy, especially in the health care industry, few assets today would be replaced with like assets. Instead, more refined or capable assets would probably be substituted. What is the replacement cost in this situation? Is it the cost of the new, improved asset or the present cost of an identical asset that would most likely *not* be purchased? Compound this question by the large number of manufacturers selling roughly equivalent items and you have some idea of the inherent difficulty and subjectivity in replacement cost valuation.

Historical cost valuation, with all its faults, is thus the basis that the accounting profession has chosen to value assets and liabilities in most circumstances. Accountants use it rather than replacement cost largely because it is more objective. There is currently some fairly strong pressure from inside and outside the accounting profession to switch to replacement cost valuation, but it is still uncertain whether this pressure will be successful.

One final, important point should be noted. At the time of initial asset valuation, the values assigned by historical cost valuation and replacement cost valuation are identical. The historical cost value is most often criticized for assets that have long useful lives, such as building and equipment. Over a period of many years, the historical cost and replacement cost values tend to diverge dramatically, partly because general inflation in our economy erodes the dollar's purchasing power. A dollar of today is simply not as valuable as a dollar of ten years ago. This problem could be remedied, without sacrificing the objectivity of historical cost measurement, by selecting a unit of purchasing power as the unit of measure: Transactions would then not be accounted in dollars but in dollars of purchasing power at a given point in time, usually the year for which the financial statements are being prepared. We will discuss this issue later when we talk about the stable monetary unit principle.

Accrual Accounting

Accrual accounting is a fundamental premise of accounting. It means that transactions of a business enterprise are recognized in the time period to which they relate, not necessarily in the time periods in which cash is received or paid.

It is quite common to hear people talk about an accrual versus a cash basis of accounting. Most of us think in cash basis terms. We measure our personal, financial success during the year by how much cash we took in. Seldom do we consider such things as wear and tear on our cars and other personal items or the differences between earned and uncollected income. Perhaps if we accrued expenses for items like depreciation on heating systems, air conditioning systems, automobiles, and furniture, we might see a different picture of our financial well-being.

The accrual basis of accounting significantly affects the preparation of financial statements in general; however, its major impact is on the preparation of the statement of revenues and expenses. The following additional transactions for Alpha Hospital illustrate the importance of the accrual principle:

- *Transaction No. 4.* Alpha Hospital bills patients $100,000 on January 16, 1987, for services provided to them.
- *Transaction No. 5.* Alpha Hospital pays employees $60,000 for their wages and salaries on January 18, 1987.
- *Transaction No. 6.* Alpha Hospital receives $80,000 in cash from patients who were billed earlier in Transaction No. 4 on January 23, 1987.
- *Transaction No. 7.* Alpha Hospital pays the $200,000 of accounts payable on January 27, 1987, for the purchase of supplies that took place on January 4, 1987.

Balance sheets prepared after each of these transactions would appear as follows:

- *Transaction No. 4*

Alpha Hospital Balance Sheet
January 16, 1987

Assets		Liabilities and Fund Balance	
Cash	$ 500,000	Accounts payable	$ 200,000
Accounts receivable	100,000	Notes payable	100,000
Supplies	200,000	Bonds payable	1,500,000
Equipment	100,000	Fund balance	1,100,000
Building	2,000,000		
Total	$2,900,000	Total	$2,900,000

Assets: Increase $100,000 (accounts receivable increase by $100,000)
Fund balance: Increases $100,000

- *Transaction No. 5*

Alpha Hospital Balance Sheet
January 18, 1987

Assets		Liabilities and Fund Balance	
Cash	$ 440,000	Accounts payable	$ 200,000
Accounts receivable	100,000	Notes payable	100,000
Supplies	200,000	Bonds payable	1,500,000
Equipment	100,000	Fund balance	1,040,000
Building	2,000,000		
Total	$2,840,000	Total	$2,840,000

Assets: Decrease by $60,000 (cash decreases by $60,000)
Fund balance: Decreases by $60,000

- *Transaction No. 6*

Alpha Hospital Balance Sheet
January 23, 1987

Assets		Liabilities and Fund Balance	
Cash	$ 520,000	Accounts payable	$ 200,000
Accounts receivable	20,000	Notes payable	100,000
Supplies	200,000	Bonds payable	1,500,000
Equipment	100,000	Fund balance	1,040,000
Building	2,000,000		
Total	$2,840,000	Total	$2,840,000

Assets: No change (cash increases by $80,000; accounts receivable decrease by
$80,000)

● *Transaction No. 7*

Alpha Hospital Balance Sheet
January 27, 1987

Assets		Liabilities and Fund Balance	
Cash	$ 320,000	Accounts payable	$ 0
Accounts receivable	20,000	Notes payable	100,000
Supplies	200,000	Bonds payable	1,500,000
Equipment	100,000	Fund balance	1,040,000
Building	2,000,000		
Total	$2,640,000	Total	$2,640,000

Assets: Decrease by $200,000 (cash decreases by $200,000)
Liabilities: Decrease by $200,000 (accounts payable decrease by $200,000)

In Transactions Nos. 4 and 5, there is an effect upon Alpha Hospital's residual interest or its fund balance. In Transaction No. 4, an increase in fund balance occurred due to the billing of patients for services previously rendered. Increases in fund balance or owner's equity resulting from the sale of goods or delivery of services are called revenues. It should be noted that this increase occurred even though no cash was actually collected until January 23, 1987, illustrating the accrual principle of accounting. Recognition of revenue occurs when the revenue is earned, not necessarily when it is collected.

In Transaction No. 5, a reduction in fund balance occurs. Costs incurred by a business enterprise to provide goods or services that reduce fund balance or owner's equity are called expenses. Under the accrual principle, expenses are recognized when assets are used up or liabilities incurred in the production and delivery of goods or services, not necessarily when cash is paid.

The difference between revenue and expense is often referred to as *net income.* In the hospital and health care industry, this term may be used interchangeably with the term *excess of revenues over expenses.*

The income statement or statement of revenues and expenses summarizes the revenues and expenses of a business enterprise over a defined period of time. If an income statement is prepared for the total life of an entity, that is, from inception to dissolution, it happens that the value for net income would be the same under both an accrual and a cash basis of accounting.

In most situations, frequent measurements of revenue and expense are demanded, creating some important measurement problems. Ideally, under the accrual accounting principle, expenses should be matched to the revenue that they helped create. For example, wage, salary, and supply costs can usually be easily associated with revenues of a given period. However, in certain circumstances, the association between revenue and expense is impossible to discover, necessitating the accountant's use of a systematic, rational method of allocating costs to a benefiting time period. In the best example of this procedure, costs such as those associated with building and equipment are spread over the estimated useful life of the assets through the recording of depreciation.

To complete the Alpha Hospital example, we will assume that the financial statements must be prepared at the end of January. Before they are prepared, certain adjustments must be made to the accounts to adhere fully to the accrual principle of accounting. The following adjustments might be recorded:

- *Adjustment No. 1.* There are currently $100,000 of patient charges that have been incurred but not yet billed.

- *Adjustment No. 2.* There is currently $50,000 worth of unpaid wages and salaries for which employees have performed services.

- *Adjustment No. 3.* A physical inventory count indicates that $50,000 worth of initial supplies have been used.

- *Adjustment No. 4.* The equipment of Alpha Hospital has an estimated useful life of ten years, and the cost is being allocated over this time period. On a monthly basis, this amounts to an allocation of $833 per month.

- *Adjustment No. 5.* The building has an estimated useful life of 40 years, and the cost of the building is being allocated equally over its estimated life. On a monthly basis, this amounts to $4,167.

- *Adjustment No. 6.* While no payment has occurred on either notes payable or bonds payable, it must be recognized that there is an interest expense associated with using money for this one-month time period. This interest expense will be paid at a later date. Assume that the note payable carries an interest rate of eight percent and the bond payable carries an interest rate of six percent. The actual amount of interest expense incurred for the month of January would be $8,167 ($667 on the note and $7,500 on the bond payable).

The effects of these adjustments on the balance sheet of Alpha Hospital, and on the ending balance sheet that would be prepared after all the adjustments were made, are presented below.

Adjustment	Amount of Change	Account(s) Increased	Account(s) Decreased
No. 1	$100,000	Fund balance	None
		Accounts receivable	None
No. 2	50,000	Wages & salaries payable	Fund balance
No. 3	50,000	None	Fund balance, supplies
No. 4	833	None	Fund balance, equipment
No. 5	4,167	None	Fund balance, building
No. 6	8,167	Interest payable	Fund balance

Alpha Hospital Balance Sheet
January 31, 1987

Assets		Liabilities and Fund Balance	
Cash	$ 320,000	Wages & salaries payable	$ 50,000
Accounts receivable	120,000	Interest payable	8,167
Supplies	150,000	Notes payable	100,000
Equipment	99,167	Bonds payable	1,500,000
Building	1,995,833	Fund balance	1,026,833
Total	$2,685,000	Total	$2,685,000

It is also possible to prepare the following statement of revenues and expenses:

Alpha Hospital
Statement of Revenues and Expenses
For month ended January 31, 1987

Revenues	$200,000
Less expenses	
Wages and salaries	$110,000
Supplies	50,000
Depreciation	5,000
Interest	8,167
Total	$173,167
Excess of revenues over expenses	$ 26,833

Note that the difference between revenue and expense during the month of January was $26,833, the exact amount by which the fund balance of Alpha Hospital changed during the month. Alpha Hospital began the month with $1,000,000 in its fund balance account and ended with $1,026,833. This illustrates an important point to remember in the reading of financial statements: *the individual financial statements are fundamentally related to one another.*

Stable Monetary Unit

The money measurement principle of accounting discussed earlier restricted accounting measures to money. In accounting in the United States, the unit of measure is the U.S. dollar. At the present time, no adjustment to changes in the general purchasing power of that unit is required in financial reports; a 1972 dollar is assumed to be equal in value to a 1987 dollar. This permits arithmetic operations, such as addition and subtraction. If this assumption were not made, addition of the unadjusted historical cost values of assets acquired in different time periods would be inappropriate, like adding apples and oranges. Current, generally accepted accounting principles incorporate the *stable monetary unit principle.*

This principle may not seem to pose any great problems. In fact, when the inflation rate was less than 2 percent annually, it did not. However, given the recent high rates of inflation, the effects of assuming a stable monetary unit can be quite dramatic. Imagine that the inflation rate in the economy is currently 100 percent, compounded monthly. The hypothetical entity under consideration is a neighborhood health center that has all its expenses, except payroll, covered by grants from governmental agencies. its employees have a contract that automatically adjusts their wages to changes in the general price level. (With a monthly inflation rate of 100 percent, it is no wonder.) Assume that revenues from patients are collected on the first day of the month following the one in which they were billed, but that the employees are paid at the beginning of each month. Rates to patients are set so that the excess of revenues over expenses will be zero. With the first month's wages set equal to $100,000, the following income and cash flow positions result for the first six months of the year:

	Income Flows			Cash Flows		
	Expense	Revenue	Net Income	Inflow	Outflow	Difference
January	$ 100,000	$ 100,000	0	$ 50,000*	$ 100,000	(50,000)
February	200,000	200,000	0	100,000	200,000	(100,000)
March	400,000	400,000	0	200,000	400,000	(200,000)
April	800,000	800,000	0	400,000	800,000	(400,000)
May	1,600,000	1,600,000	0	800,000	1,600,000	(800,000)
June	3,200,000	3,200,000	0	1,600,000	3,200,000	(1,600,000)
	$6,300,000	$6,300,000	0	$3,150,000	$6,300,000	(3,150,000)

*$50,000 is equal to the revenue billed in December.

Note the tremendous difference between income and cash flow. While the income statement would indicate a break-even operation, the cash balance at the end of June would be a negative $3,150,000. Obviously, the health center's operations cannot continue indefinitely in light of the extreme cash hardship position imposed.

Fortunately, the rate of inflation in our economy is not 100 percent. However, smaller rates of inflation compounded over long periods of time could create similar problems. For example, setting rates equal to historical cost depreciation of fixed assets leaves the entity with a significant cash deficit when it is time to replace the asset. Yet, currently many third party payers do in fact limit reimbursement to unadjusted historical cost depreciation, and few health care organizations actually set rates at levels necessary to recover replacement cost.

Fund Accounting

Fund accounting is a system in which an entity's assets and liabilities are segregated in the accounting records. Each fund may be thought of as an independent entity with its own self-balancing set of accounts. The basic accounting equation discussed under the duality principle must be satisfied for each fund—assets must equal liabilities plus fund balance for the particular fund in question. This is, in fact, how the term *fund balance* developed; a fund balance originally represented the residual interest for a *particular fund.*

Fund accounting is widely employed by nonprofit, voluntary health care facilities, especially hospitals. It is not a basic concept or principle of accounting like those previously discussed, but it is a feature peculiar to accounting for many health care organizations. It evolved primarily for use in stewarding funds donated by external parties who imposed stipulations on the usage of those monies.

Two major categories of funds are presently used in the hospital industry and in other health care facilities: They are restricted and unrestricted. A restricted fund is one in which a third party, outside the entity, has imposed certain restrictions on the use of donated monies or resources. There are three common types of restricted funds:

1. specific purpose funds
2. plant replacement and expansion funds
3. endowment funds

Specific purpose funds are donated by individuals or organizations and restricted for purposes other than plant replacement and expansion or endowment. Monies received from government agencies to perform specific research or other work are examples of specific purpose funds.

Plant replacement and expansion funds are restricted for use in plant replacement and expansion. Assets purchased with these monies are not recorded in the fund. When the monies are used for plant purposes, the amounts are transferred to the unrestricted fund. For example, if $200,000 in cash from the plant replacement fund were used to acquire a piece of equipment, the equipment and fund balance of the unrestricted fund would be increased.

Endowment funds are contributed to be held intact for generating income. The income may or may not be restricted for specific purposes. Some endowments are classified as "term" endowments. That is, after the expiration of some time period, the restriction on use of the principal is lifted. The balance is then transferred to the unrestricted fund.

Unrestricted funds have no third party donor restrictions imposed upon them. In some cases, the governing board of the organization may restrict use, but, since this is not an external or third party restriction, the funds are still classified as unrestricted. Sometimes, the unrestricted fund is referred to as the general or operating fund.

CONVENTIONS OF ACCOUNTING

The accounting principles discussed up to this point are important in the preparation of financial statements. However, several widely accepted conventions modify the application of these principles in certain circumstances. We shall discuss three of the more important conventions:

1. conservatism
2. materiality
3. consistency

Conservatism affects the valuation of some assets. Specifically, accountants use a "lower of cost or market rule" for valuing inventories and marketable securities. The "lower of cost or market" rule means that the value of a stock of inventory or marketable securities would be its actual cost or market value, whichever is less. For these resources, there is a deviation from cost valuation to market valuation whenever market value is lower.

Materiality permits certain transactions to be treated out of accordance with generally accepted accounting principles. This might be permitted because the transaction does not materially affect the presentation of financial position. For example, theoretically, paper clips have an estimated useful life greater than one year. However, the cost of capitalizing this item and systematically and rationally allocating it over its useful life is not justifiable; the difference in financial position that would be created by not using generally accepted accounting principles would be immaterial.

Consistency limits the accounting alternatives that can be used. In any given transaction, there is usually a variety of available, generally acceptable accounting treatments. For example, generally accepted accounting principles permit the use of double declining balance, sum of the year digits, or straight-line methods for allocating the costs of depreciable assets over their estimated useful life; but the consistency convention limits an entity's ability to change from one acceptable method to another. Recall that the opinion paragraph in a CPA's audit report assures that generally accepted accounting principles have been applied on a basis *consistent* with that of the previous year.

SUMMARY

In this chapter we have discussed the importance of generally accepted accounting principles in deriving financial information. Though these principles are formally required only in the preparation of audited financial statements, they influence the derivation of most financial information. An understanding of some of the basic principles is critical to an understanding of financial information in general.

Six specific principles of accounting were discussed in some detail:

1. accounting entity
2. money measurement
3. duality
4. cost valuation
5. accrual accounting
6. stable monetary unit

In addition to these, the general importance of fund accounting, as it relates to the hospital and health care industry, was discussed. The chapter concluded with a discussion of three conventions that may modify the application of generally accepted accounting principles in specific situations.

ASSIGNMENTS

1. ABC Medical Center has undergone a recent corporate reorganization. The following structure resulted:

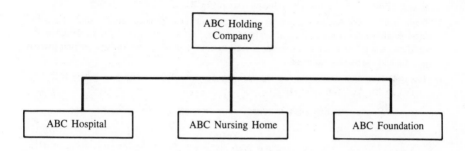

What difficulties might be experienced in preparing financial statements for the ABC Hospital?

2. Does the value of total assets represent the economic value of the entity?

3. What is the difference between stockholders' equity and fund balance?

4. A home health care firm has purchased five automobiles for use in treating its patients. Each car cost $12,000 and has an estimated useful life of three years. Each year, the replacement cost of the automobiles is expected to increase ten percent. At the end of the third year, replacement cost would be $15,972. The firm anticipates that each car will be used to make 1,500 patient visits per year. If the firm prices each visit to recover just the historical cost of the cars, it will include a capital cost of $2.67 per visit ($12,000/4,500 total visits). Assuming the revenue generated from this capital charge is invested at ten percent, will the firm have enough funds available to meet its replacement cost? How would this situation change if price level depreciation were used to establish the capital charge?

5. A health maintenance organization (HMO) has just been formed. During its first year of operations, the organization reported an accounting loss of $500,000. Cash flow during the same period was a positive $500,000. How might this situation exist, and which measure better describes financial performance?

6. What is the difference between restricted and unrestricted funds?

7. Why is consistency in financial reporting critical to fairness in financial representation?

SOLUTIONS AND ANSWERS

1. It may be difficult to associate specific assets and liabilities for the ABC Hospital. For example, debt may have been issued by the holding company to finance projects for both the hospital and the nursing home. In addition, commonly used assets may be involved, such as a dietary department providing meals for both hospital and nursing home patients. Some expenses may also be difficult to trace to either the hospital or the nursing home. For example, how should expenses that are common to the hospital, the nursing home, and the foundation, such as

administrative expenses of the holding company, be allocated? Thus, many problems of jointness may make preparation of the financial statements for the hospital difficult, but such statements are still likely to be a necessity for adequate planning and control.

2. Only coincidentally would the value of total assets equal the economic value of the entity. Total assets, as reported in the balance sheet, represent the undepreciated historical cost of assets acquired by the entity. Economic value of an entity is related to the discounted value of future earnings or the market value of the entity if sold.

3. Both stockholders' equity and fund balance represent the difference between total assets and total liabilities. Stockholder's equity is used in investor-owned corporations to designate the residual owners' claims. Fund balance is used in not-for-profit corporations in which there is no residual ownership interest.

4. The following data are relevant to the pricing decision of the home health care firm with regard to the five automobiles:

Funds available with historical cost depreciation/car:

	Depreciation	Years Invested (10%)	Future Value (10%)
Year 1	$ 4,000	2	$ 4,840
Year 2	4,000	1	4,400
Year 3	4,000	0	4,000
	$12,000		$13,240

Shortage = $15,972 − $13,240 = $2,732/car

Funds available with price level depreciation/car:

	Depreciation	Years Invested (10%)	Future Value (10%)
Year 1	$ 4,400	2	$ 5,324
Year 2	4,840	1	5,324
Year 3	5,324	0	5,324
	$14,564		$15,972

Shortage = $15,972 − 15,972 = 0

Thus, the prices should be set equal to expected replacement cost. Clearly, pricing services to recover capital costs is critical to long-term financial survival.

5. The HMO could have received large payments in advance for providing health services to major employers. This would mean that a liability to provide future services exists. Both accounting loss and cash flow are important in assessing financial performance. The accounting loss is symbolic of a critical operational problem with regard to revenue and expense relationships. The positive cash flow may be temporary unless revenue exceeds expenses in future periods.

6. A restricted fund is one that has a third party donor restriction placed upon the utilization of the funds. An unrestricted fund has no such restriction.

7. Changes in financial reporting can impair the comparability of financial results between years for a given firm.

Chapter 4

Financial Statements

Understanding the principles of accounting is a critical first step in understanding financial statements. However, the format and language of financial statements may be unintelligible to the occasional reader. In this chapter we discuss in some detail the four major general purpose financial statements:

1. balance sheet
2. statement of revenues and expenses
3. statement of changes in financial position
4. statement of changes in fund balances

In addition, we examine the footnotes to the financial statements.

The balance sheet and statement of revenues and expenses are more widely published and used than the other two statements. Understanding them enables a reader to use the other two financial statements and financial information in general. Therefore, in the following discussion, we pay major attention to the balance sheet and statement of revenue and expenses.

The balance sheets examined in the following two sections illustrate the separation of funds into restricted and unrestricted categories. Restricted funds are not available for general operating purposes. The duality principle can also be seen operating in these balance sheets. Assets equal liabilities plus fund balance in both restricted and unrestricted balance sheets. In both cases, the entity being accounted for is Omega Hospital.

BALANCE SHEET: UNRESTRICTED FUNDS

Current Assets

Assets that are expected to be exchanged for cash or consumed during the operating cycle of the entity (or one year, whichever is longer) are classified as current assets on the balance sheet. The operating cycle is the length of time between acquisition of materials and services and collection of revenue generated by them. Since the operating cycle for most health care organizations is significantly less than one year (perhaps three months or less), current assets are predominantly those that may be expected to be converted into cash or used to reduce expenditures of cash within one year.

Cash

Cash represents the funds on hand in bill or coin form or in savings or checking accounts. It does not include funds restricted in some way, for example, cash funds restricted for investment in retirement plans or self-insurance plans.

Marketable Securities

Marketable securities, or short-term investments, comprise another major category of current assets that often shows up on balance sheets, although it is not shown in Exhibit 4–1. In some cases, cash and marketable securities are combined. This is not considered bad reporting because the liquidity of marketable securities allows them to be treated as cash for most purposes. Marketable securities are short-term investments that meet two criteria. First, management must intend to sell or convert them to cash within a year's time. This is guaranteed if the maturity of the investment is less than one year. Second, they must have a readily available and active market. Marketable securities are valued at their cost or market value, whichever is lower. This is one of the few exceptions to the cost valuation principle.

Accounts Receivable

Accounts receivable represent legally enforceable claims on customers for prior services or goods. In Omega Hospital, there are two categories of accounts receivable: patient and other. Other accounts receivable in a health care organization imply revenue derived from sources other than patient

Exhibit 4–1 Balance Sheet for Omega Hospital, Unrestricted Funds

Omega Hospital Balance Sheet
Unrestricted Funds June 30, 1987
(with comparative figures for 1986)

	June 30	
	1987	1986
Assets		
Current assets		
Cash	$ 376,766	$ 46,073
Accounts receivable		
Patients (less contractual allowances from third party payers of $278,000 in 1987 and $248,000 in 1986, and allowance for doubtful accounts of $330,000 in 1987 and $295,000 in 1986)	3,675,531	2,846,266
Other	272,144	260,070
Inventories	325,720	255,176
Prepaid expenses	343,640	289,806
Total current assets	4,993,801	3,697,391
Property and equipment		
Land and improvements	413,809	408,557
Buildings and equipment	11,191,834	10,776,959
Building additions in progress	25,741,801	18,199,040
Other construction in progress	377,317	36,502
	37,724,761	29,421,058
Allowances for depreciation	6,745,307	6,106,815
Total property and equipment	30,979,454	23,314,243
Other assets		
Board-designated investments	98,328	102,470
Total	$36,071,583	$27,114,104
Liabilities reserve and fund balance		
Current liabilities		
Accounts payable—trade	$ 797,966	$ 760,920
construction contractor	1,665,797	1,724,878
Advances from third party payers	142,051	—
Loan payable—restricted fund	—	554,689
Accrued expenses	1,341,393	868,091
Payroll deductions	127,478	143,017
Current maturities or mortgages payable	222,386	—
Total current liabilities	4,297,071	4,051,595
Mortgages payable	21,515,300	14,440,202
Loan payable—restricted fund	1,390,905	—
Total liabilities	27,203,276	18,491,797
Deferred revenue	56,000	76,000
Fund balance	8,812,307	8,546,307
Total	$36,071,583	$27,114,104

services. For example, Omega Hospital has a physician's office building, a parking ramp, and a number of educational programs. Accounts receivable may exist in one or all of those areas.

Patient accounts receivable are usually the largest accounts receivable item, and, for that matter, the largest single current asset item in the balance sheet. Omega Hospital is no exception—it has an estimated $3,675,531 in accounts receivable that will eventually result in cash. The actual dollar amount of accounts receivable is higher but is reduced by estimated allowances.

A characteristic of hospitals and other health care organizations that makes their accounts receivable different from those of most other organizations is that the charges actually billed to patients are quite often settled for substantially less than the amounts charged. The differences are also known as allowances. Four major categories of allowances are used to restate accounts receivable to expected, realizable value:

1. charity allowances
2. courtesy allowances
3. doubtful account allowances
4. contractual allowances

A charity allowance is the difference between established service rates and amounts actually charged to indigent patients. Many health care facilities, especially clinics and other ambulatory care settings, have a policy of scaling the normal charge by some factor based on income. A courtesy allowance is the difference between established rates for services and rates billed special patients, such as employees, doctors, and clergy. A doubtful account allowance is the difference between rates billed and amounts expected to be recovered. For example, a medically indigent patient might actually receive services that have an established rate of $100, but be billed only $50. If it is anticipated that the patient will not pay even the $50, then that $50 will show up as a doubtful account allowance.

In most situations, contractual allowances represent the largest deduction from accounts receivable. A contractual allowance is the difference between rates billed to a third party payer, such as Medicare, and the amount that will actually be paid by that third party payer. For example, a Medicare patient may receive hospital services priced at $4,000 but actually pay the hospital only $3,000 for those services, based upon the patient's DRG classification. If this account is unpaid at the fiscal year end, the financial statements would include the net amount to be paid, $3,000, as an account receivable. Accounts receivable represent the amount of cash expected to be received, not the gross prices charged. Since most major payers—such as Medicare, Medicaid, and Blue Cross—have a contractual relationship that permits payment on a basis other than charges, contractual allowances can be, and usually are, very large.

It is important to note that the allowances are estimates and will, in all probability, differ from the actual value of accounts receivable that will eventually be written off. For example, Omega Hospital shows an expected value of accounts receivable to be collected as $3,675,531 in 1987, but it actually has $4,283,531 of outstanding accounts receivable.

Net accounts receivable	$3,675,531
Contractual allowances	278,000
Doubtful account allowance	330,000
Accounts receivable gross	$4,283,531

Since estimation of allowances is so critical to the reported value of accounts receivable, the methodology should be scrutinized. Just how was the estimate developed? Has the estimating method been used in the past with any degree of reliability? An external audit performed by an independent CPA can usually provide the required degree of reliability and assurance.

Inventories

Inventories in a health care facility represent items that are to be used in the delivery of health care services. They may range from normal business office supplies to highly specialized chemicals used in a laboratory.

Prepaid Expenses

Prepaid expenses represent expenditures already made for future service. In Omega Hospital, they may represent prepayment of insurance premiums for the year, rents on leased equipment, or other similar items. For example, an insurance premium for a professional liability insurance policy may be $600,000 per year, due one year in advance. If this amount were paid on January 1st, then on June 30th, $300,000, or one-half the total, would be shown as a prepaid expense.

Property and Equipment

This category is sometimes called fixed assets or shown more descriptively as plant property and equipment. Items in this category represent investment in tangible, permanent assets; they are sometimes referred to as the capital assets of the organization. These items are shown at the historical cost or acquisition cost, reduced by allowances for depreciation.

Land and Improvements

Land and improvements represent the historical cost of the earth's surface owned by the health care facility and the historical cost of any improvements erected on it. Such improvements might include water and sewer systems, roadways, fences, sidewalks, shrubbery, and parking lots. While land may not be depreciated, land improvements may. Land held for investment purposes are not shown in this category but will appear as an investment in the other assets section.

Buildings and Equipment

Buildings and equipment represent all buildings and equipment owned by the entity and used in the normal course of its operations. These items are also stated at historical cost. Buildings and equipment not used in the normal course of operations should be reported separately. For example, real estate investments would not be shown in the fixed asset or plant property and equipment section but in the other assets section. Equipment in many situations is classified into three categories: (1) *fixed equipment*—affixed to the building in which it is located, including items such as elevators, boilers, and generators; (2) *major movable equipment*—usually stationary but capable of being moved, including reasonably expensive items such as automobiles, laboratory equipment, and x-ray apparatus; and (3) *minor equipment*—usually low in cost with short estimated useful lives, including such items as wastebaskets, glassware, and sheets.

Construction in Progress

Construction in progress represents the amount of money that has been expended on projects that are still not complete at the date the financial statement is published. In Omega Hospital, there are currently $25,741,801 of building additions in progress and $377,317 of other construction in progress. When these projects are completed, the values will be charged to buildings and equipment.

Allowance for Depreciation

Allowance for depreciation represents the accumulated depreciation taken on the asset to the date of the financial statement. The concept of depreciation is important and useful in a wide variety of decisions. The following example illustrates the depreciation concept: A $500 desk is purchased and depreciated over a five-year life. The balance sheet values are presented below.

	Year				
	1	2	3	4	5
Historical equipment cost	$500	$500	$500	$500	$500
Allowance for depreciation	100	200	300	400	500
Net	$400	$300	$200	$100	$ 0

In the case of Omega Hospital, there is $6,745,307 of accumulated depreciation at June 30, 1987. The historical cost base for this amount is probably fairly close to $11,191,834, the historical cost value of buildings and equipment. In reality, the figure is slightly higher because land improvements are also depreciated and would be included in the accumulated depreciation total. This means that 60.26 percent of the historical cost of present facilities has been depreciated in prior years. As the ratio of allowance for depreciation to building and equipment increases, it usually signifies that a physical plant will need replacement in the near future. Omega Hospital appears to be in such a situation, which may partially explain the current construction.

Other Assets

Other assets are assets that are neither current nor involve plant and equipment. Typically, they are either investments or intangible assets. In the case of Omega Hospital, all other assets consist of investments that have been board-restricted; they must be shown in the unrestricted balance sheet because the board restriction does not qualify as a third party restriction. However, they are shown separately in the unrestricted balance sheet to identify the restriction.

Two major intangible asset items that show up in some health care facility balance sheets are goodwill and organization costs. Goodwill represents the difference between the price paid to acquire another entity and the fair market value of the acquired entity's assets, less any related obligations or liabilities. Goodwill shows up mainly in proprietary facilities, although it is also being increasingly seen in voluntary not-for-profit organizations as they acquire other health care entities. Organization costs are expended for legal and accounting fees and other items incurred at the formation of the entity. The cost of these items is usually amortized over some allowable life.

Current Liabilities

Current liabilities are obligations that are expected to require payment in cash during the coming year or operating cycle, whichever is longer. Like current assets, they are generally expected to be paid in one year's time.

Accounts Payable

Accounts payable may be thought of as the counterpart of accounts receivable. They represent the entity's promise to pay money for goods or services it has received. In the Omega Hospital example, two types of accounts payable appear, one resulting from normal activity, called accounts payable—trade, the other due to the construction contractor for work in process, referred to as accounts payable—construction contractor.

Advances from Third Parties

Advances from third parties constitute an account that is somewhat peculiar to the health care industry. In some situations, a third party payer, Blue Cross particularly, will pay a health care entity a sum in advance of the provision of services. Since the entity must generally invest its resources prior to payment, this advance partially offsets the entity's requirement for a cash outflow and helps meet the financial requirements of the health care facility. An additional advantage is that the advance may reduce the amount of money a health care provider must borrow; this in turn reduces interest expense and thereby keeps costs down in the long run.

Accrued Expenses

Accrued expenses are obligations that result from prior operations. They are thus a present right or enforceable demand. The accruing of interest expense with the passage of time, discussed in Chapter 3, is an example. Other examples of accrued expenses are payroll, vacation pay, tax deductions, rent, and insurance. In some cases, especially payroll, accrued expenses are disaggregated to show material categories. Omega Hospital does not do this, but it does show a separate listing of payroll deductions.

Payroll Deductions

Payroll deductions represent amounts withheld from employees' wages to meet a variety of federal, state, and local obligations, for example, social security contributions and income taxes.

Current Maturities of Long-Term Debt

Current maturities of long-term debt represent the amount of principal that will be repaid on the indebtedness within the coming year. It does not equal the total amount of the payments that will be made during that year. Total payments include both interest and principal; current maturities of long-term debt include just the principal portion. For example, if at the June 30th fiscal year close, a total of $360,000 ($30,000 per month) will be paid on long-term indebtedness during the coming year and, of this amount, only $120,000 is principal payment, then $120,000 would be shown as a current maturity of long-term debt.

Noncurrent Liabilities

Noncurrent liabilities include obligations that will not require payment in cash for at least one year or more. Omega Hospital shows two types of noncurrent liabilities, mortgage payable and loan payable from restricted fund.

Mortgage Payable

Mortgage payable is one source of long-term indebtedness. The adjective mortgage implies that the indebtedness is collateralized by a lien on some set of the entity's assets. Other examples of long-term debt are bonds payable and notes payable.

Loan Payable—Restricted Fund

Omega Hospital also has a noncurrent liability described as a loan payable from restricted funds. This brings up an important issue. Just how valid is this liability? The debt is, after all, owed to the entity itself. Note that at June 30, 1986, the indebtedness of $554,689 is classified as a current liability, but on June 30, 1987, the indebtedness of $1,390,905 is classified as noncurrent. This transfer from current liabilities to noncurrent liabilities causes some speculation about the validity of the indebtedness. However, it must be remembered that a restricted fund is one in which a third party has imposed some restrictions on use. The validity of the loan, as well as the separation of funds, depends upon the legitimacy of those restrictions.

Deferred Revenue

Deferred revenue is not classified as liability or fund balance. Deferred revenue means cash or other assets received prior to the actual recognition of the amount as revenue. Typically, in the health care industry, the deferred revenue account is used to recognize timing differences between the receipt of cash and the recognition of it as revenue. For example, Omega Hospital may have used some form of accelerated depreciation for cost-reimbursement purposes but used straight-line depreciation for financial reporting. Specifically, in the desk illustration discussed earlier, straight-line depreciation in the first year would be $100. If the sum of the year's digits depreciation method were used for reimbursement purposes, first year depreciation would be $167. The difference ($67) would be recorded as deferred revenue. At the conclusion of the useful life of this asset, the deferred revenue account would be zero.

Fund Balance

Fund balance, as discussed earlier, represents the difference between assets and the claim to those assets by third parties or liabilities. Increases in this account balance usually arise from one of two sources: (1) contributions or (2) earnings.

In the nonprofit health care industry, there is usually no separation in the fund balance account to recognize these two sources. Thus, there is no indication of how much of Omega Hospital's fund balance of $8,812,307 was earned and how much was contributed. Financial statements prepared for proprietary entities do show this breakdown. Earnings of prior years, reduced by dividend payments to stockholders, are shown in an account labeled retained earnings.

In any given year, however, it is possible to determine the sources of change in fund balance by examining the statement of changes in fund balance (see Exhibit 4–5). For example, in fiscal year 1987, transfers from the plant replacement and renovation fund, a restricted fund, accounted for all the increase in fund balance. These transfers more than offset the operating loss of $226,247 for the period.

The value of the fund balance account at any point in time is often confused with the cash position of the entity. However, cash and fund balance will hardly ever be equal. In most situations, the cash balance will be far less than fund balance. For example, Omega Hospital has $8,812,307 in fund balance at June 30, 1987, but only $376,766 in cash at the same date. Thus, the assumption that the $8,812,307 reported as fund balance can be converted into cash is a false assumption.

BALANCE SHEET: RESTRICTED FUNDS

The balance sheet of Omega Hospital has a separate accounting for four funds that third parties have restricted (see Exhibit 4–2):

1. special purpose fund
2. research fund
3. endowment fund
4. plant replacement and renovation fund

It is possible to think of these four funds as separate balance sheets, each satisfying the basic accounting equation of

$$assets = liabilities + fund\ balance.$$

For example, Omega Hospital's plant replacement and renovation fund has a balance of $3,378,408, which must equal its assets because no liabilities exist. The assets of the plant replacement and renovation fund consist of $1,681,258 in cash and money market investments, $306,245 in pledges receivable, and $1,390,905 in loans receivable from unrestricted funds.

Omega Hospital Balance Sheet
Plant Replacement and Renovation Fund

Assets		Fund Balance	
Cash and money market investments	$1,681,258		
Pledges receivable	306,245		
Loan receivable—unrestricted fund	1,390,905		$3,378,408
Total	$3,378,408	Fund balance	$3,378,408

This arithmetic is also representative of the other three funds.

The use of the cost valuation principle can be seen clearly in the investments of the endowment fund. In 1986 and 1987, the market value of the investments was less than their historical cost, but cost valuation

Exhibit 4–2 Balance Sheet for Omega Hospital, Restricted Funds

Omega Hospital
Balance Sheet
Restricted Funds
June 30, 1987
(with comparative figures for 1986)

	June 30	
	1987	1986
Assets		
Cash and money market investments		
Specific-purpose funds	$ 117,889	$ 92,156
Research funds	57,848	46,347
Endowment funds	62,161	52,096
Plant replacement and renovation fund	1,681,258	2,248,863
Investments—endowment funds, at cost (approximate market value $575,431 in 1987 and $538,000 in 1986)	685,815	685,815
Plant replacement and renovation fund		
Pledges receivable	306,245	678,662
Loan receivable from unrestricted fund	1,390,905	554,689
	$4,302,121	$4,358,628
Fund balance		
Specific-purpose funds	$ 117,889	$ 92,156
Research funds	57,848	46,347
Endowment funds		
Free care	598,426	598,426
Scholarships	111,529	112,212
Other	38,021	27,273
Plant replacement and renovation fund	3,378,408	3,482,214
	$4,302,121	$4,358,628

continued to be used. In reality, Omega Hospital does not have $685,815 in endowment fund investments; it has only a realizable value of $575,431. This difference could be caused by poor investment management or external limitations on investment, imposed by the stipulations of the initial gift. Regardless of the reason, the hospital has seen a decline in its initial donated value of $110,384 (see Exhibit 4–2).

Pledges receivable is an account that may be unfamiliar to many individuals. It represents a legally enforceable commitment from a third party. In the case of Omega Hospital, $306,245 of pledges are currently outstanding as of June 30, 1987. These pledges are restricted and must be used for plant replacement and renovation. Restricted in this way, they will never have to be reported as income by Omega Hospital. Depending upon management's objectives, it may or it may not be advantageous to restrict the majority of gifts. For example, a hospital faced with regulatory controls on income may wish to restrict all pledges so that it will not have to report them as income. Nonetheless, it is important to recognize such sources of unreported income in the assessment of a health care entity's financial strength.

STATEMENT OF REVENUE AND EXPENSE

The statement of revenue and expense (Exhibit 4–3) has become a financial statement of increasing importance, both in the proprietary and nonproprietary sector. It gives a better picture of operations in a given time period than a balance sheet does. A balance sheet summarizes the wealth position of an entity at a given point in time by delineating its assets, liabilities, and fund balance. An income statement provides information concerning *how* that wealth position was changed through operations.

An entity's ability to earn an excess of revenue over expenses is an important variable in many external and internal decisions. A series of income statements indicates this ability well. Creditors use income statements to determine the entity's ability to pay future and present debts; management and rate regulating agencies use them to assess whether current and proposed rate structures are adequate.

The *entity principle* is an important factor in analyzing and interpreting the statement of revenue and expense. Income, the excess of revenue over expenses, comes from a large number of individual operations within a health care entity and is aggregated in the statement of revenue and expense. For example, reports on minor breakdowns may be required on a departmental basis for some decisions; little can be said about specific rates and their adequacy within a health care facility if departmental statements of revenue and expense are not available. Such statements are in fact frequently available and should be used. Here, however, our focus is on the general purpose

Exhibit 4–3 Statement of Revenues and Expenses for Omega Hospital

Omega Hospital
Statement of Revenue and Expense
Year Ended June 30, 1987
(with comparative figures for 1986)

	Year Ended June 30	
	1987	1986
Hospital services		
Patient service revenue	$23,448,220	$19,814,924
Allowances and uncollectible accounts	1,208,376	751,475
Patient service revenue, before contractual allowances	22,239,844	19,063,449
Other operating revenue	665,160	614,834
Total operating revenue	22,905,004	19,678,283
Operating expenses		
Nursing services	7,331,032	6,329,254
Other professional services	7,273,611	6,303,910
General services	3,769,307	3,086,584
Fiscal services	1,002,768	869,857
Administrative services	2,871,246	1,902,813
Provision for depreciation	549,799	470,609
Interest expense	156,695	85,266
Total operating expenses	22,954,458	19,048,293
Excess (deficiency) of operating revenues over operating expenses	(49,454)	629,990
Nonoperating revenues	11,126	67,989
Excess (deficiency) of revenues over expenses	(38,328)	697,979
Professional office building services		
Excess of expenses over revenues	(80,420)	—
Parking ramp service		
Excess of expenses over revenues	(107,499)	—
Excess (deficiency) of revenues over expenses	$(226,247)	$ 697,979

statement of revenue and expense, which is an aggregate of individual departments' income.

Revenue

Generally speaking, revenue in a health care facility comes from three sources:

1. operations related to patient services
2. operations not related to patient services
3. nonoperating sources

Patient Service Revenue

Patient service revenue in most facilities is by far the largest source of revenue. Omega Hospital reported $23,448,220 of patient service revenue in 1987. This amount is stated at its gross or billed value and does not reflect what amounts were actually collected or expected to be collected. To determine what was or will be collected, the gross figure must be reduced by estimates of the four categories of allowances discussed earlier in the chapter. Omega Hospital had $1,208,376 of allowances and uncollectible accounts in 1987, which yielded a net patient service revenue of $22,239,844. Net patient service revenue reflects the amount of revenue that will be realized in cash payments; it measures what is or will be collected, not what was charged.

Earlier discussion of accounts receivable briefly mentioned the four categories of allowances (charity, courtesy, contractual, and uncollectible) that must be estimated to state accounts receivable properly in terms of realizable cash value. Note that the value of the estimated allowances for accounts receivable in 1987 (see Exhibit 4–1) is

$$\$278,000 + \$330,000 = \$608,000.$$

This figure is significantly less than the amount shown in the statement of revenue and expenses for allowances, $1,208,376. This kind of difference is quite common. Remember that the balance sheet value reflects the estimated allowances for accounts still outstanding, whereas the statement of revenue and expenses reflects the allowance for all patient service revenue billed during the year.

Certain categories of patient service revenue are important in decision making. Payment source is especially important. Some common categories of payment sources are—

- Medicare
- Medicaid
- Blue Cross
- commercial insurance
- self-pay
- other

Identification of these categories is critical to setting rates and making many other financial decisions, such as in the projection of short-term cash flow and collection efforts. Ordinarily, this information is available within the entity, though it is not usually published in general-purpose financial statements. Departmental breakdowns of data are also useful in many decisions and are available internally, but they are not usually published in general-purpose financial statements.

Other Operating Revenue

Other operating revenue is generated from normal, day-to-day operations not directly related to patient care. It is usually classified by source into three categories: (1) educational programs, (2) grants, and (3) miscellaneous. Revenue from such educational programs as nursing, medicine, laboratory, and x-ray technology may generate tuition and other fees that show up in this category. Omega Hospital has a relatively large dollar amount of other operating revenue—$665,160 in 1987—much of it representing tuition from educational programs.

Grants from research projects or projects run by federal or other agencies are also reported as other operating revenue. Omega Hospital has some monies in this category, as shown in the statement of changes in fund balances (see Exhibit 4–5). A transfer of $75,775 as other operating revenue was made from the restricted research fund to the unrestricted fund in 1987.

Miscellaneous sources of other operating revenue include such items as revenue from office rentals, cafeteria and gift shop sales, and parking lot fees. It is important to note that this revenue is not always offset against its related expenses. As a result, it is sometimes impossible to determine whether the operations were profitable or not. If they are minor or immaterial, their value determination is not an important problem. However, Omega Hospital believes that its parking lot and professional office building operations are significant enough to warrant separate reporting. Therefore, in Omega's statement of revenue and expenses, this revenue is netted against related expenses, rather than appearing just as other operating revenue.

Nonoperating Revenue

Nonoperating revenue is revenue not related to patient care or to normal day-to-day operations. Major categories of nonoperating revenue are (1) unrestricted gifts, (2) unrestricted income from endowments, and (3) miscellaneous.

Unrestricted gifts—gifts with no restrictions on use—are treated as nonoperating revenue. Omega Hospital had relatively few of these gifts in the two years for which we have information. However, it did receive a large dollar amount of gifts restricted for plant replacement and renovation in the past, as evidenced by the values for pledges receivable shown in the restricted balance sheet.

If income from an endowment is not restricted, it may be used for general operating purposes and treated as nonoperating revenue. The statement of changes in fund balances (see Exhibit 4–5) shows that only $2,018 of income was designated as nonoperating revenue in 1987. Revenue from miscellaneous sources includes income from unrestricted funds; rentals of facilities not used in operations, such as farm land or apartments; and, in some cases, the fair market value of services donated by volunteers.

Operating Expenses

In these days of increasing concern over health care costs, decision makers are paying more attention to health care facilities' operating expenses. Generally speaking, there are two ways that expenses may be categorized: (1) by cost or responsibility center or (2) by object or type of expenditure.

In most general-purpose financial statements, costs are reported by cost center or department. Omega Hospital breaks down expenses into five major categories of departments:

1. nursing service areas
2. other professional service areas
3. general service areas
4. fiscal service areas
5. administrative service areas

Nursing service and other professional services could also be classified as revenue departments. They provide services directly to patients, for which there is a charge. General, fiscal, and administrative services are indirect or support-area services; they are not direct patient services, but rather support the nursing and other professional service areas.

Two expenses, depreciation and interest, are listed by object or type of expense category. As explained in the next chapter, these two expense categories are critical to many decisions and require separate reporting.

It should be noted that expense and expenditure (or payment and cash) may not be equivalent in any given period. For example, a health care facility may incur an expenditure of $1,000,000 to buy a piece of equipment, but may only charge $200,000 as depreciation expense in a given year. In general, expenditure reflects the payment of cash, while expense recognizes prior expenditure that has produced revenue. In general, there are three major categories of expenditures that are not treated as expenses:

1. retirement or repayment of debt
2. investment in new fixed assets
3. increases in working capital or current assets

One major category of expense—depreciation on fixed assets—does not involve a cash expenditure. In addition, other normal accruals, such as vacation and sick leave benefits, may be recognized as expense but involve no immediate cash outlay.

STATEMENT OF CHANGES IN FINANCIAL POSITION

The statement of changes in financial position is designed to give additional information on the flow of funds within an entity. As we have noted, the concept of expense does not necessarily give decision makers information on funds flow. The statement of changes in financial position is designed to give information on the flow of funds within an entity and to summarize the sources that make funds available and the uses for those funds during a given period.

Funds are usually defined as working capital. This is true for Omega Hospital, as shown in its statement of changes in financial position (see Exhibit 4–4). Major categories of fund sources include:

• income-related sources
• debt financing
• sale of assets

Major uses of funds include:

• purchase of fixed assets
• repayment of debt
• increases in working capital

Income-related sources represent the difference between revenue and expenses, plus the related depreciation expense. Depreciation is added back to income because depreciation does not involve an actual expenditure of cash or funds. Many financial analysts refer to the sum of depreciation and net

Exhibit 4–4 Statement of Changes in Financial Position for Omega
Hospital, Unrestricted Funds

Omega Hospital
Statement of Changes in Financial Position
Unrestricted Funds
Year Ended June 30, 1987

	12 Months to June 30, 1987
Source of funds	
Net operating income before depreciation	$ 500,345
Nonoperating income	11,126
Professional office building income before depreciation	(2,883)
Parking ramp income before depreciation	31,253
Loan from restricted funds	1,390,905
Increase in mortgage payable	7,075,098
County construction grant	128,000
Decrease in other assets	4,142
Transferred from restricted fund for plant renovation and equipment	364,247
Total sources of funds	$9,502,233
Uses of funds	
Purchase of fixed assets	888,538
Construction of new facilities	7,542,761
Decrease in deferred revenue	20,000
Increase in working capital	1,050,934
Total uses of fund	$9,502,233
Changes in working capital	
Increase in current assets	$1,296,410
Less increase in current liabilities	245,476
Increase in working capital	$1,050,934

income as cash flow. In Omega Hospital, net operating income before
depreciation was $500,345, which equals $549,799 of depreciation less the
$49,454 operating loss.

STATEMENT OF CHANGES IN FUND BALANCE

The statement of changes in fund balance for both unrestricted and
restricted funds merely accounts for the changes in fund balance during the
year. Information on flows between restricted and unrestricted funds and
flows into the entity that are restricted can be obtained from this statement.

In fical years 1986 and 1987, Omega Hospital had a lot of activity in the plant replacement and renovation fund (see Exhibit 4–5). The fund received $363,000 in county construction grants, earned $412,530 in interest on its investment, and received $174,383 in pledges. Such transactions are never reported as income in a statement of revenues and expenses, but they did have a very positive effect on the Omega Hospital's financial position. Close scrutiny of the statement of changes in fund balance can detect many of these flows.

Exhibit 4–5 Statement of Changes in Fund Balance for Omega Hospital

Omega Hospital
Statement of Changes in Fund Balances
Year Ended June 30, 1987,
with Comparative Figures for 1986

	Year Ended June 30	
	1987	1986
Unrestricted funds		
Balance at beginning of year	$8,546,307	$7,129,625
Excess (deficiency) of revenues over expenses	(226,247)	697,979
Transfers from plant replacement and renovation fund to purchase property and equipment		
County construction grant	128,000	235,000
Renovation construction	302,032	450,110
Other donations and bequests	62,215	33,593
Balance at end of year	$8,812,307	$8,546,307
Restricted funds		
Specific purpose funds		
Balance at beginning of year	$ 92,156	$ 83,586
Increases		
Contributions	40,019	30,472
Grants	28,397	10,478
Nursing school tuition and fees	57,851	47,312
Nursing student loan repayments	4,585	5,404
Transfer from endowment funds	3,781	3,912
Total increases	134,633	97,578

Exhibit 4–5 continued

	Year Ended June 30	
	1987	1986
Decreases		
Specific purpose disbursements	24,512	19,482
Transfers to unrestricted fund		
Operating revenue or expense	51,037	42,085
Nursing student scholarships	13,148	12,116
Property and equipment	14,134	—
Transfer to plant replacement and renovation fund	—	8,079
Student loan cancellation and repayment of government student loan advances and contraadjustments	6,069	7,246
	108,900	89,008
Balance at end of year	$ 117,889	$ 92,156
Research funds		
Balance at beginning of year	$ 46,347	$ 44,942
Increases		
Contributions and bequests	3,688	1,584
Grants	83,588	151,208
Total increases	87,276	152,792
Decreases		
Transfers to unrestricted funds (operating revenues)	75,775	151,387
Balance at end of year	$ 57,848	$ 46,347
Endowment funds		
Balance at beginning of year	$ 737,911	$ 741,133
Increases		
Income from investments	43,898	49,430

Exhibit 4–5 continued

	Year Ended June 30	
	1987	1986
Decreases		
Transfers to unrestricted funds		
Operating revenue	22,311	36,497
Nonoperating revenue	2,018	2,022
Endowment fund disbursements	5,723	10,221
Transfers to specific purpose funds	3,781	3,912
Total decreases	33,833	52,652
Balance at end of year	$ 747,976	$ 737,911
Plant replacement and renovation fund		
Balance at beginning of year	$3,482,214	$3,539,497
Increases		
Contributions	2,125	2,015
County construction grant	128,000	235,000
Interest earned	187,667	224,863
Donated equipment	62,215	25,514
Transfer from specific purpose funds	—	8,079
Pledges receivable from building fund campaign	8,434	165,949
Total increases	388,441	661,420
Decreases		
Transfers to unrestricted fund		
County construction grant	128,000	235,000
Renovation construction	302,032	450,110
Donated property and equipment	62,215	33,593
Total decreases	492,247	718,703
Balance at end of year	$3,378,408	$3,482,214

SUMMARY

In this chapter we have discussed the contents of four general purpose financial statements:

- balance sheet
- statement of revenues and expenses

- statement of changes in financial position
- statement of changes in fund balances

Primary attention was directed at the first two, Balance Sheet and Statement of Revenues and Expenses, which provide a basis for most financial information.

Our attention in this chapter was directed at understanding the basic information available in these four financial statements. The next two chapters will discuss how that information can be interpreted and used in actual decision making.

FOOTNOTES TO FINANCIAL STATEMENTS

The footnotes to financial statements are an integral part of the total financial report. There is usually a wealth of information contained in them, and they should never be ignored. Some of the major categories of information in such footnotes are:

- summary of significant accounting policies
- description of long-term debt
- description of leases
- discussion of pension plans
- discussion of contingent liabilities and professional liability arrangements

A set of footnotes to an actual financial report is shown in Exhibit 4–6 (they do not relate to the financial statements of Omega Hospital). These notes provide detail in all of the areas listed above, plus several others.

Exhibit 4–6 Notes to Financial Statements

Notes to Financial Statements
ABC Medical Center
June 30, 1987

- Note A—Significant accounting policies

Inventories: Inventories are stated at the lower of first-in, first-out cost or market value.

Property and equipment: Property and equipment are stated on the basis of cost or approximate fair value at date of donation. Depreciation, which includes amortization of assets under capital leases, is computed principally by the straight-line method, using rates designed to amortize the cost of such assets over their estimated useful lives.

Expenditures for maintenance, repairs, and renewals are charged to operations as they are incurred and betterments are capitalized. The ABC Medical Center eliminates from the accounts the cost and related allowances for property and equipment sold or retired, and any resulting gains or losses are included in operations concurrently.

Exhibit 4–6 continued

Investments: Investments in marketable securities are generally stated at cost or fair market value at date of donation.

Cost reimbursement activities with third party payers: A significant portion of the medical center's revenues is received under contractual arrangements with the Medicare, Medicaid, and Blue Cross programs, whereby the medical center is paid based on allowable costs, as defined. Amounts received under these programs are generally less than at the established billing rates, and the difference is accounted for as a contractual adjustment. Preliminary settlements are subject to redetermination by the responsible agency. The medical center's management believes that adequate provision for anticipated adjustments has been made in the financial statements.

The provision for contractual adjustments is based on revenues and expenses reported for financial statement purposes. The medical center's deferred revenue results from timing differences between expenses reported in the financial statements and currently allowable cost, as defined by third party payers. The timing differences result primarily from recognizing sick pay on the accrual basis and computing depreciation by the straight-line method for financial reporting, whereas the cash basis and accelerated depreciation accounting methods, respectively, are used for certain reimbursement programs.

Income taxes: The medical center is a nonprofit corporation and has been granted an exemption from the payment of income taxes.

Specific-purpose and endowment funds: The medical center recognizes these resources as revenue during the period in which the expenditures are made for the purpose intended by the donor.

Reclassifications: Certain amounts reported for 1986 have been reclassified to conform with the current year's presentation, with no impact on financial condition.

• Note B—Restatement of 1986 financial statements

The 1986 financial statements for the ABC Medical Center have been restated to reflect proper application of a cost-reimbursement principle that was clarified in connection with an intermediary audit of the medical center's 1986 third party cost reports. The provision for contractual adjustments has been increased by $600,000 for 1986, resulting in a reduction of revenues in excess of expenses in the same amount.

During 1987, the medical center elected to change the reporting treatment of the plant replacement and renovation fund and the loan repayment sinking fund, which had been established to comply with related loan agreements. Previously, these funds had been reported as restricted funds in the medical center's financial statements. Current industry financial reporting practice indicates that funds such as these, established by requirements of nondonor third parties, should be reported in the unrestricted fund. Balances in these funds are now reported in the unrestricted fund as noncurrent assets. 1986 balances have been restated to conform with 1987 presentation, including nonoperating income, which has been increased by $270,000, representing investment earnings on these funds during 1986.

• Note C—Construction in progress

Construction in progress includes expenditures relating to the renovation of existing facilities. The remaining estimated costs to complete, $7,006,980, will be financed through the proceeds from revenue bonds issued in July of 1986 (see Note D).

• Note D—Long-term debt

Exhibit 4–6 continued

On July 15, 1986, the XYZ Hospital Finance Authority issued Series A Revenue Bonds on behalf of the ABC Medical Center in the principal amount of $11,565,000 to finance the renovation of the center's facilities. The proceeds from the bonds were placed with a trustee. The medical center received from the trustee $10,859,500 in exchange for an FHA-insured mortgage note. The mortgage, together with revenues from the project, secure the bonds. The trustee placed the remaining proceeds into a debt service fund, which will be used along with payments on the mortgage by the medical center to make principal and interest payments to the bondholders. The loan agreement requires the medical center to maintain a mortgage reserve fund for use in the event of default. This fund had a balance of $227,148 at June 30, 1987. It is the obligation of the medical center to make loan repayments and any other payments required to pay the interest, principal, and redemption premium, if any, on the bonds.

Long-term debt at June 30, 1987 and 1986, consisted of the following:

	1987	1986
FHA-insured mortgage note, payable in monthly installments of $131,403, including interest at 8.1% plus .5% insurance fee secured by first mortgage on all property, due on December 31, 2004	$14,695,319	$15,065,393
HHS-guaranteed loan, payable in monthly installments of $79,980, including interest at 7.9% with an interest subsidy of 3% (effective interest rate of 4.9%), secured by second mortgage on all property, due on October 1, 2002	8,193,082	8,492,616
FHA-insured mortgage note, payable in equal monthly installments commencing May 1, 1990, including interest at 11%, secured by third mortgage on all property, due April 1, 2010	10,859,500	
Notes payable to the State Hospital Finance Authority, payable in varying monthly installments including interest ranging from 8.75% to 10.95%, secured by equipment with a carrying value of $2,416,937 at June 30, 1987	2,286,732	1,254,913
Note payable with monthly installments of $12,849, including interest at 15%, secured by certain equipment with a carrying value of $352,114 at June 30, 1987	337,164	
Capitalized lease obligations		24,280
	36,371,797	24,837,202
Less current maturities	1,331,951	926,361
Totals	$35,039,846	$23,910,841

Exhibit 4–6 continued

The FHA loan due 2005 and HHS loan agreements require that, among other things, the medical center maintain a loan repayment fund to be accumulated from that part of its revenue attributable to depreciation expense. The fund is to be sufficient to pay the principal amounts due on the loans and the cost of certain equipment replacement. Such amount must be deposited not less than annually in a separate fund to ensure the accumulation of interest. Withdrawals from the fund may be made only as prescribed in the agreements.

Principal maturities of long-term debt for the four years subsequent to June 30, 1988, are as follows: 1989—$1,488,583; 1990—$1,705,082; 1991—$1,568,827; 1992—$1,375,734.

Interest cost of $124,000 was capitalized in 1987 in connection with the medical center's construction and renovation program.

● Note E—Leases

Future minimum payments, by year and in the aggregate, under noncancelable operating leases with initial or remaining terms of one year or more, consisted of the following at June 30, 1987:

1988	$412,926
1989	107,190
1990	83,488
1991	65,659
1992	7,500
Total minimum lease payments	$676,763

Rental expense under the operating leases, all of which constituted minimum rentals, aggregated $415,000 in 1987 and $407,000 in 1986.

● Note F—Pension plan

The ABC Medical Center has a pension plan covering substantially all of its employees. Pension expense was $1,013,982 in 1987 and $1,188,746 in 1986. The medical center's policy is to fund pension cost accrued, including amortization of past service cost over 30 years.

Accumulated plan benefit information, as estimated by consulting actuaries, and plan net assets for the medical center's plan are as follows:

	January 1	
	1987	1986
Actuarial present value of accumulated plan benefits:		
Vested	$3,930,249	$6,735,207
Nonvested	441,289	833,814
	$4,371,538	$7,569,021
Net assets available for benefits	$8,261,777	$8,354,398

The reduction in the actuarial present value of accumulated plan benefits is due primarily to the actuary's use of different mortality tables in the 1987 computation. In addition, on July 1, 1986, annuities were purchased for all retirees of record on that date by the plan's previous trustee. Therefore, there is no liability remaining for that group of participants.

Exhibit 4–6 continued

The actuarial present value of accumulated plan benefits for the plan is estimated by the consulting actuaries using an assumed rate of return of 7½ percent.

• Note G—Liability risk insurance

The ABC Medical Center maintains a program of self-insurance for all professional liability and patient general liability risks for claims up to $100,000 per claim and $800,000 in the aggregate. The program is supplemented with a comprehensive excess insurance policy up to $11,000,000 per claim and $13,000,000 in the aggregate. Provision for self-insurance charged to operations was $268,452 in 1987 and $102,897 in 1986. Comprehensive excess insurance premiums were $562,740 and $548,538 in 1987 and 1986, respectively.

The medical center is aware of certain incidents that may result in the assertion of additional claims, and other claims may be asserted arising from services provided to patients in the past. An estimate of the ultimate cost of such potential claims has been provided in the financial statements. The medical center's management believes that the provision for potential claims is adequate.

• Note H—Commitments

The medical center utilized funds from the Hill-Burton program in 1973 and, consequently, must provide a certain volume of uncompensated services each year through 1993. The medical center has provided uncompensated services (1987—$719,069; 1986—$882,211) which exceed the requirements for each of the years ended June 30, 1987 and 1986.

ASSIGNMENTS

1. Determine the amount of net operating income that would result for a hospital whose payer mix and expected volume (100 cases) is as follows:

30 Medicare cases	pay $2,000 per case
30 Blue Cross cases	pay average cost
20 commercial cases	pay 100 percent of charges
10 Medicaid cases	pay average cost
8 self-pay cases	pay 100 percent of charges
2 charity cases	pay nothing

Average cost per case is expected to be $2,200, and the average charge per case is $2,500.

2. How could you determine the amount of debt principal that will be retired during the next year through an examination of the financial statements?

3. What are the titles of the four financial statements that are usually included in an audited financial report?

4. Shady Rest nursing home has just acquired a home health firm for $850,000 in cash. The balance sheet of the home health firm looked as follows just prior to the acquisition:

Current assets	$200,000
Net fixed assets	100,000
Total	$300,000
Current liabilities	$100,000
Shareholder's equity	200,000
Total	$300,000

Describe how this acquisition might be reflected on the balance sheet of Shady Rest.

5. Describe several items that are treated as expenses in the income statement but do not require any expenditure of cash in the present period.

6. A major medical supplier has donated $45,000 worth of medical supply items to your firm. These items are then used in the treatment of patients. Explain how this transaction would be recorded in your firm's financial statements.

7. Your local Blue Cross plan reimburses you on the basis of average cost per patient day. An interim rate of $400 per day has been established. Charges to Blue Cross patients have been averaging $465 per day. At the end of the year, an audit was conducted and the actual cost per Blue Cross patient day was found to be $415. During the year, 45,000 Blue Cross patient days were billed and paid for at the interim rate. There are 3,000 Blue Cross patient days that were not billed at the end of the fiscal year. With this information, determine the following amounts:

- gross Blue Cross revenue
- Blue Cross contractual adjustment from revenue
- net Blue Cross revenue
- net receivable due from Blue Cross

8. Your HMO is experiencing a critical shortage of funds. Using the statement of changes in financial position as a framework for discussion, explain how you might attempt to reduce the need for additional funds.

9. Your hospital has experienced negative levels of expenses over revenues for the last five years. The total amount of accumulated deficits is $5 million, but you have noticed that your fund balance has increased $2 million during the same period. How might this situation be explained?

10. You have been reading the footnotes to your hospital's financial statements and were surprised to see that the actuarial present value of accumulated pension plan benefits is $4,500,000. A footnote cites a fund of $8,500,000 that has been established to pay these benefits. However, you can find no mention of either the liability or the fund in the balance sheet. What might explain this situation?

SOLUTIONS AND ANSWERS

1. The calculations to determine the hospital's net operating income would be as follows:

Gross patient revenue:

Medicare (30 × $2,500)	$ 75,000
Blue Cross (30 × $2,500)	75,000
Commercial (20 × $2,500)	50,000
Medicaid (10 × $2,500)	25,000
Self-pay (8 × $2,500)	20,000
Charity (2 × $2,500)	5,000
Total	$250,000

Deductions from gross patient revenue:

Medicare (30 × ($2,500 − $2,000))	$ 15,000
Blue Cross (30 × ($2,500 − $2,200))	9,000
Commercial (20 × ($2,500 − $2,500))	0
Medicaid (10 × ($2,500 − $2,200))	3,000
Self-pay (8 × ($2,500 − $2,500))	0

Charity (2 × ($2,500 − 0))	5,000
Total	$ 32,000
Net patient revenue	$218,000
Total expenses (100 × $2,200)	$220,000
Excess of revenues over expenses	($2,000)

2. The value reported for current maturities of long-term debt in the balance sheet should represent the value of debt principal that will be retired during the next fiscal year.

3. The four financial statements are:

   • balance sheet

   • statement of revenues and expenses

   • statement of changes in fund balance

   • statement of changes in financial position

4. First, fair market value of the assets acquired by Shady Rest would be determined. In this example, we will assume that the current asset value would not change but the fixed assets would be restated to $300,000 at fair market value. Shady Rest is thus acquiring total assets worth $500,000 and assuming liabilities of $100,000 for a net book value of $400,000. Since they are paying $850,000 for these assets, there would be a goodwill account of $450,000 created for the residual. The following account changes would occur:

   • cash—decrease of $850,000

   • current assets—increase of $200,000

   • net fixed assets—increase of $300,000

   • goodwill—increase of $450,000

   • current liabilities—increase of $100,000

   The goodwill value would be charged to expense in future time periods.

5. Pension expense would not require an actual expenditure of cash at the present time, although a payment may be made to a trustee for investment. Other accruals—such as vacation benefits, sick leave benefits, and FICA accruals—may not require immediate cash expenditures.

6. The fair market value of the items donated would be treated as other operating revenue. In this case, if $45,000 is the fair market value, that amount would be shown as other operating revenue.

7. The following values for the four sources of revenue would result:

Gross revenue (48,000 × $465)	$22,320,000
Contractual adjustment (48,000 × $465−$415))	2,400,000
Net revenue (48,000 × $415)	$19,920,000
Net receivable ((3,000 × $415) + (45,000 × $15))	$ 1,920,000

8. The major categories of fund usage in the statement of changes in financial position are.

   • repayment of debt

   • purchase of fixed assets

   • increase in working capital

   Conservation of funds could occur in any one of these three areas. For example, the HMO could postpone or delay new fixed asset acquisitions. It could also try to restructure its debt, especially in situations where a large proportion of the debt is short-term. Finally, it could attempt to reduce the amount of funds necessary for working capital increases. This could be accomplished through a reduction in the HMO's receivable cycle or through an increase in its payable cycle.

9. In this example, the hospital has increased its total equity by $7 million through sources other than income. The most likely sources of these funds are transfers from restricted funds, such as from plant replacement, or from direct equity transfers from related parties, such as a holding company. It is important to note that the funds were not derived from unrestricted contributions. Unrestricted contributions would have been shown as nonoperating revenue and thus included in the computation of excess of revenues over expenses.

10. Pension funds in a defined benefit plan are often held by a trustee and are not shown on the firm's financial statements. This is most likely the situation here. It is important to examine periodically the relationship between the pension fund and the actuarial present value of the pension fund liability. Changes in actuarial assumptions—for example, in mortality, investment yield, or inflation rates—can have a dramatic influence over the size of the liability. The relevant information can be found in the footnotes to the financial statements.

Chapter 5

Accounting for Inflation

To adjust for the effects of changing price levels, the Financial Accounting Standards Board (FASB), in September 1979, issued the "Statement of Financial Accounting Standards No. 33." The major provisions of this statement require supplementary information in the following five areas for fiscal years ended on or after December 25, 1979:

1. income from continuing operations adjusted for the effects of general inflation
2. purchasing power gain or loss
3. income from continuing operations on a current cost basis
4. current cost amounts of inventory and property, plant, and equipment at the end of the fiscal year
5. increases or decreases in current cost amounts of inventory and property, plant, and equipment, net of inflation

The FASB statement applies to public enterprises that either have total assets in excess of $1 billion or have inventory and property, plant, and equipment (before deducting accumulated depreciation) of more than $125 million. It is likely that the reporting requirements of the FASB Statement No. 33, perhaps in a modified form, will be extended to a much larger set of business organizations in the future.

The rationale for these changes in financial reporting stems from the inaccuracy and inability of present unadjusted historical cost reports to measure financial position accurately in an inflation-riddled economy. Unless inflationary pressures in the economy are removed, it seems logical to assume that alternative financial reporting systems that can account for the effects of changing price levels will be adopted. It also seems logical to expect that the accounting profession will eventually extend alternative reporting requirements to all business organizations. Hospitals and other health care organizations will, in all probability, be included.

At present, the effect of these financial reporting changes has not been clearly demonstrated. Thus, many individuals have formed beliefs and expectations about financial reporting changes that may not be accurate.

The major purpose of this chapter is to discuss and describe the major alternatives for reflecting the effects of inflation in financial statements. Specific methods are described, and the adjustments that need to be made to convert historical cost statements are illustrated. This discussion should provide a basis for understanding and using financial statements that have been adjusted for inflation.

REPORTING ALTERNATIVES

Methods of financial reporting can be categorized along two dimensions: (1) the method of asset valuation and (2) the unit of measurement. Two major methods of asset valuation are (1) acquisition (or historical) cost and (2) current (or replacement) value.

Asset valuation at acquisition cost means that the value of the asset is not changed over time to reflect changing market values. Amortization of the value may take place, but the basis is the acquisition cost. Depreciation is recorded, using the acquisition, or historical, cost of the asset. Utilizing an acquisition cost valuation method postpones the recognition of gains or losses from holding assets until the point of sale or retirement. Current valuation of assets revalues the assets in each reporting period. The assets are stated at their current value rather than their acquisition cost. Likewise, depreciation expense is based on the current value, not the historical cost. Current valuation recognizes gains or losses from holding assets prior to sale or retirement.

There are also two major alternative units of measurement in financial reporting: (1) nominal, or unadjusted, dollars and (2) constant dollars measured in units of general purchasing power. Use of a nominal dollar unit of measurement simply means that the attribute being measured is the number of dollars. From an accounting perspective, a dollar of one year is no different from a dollar of another year. No recognition is given to changes in the purchasing power of the dollar, because the attribute is not measured. The major outcome associated with the use of this measurement unit is that gains or losses, regardless of when they are recognized, are not adjusted for changes in purchasing power. For example, if a piece of land that was acquired for $1 million in 1967 were sold for $5 million in 1987, it would have generated a $4 million gain, regardless of changes in the purchasing power of the dollar during the 20-year period.

A constant dollar measuring unit reports the effects of all financial transactions in terms of constant purchasing power. The units that are usually used are the purchasing power of the dollar at the end of the reporting period or the average during the fiscal year. The measurement is made by multiplying the unadjusted, or nominal, dollars by a price index to convert to a measure of constant purchasing power. In periods of inflation, when using a constant dollar measuring unit, gains from holding assets are reduced, while losses are increased. Thus, in the above land sale example, the initial acquisition cost would be restated to 1987 dollars to reduce the gain:

Sale price of land (1987 dollars)	$5,000,000
Less acquisition cost restated (1987 dollars)	2,038,504
Gain on sale	$2,961,496

Constant dollar measurement has a further significant effect upon financial reporting: The gains or losses created by holding monetary liabilities or assets during periods of purchasing power changes are recognized in the financial reporting. For example, an entity that owed $25 million during a year when the purchasing power of the dollar decreased by ten percent would report a $2.5 million (0.10 × $25 million) purchasing power gain. All gains or losses would be recognized, regardless of the valuation basis used.

Monetary assets and liabilities are defined as those items that reflect cash or claims to cash that are fixed in terms of the number of dollars, regardless of changes in prices. Almost all liabilities are monetary items, whereas monetary assets consist primarily of cash, marketable securities, and receivables. Purchasing power gains or losses are recognized on monetary items because there is an assumption that the gains or losses are already realized, since repayments or receipts are fixed.

The interfacing of the valuation basis and the unit of measurement basis produces four alternative financial reporting methods (see Table 5–1). Each of the four methods is a possible basis for financial reporting. The unadjusted historical cost (HC) method represents the present method used by accountants; the other three methods are alternatives that would provide some degree of inflationary adjustment not present in the HC method. Both of the constant dollar methods, historical cost–general price level adjusted (HC–GPL) and current value–general price level adjusted (CV–GPL), are required by FASB Statement No. 33. The HC–GPL method is referred to as historical cost/constant dollar accounting, while the CV–GPL method is referred to as current cost accounting.

Table 5–1 Alternative Financial Reporting Bases

Unit of measurement	Asset Valuation Method	
	Acquisition Cost	Current Value
Nominal dollars	Unadjusted Historical Cost (HC)	Current Value (CV)
Constant dollars	Historical Cost-General Price Level Adjusted (HC-GPL) (FASB #33 Constant Dollar Accounting)	Current Value-General Price Level Adjusted (CV-GPL) (FASB #33 Current Cost Accounting)

Table 5–2 summarizes the effects the four reporting methods would have upon three major income statement items: (1) depreciation expense, (2) purchasing power gains or losses, and (3) unrealized increases in replacement values. However, the net effect of the changes in these items upon net income for an individual institution cannot be predicted; the composition and age of the assets, as well as the prior patterns of financing, will determine whether the net effect will be positive or negative, and to what degree.

USES OF FINANCIAL REPORT INFORMATION

The measurement of financial position is an important function, and its results are useful to a great variety of decision makers, both internal and external to the organization. Changes in financial reporting methods will unquestionably alter the resulting measures of financial position reported in financial statements. These changes are quite likely to produce changes in the decisions that are based on the financial reports (see Figure 5–1).

Lenders represent an important category of financial statement users who may change their decisions on the basis of a new financial reporting method. The lender's major concern is the relative financial position of both the individual firm and the industry. A decrease in the relative financial position of the industry could seriously affect both the availability and the cost of credit. If, for a variety of reasons, new measurements of financial position make the health care industry appear weaker than other industries, financing terms could change. Particularly for the health care industry, which is increasingly dependent upon debt financing, the importance of financial reporting method changes cannot be overstated. Research on the results of

Table 5–2 Major Effects of Alternative Reporting Methods upon Net Income Measurement

Reporting Methods	Impact Variables		
	Depreciation Expense	*Purchasing Power Gains/Losses*	*Unrealized Gains in Replacement Value*
Unadjusted historical cost (HC)	No change	No change/Not recognized	No change/Not recognized
General price level, adjusted historical cost (HC-GPL)	Increase/GPL depreciation is recognized	Gain or loss/ Depends upon the *net* monetary asset position	No change/Not recognized
Current value (CV)	Increase/Will recognize current replacement cost	No change/Not recognized	Gain/Will recognize increase in replacement cost
General price level, adjusted current value (CV-GPL)	Increase/Will recognize current replacement cost	Gain or Loss/ Depends upon the *net* monetary asset position	Gain/Will recognize increase in replacement cost but will reduce the amount by changes in the GPL

changing to an HC–GPL method has shown that the relative financial positions of individual firms and industries are also likely to change

Changes in financial reporting methods could also have an effect upon decisions reached by regulatory and rate-setting organizations. As a result of such changes, comparisons of costs across institutions may be more meaningful than they were before. For example, the capital costs of institutions that operate in relatively new physical plants may not be compared with the unadjusted historical capital costs of older facilities. Without these adjustments, new facilities may appear to have higher costs and thus be less efficient, whereas in fact the opposite may be true.

The actions of interested community leaders who have access to, and make decisions based on, financial statements might also be affected by reporting method changes. For example, suppose that individual, corporate, and public agency giving is in part affected by reported income. Many in fact regard reported income as a basic index of need, and the relationship between income and giving seems logical. Thus, since each of the alternative financial reporting methods we have discussed will produce a different measure of income, total giving in each case could be affected.

Internal management decisions might also change with a new financial reporting method. Perhaps the most obvious example of such a change would

Figure 5–1 Financial Data in Decision Making

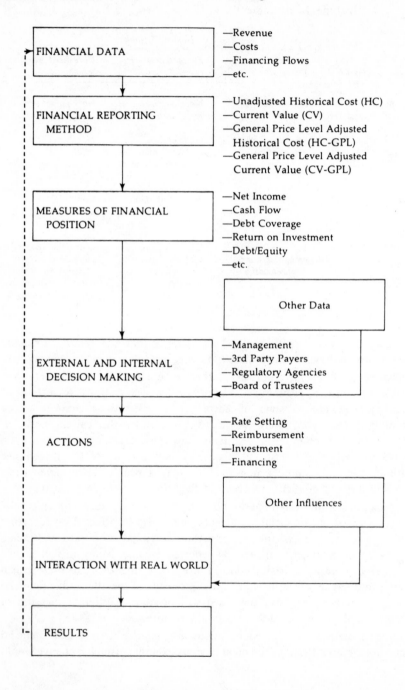

be in rate setting. Studies have shown that, in the nonprofit hospital industry, rates are closely aligned with reported costs. Thus, changes in costs produced by a financial reporting change are likely to affect rates.

CASE EXAMPLE: WILLIAMS CONVALESCENT CENTER

In the remainder of this chapter, we show how adjustments are made in the income statement and balance sheet of Williams Convalescent Center, a 120-bed skilled and intermediate care facility, to take into account the effects of inflation. The center's two financial statements are shown in Exhibits 5–1 and 5–2. You will note that values are reported for each of three reporting methods:

1. unadjusted historical cost (HC)
2. historical cost—general price level adjusted (HC–GPL)
3. current value—general price level adjusted (CV–GPL)

In this discussion, we do not describe or apply the current value (CV) method. This method is not being seriously considered by the accounting profession at this time, and it is not likely to be considered in the future. The CV method suffers from a serious flaw: It does not recognize the effects of changing price levels upon equity. In short, the CV method would treat increases in the replacement cost of assets as a gain and not restate them for changes in purchasing power.

Table 5–3 presents a table of values for the Consumer Price Index (CPI). The CPI is the price index that is used by the accounting profession at the present time to adjust financial statements for the effects of inflation.

Price Index Conversion

The two methods (HC and HC–GPL) we have selected to adjust the financial statements of the Williams Convalescent Center both utilize a constant dollar as the unit of measurement. This means that purchasing power, not the dollar, is the unit of measurement. That is, all reported values in the financial statements are expressed in dollars of a specified purchasing power. Usually the purchasing power used is the period end value. In our case example, Williams Convalescent Center uses the purchasing power as of December 31, 1984.

Restatement of nominal or unadjusted dollars to constant dollars is a relatively simple process, at least conceptually. All that is required is three pieces of information:

Exhibit 5–1 Statement of Income for the Williams Convalescent Center

	Historical Cost 1984	Constant Dollar (Historical Cost–General Price Level Adjusted) 1984	Current Cost (Current Value–General Price Level Adjusted) 1984
Williams Convalescent Center Statement of Income (000s Omitted)			
Operating revenues	$3,556	$3,625	$3,625
Operating expenses	3,253	3,316	3,316
Depreciation	74	177	185
Interest	102	104	104
Net income	$ 127	$ 28	$ 20
Purchasing power gain from holding net monetary liabilities during the year	—	$ 43	$ 43
Increase in specific prices of property, plant, and equipment during the year	—	—	$ 136
Less effect of increase in general price level	—	—	$ 144
Increase in specific prices over (under) increase in the general price level	—	—	$ (8)
Change in equity due to income transactions	$ 127	$ 71	$ 55

1. unadjusted value of the account in historical or nominal dollars
2. a price index that reflects the purchasing power in which the unadjusted value is currently expressed
3. a price index that reflects the purchasing power at the date the account is to be restated

For example, Williams Convalescent Center's long-term debt at December 31, 1983, is $1,203 (see Exhibit 5–2) (000s omitted). To express that amount .

Exhibit 5–2 Balance Sheet for the Williams Convalescent Center

	Historical Cost		Constant Dollar (Historical Cost–General Price Level Adjusted)	Current Cost (Current Value–General Price Level Adjusted)
Williams Convalescent Center Balance Sheets (000s omitted)				
	December 31			
	1983	1984	1984	1984
Current assets				
Cash	$ 98	$ 21	$ 21	$ 21
Accounts receivable	217	249	249	249
Supplies	22	27	27	27
Prepaid expenses	36	36	36	36
Total Current Assets	$ 373	$ 333	$ 333	$ 333
Property and equipment				
Land	200	200	530	525
Building and equipment	2,102	2,228	5,333	5,570
	2,302	2,428	5,863	6,095
Less accumulated depreciation	783	844	2,020	2,186
	1,519	1,584	3,843	3,909
Investments	161	596	596	596
Total Assets	$2,053	$2,513	$4,772	$4,838
Current liabilities	412	493	493	493
Long-term debt	1,203	1,478	1,478	1,478
Partners' equity	438	542	2,801	2,867
	$2,053	$2,513	$4,772	$4,838

in constant dollars as of December 31, 1984, the following adjustment would be made:

$$\text{Unadjusted amount} \times \frac{\text{Price index converting to}}{\text{Price index converting from}} = \text{Constant dollar value}$$

$$\$1,203 \times \frac{315.5}{303.5} = \$1,251$$

Table 5–3 Consumer Price Index, Year-End Values

Year	CPI
1970	119.1
1971	123.1
1972	127.3
1973	138.5
1974	155.4
1975	166.3
1976	174.3
1977	186.1
1978	202.9
1979	229.9
1980	258.4
1981	283.4
1982	292.4
1983	303.5
1984	315.5

Source: United States Department of Labor, Bureau of Labor Statistics

The value of the beginning long-term debt for the center would be $1,251 expressed in purchasing power as of December 31, 1984. The adjustment method described above is the same for all other accounts. The price index to which the conversion is made is usually the price index at the ending balance sheet date (December 31, 1984, in our example). The price index from which the conversion is made represents the purchasing power in which the account is currently expressed. This value will vary depending upon the classification of the account as either monetary or nonmonetary.

Monetary versus Nonmonetary Accounts

When restating financial statements from one based on a historical cost method to one based on a constant dollar method, it is critical to distinguish between monetary accounts and nonmonetary accounts. Monetary accounts are automatically stated in current dollars and therefore require no price-level adjustments. Monetary items, discussed earlier in this chapter, consist of cash or claims to cash or promises to pay cash that are fixed in terms of dollars, regardless of price level changes. Nonmonetary accounts require price-level adjustments in order to be stated in current dollars.

Because of the fixed nature of monetary items, holding them during a period of changing price levels creates a gain or loss. This can be seen in the following data from the Williams Convalescent Center (000s omitted):

	Unadjusted	Conversion Factor	Constant Dollars
Beginning long-term debt (12/31/83)	$1,203	315.5/303.5	$1,251
–Repayment (6/30/84)	152	315.5/309.5	155
+New debt (6/30/84)	427	315.5/309.5	435
Ending long-term debt (12/31/84)	$1,478		$1,531
–Actual ending long-term debt (12/31/84)			$1,478
Purchasing power gain			$ 53

The above data assume that a repayment and new issue occurred at the midpoint of the year, June 30, 1984. The price index at that point would have been approximately 309.5. This resulted from taking the average of the beginning and ending values, (303.5 + 315.5)/2. In constant dollars, the Williams center would have reported $1,531 of long-term debt at December 31, 1984. However, the actual value of the long-term debt at that date was $1,478. The difference of $53 represents a purchasing power gain to the center during the year. Because the price level increased during 1984, the value of the long-term debt actually owed by the center declined when measured in constant purchasing power.

Nonmonetary asset accounts must always be restated to purchasing power at the current date. The price index at the time of acquisition represents the price index from which the conversion is made. The price index at the current date represents the index to which the conversion is made. To illustrate the adjustment, assume that the building and equipment account of Williams Convalescent Center has the following age distribution:

Year Acquired	Cost	Conversion Factor	Constant Dollar Cost (12/31/84)
1970	$1,500	315.5/119.1	$3,974
1978	401	315.5/202.9	624
1981	201	315.5/283.4	224
1984	126	315.5/315.5	126
	$2,228		$4,948

The above data show that assets with a historical cost of $2,228 represent $4,948 of cost when stated in dollars as of December 31, 1984. The latter value is much more meaningful than the former as a measure of actual asset cost in 1984. It provides the center with a measure of cost that is expressed in dollars as of the current date and thus better represents its actual investment. Depreciation expense should also be restated in 1984 dollars in order to portray accurately the center's actual cost of using its building and equipment in the generation of current revenues.

Adjusting the Income Statement

Operating Revenues

If one assumes that revenues are realized equally throughout the year, it simplifies the restatement significantly. If the assumption is valid, and in most cases it is, it means that the revenues can be considered realized at the midpoint of the year, in our case, June 30, 1984. As already noted, the price index at June 30, 1984, can be assumed to be the average of the beginning and ending price index, or 309.5. The restated operating revenue would be calculated as follows:

$$\$3,556 \times 315.5/309.5 = \$3,625$$

Operating Expenses

Based on the same assumption that we used with operating revenues, the adjustment for operating expenses would be:

$$\$3,253 \times 315.5/309.5 = \$3,316$$

It should be noted that operating expenses do not include depreciation or interest. Separate adjustments for these two items may be required.

Depreciation

The depreciation expense adjustment is different from the earlier adjustments in two ways. First, depreciation expense represents an amortization of assets purchased over a long period of time, usually many years. This means that the midpoint conversion method used for operating revenues and operating expenses is clearly not appropriate. Second, the adjustment methods for the constant dollar and current cost methods diverge. Depreciation expense may vary considerably because the current cost of the assets may differ dramatically from the constant dollar cost. Remember, a price index represents price changes for a large number of goods and services; specific price changes of individual assets may vary significantly from that index.

Constant dollar adjustment. There are two methods that can be used to adjust depreciation expense to a constant dollar amount. The most accurate method is to perform an adjustment for each individual asset. This can be a time-consuming process, however, and may not be worth the effort.

Alternatively, an average acquisition date can be estimated by first determining the average age of the assets, as follows:

$$\text{Average age} = \frac{\text{Accumulated depreciation}}{\text{Depreciation expense}} = \frac{\$844}{\$74} = 11.4 \text{ years}$$

If one uses straight-line depreciation, this way of estimating average age is reasonably reliable. For the Williams Convalescent Center, an average of 11.4 years would imply that the assets were purchased sometime in 1973. Interpolation would yield a price index of 131.8. Depreciation expense in 1984 expressed in constant dollars thus would be:

$$\$74 \times 315.5/131.8 = \$177$$

Current cost adjustment. The identification of the current cost of existing physical assets is a subjective and complex process. To many individuals, the current cost method provides little additional value, compared with the constant dollar method. Whether it will be eventually eliminated and replaced by the constant dollar method is not clear at this time.

The first issue to address in the adjustment is the definition of current cost. By and large, current cost can be equated to the replacement cost of the assets. In short, we must determine what the cost of replacing assets in today's dollars would be. This could be estimated through a variety of techniques, using, for example, insurance appraisals or specific price indexes. In the case of the Williams Convalescent Center, we will assume a recent insurance appraisal indicated a replacement cost of $5,570 for buildings and equipment. With this estimate, depreciation expense could be adjusted as follows:

$$\frac{\text{Appraisal cost}}{\text{Historical cost}} \times \text{Depreciation expense} = \text{Restated depreciation expense}$$

$$\frac{\$5,570}{\$2,228} \times \$74 = \$185$$

Interest Expense

We will again assume that interest expense is paid equally throughout the year. This assumption would produce the following interest expense adjustment:

$$\$102 \times 315.5/309.5 = \$104$$

Purchasing Power Gains or Losses

A purchasing power gain results if one is a net debtor during a period of rising prices, while a purchasing power loss results if one is a net creditor during such a period. In most health care firms, purchasing power gains result because liabilities exceed monetary assets. A firm is thus paying its debts with dollars that are cheaper than the ones it received.

To calculate purchasing power gains or losses, net monetary asset positions must first be calculated. The net monetary position for the Williams Convalescent Center is presented below:

Monetary assets	Beginning (12/31/83)	Ending (12/31/84)
Cash	$ 98	$ 21
Accounts receivable	217	249
Prepaid expenses	36	36
Investments	161	596
Monetary assets	$ 512	$ 902
Monetary liabilities		
Current liabilities	$ 412	$ 493
Long-term debt	1,203	1,478
Monetary liabilities	$ 1,615	$ 1,971
Net monetary assets	$(1,103)	$(1,069)

The actual calculation of the purchasing power gain for the Williams Convalescent Center is as follows:

	Actual Dollars	Conversion Factor	Constant Dollars
Beginning net monetary liabilities	$1,103	315.5/303.5	$1,147
–Decrease	34	315.5/309.5	35
Ending net monetary liabilities	$1,069		$1,112
–Actual			$1,069
Purchasing power gain			$ 43

Because the center was in a net monetary liability position during the year, it experienced a purchasing power gain of $43. This value is not an element of net income; it is rather shown below the net income line in Exhibit 5–1. It thus affects the change in equity.

Increase in Specific Prices over General Prices

The adjustment to take into account an increase in specific prices over general prices is made only in the current cost method. The constant dollar method does not recognize any increases (or reductions) in prices that are different from the general price level. In short, no gains or losses from holding assets are permitted in the constant dollar method.

The calculations involved in this adjustment can be terribly complex. In our Williams Convalescent Center example, we will make some assumptions to simplify the arithmetic without impairing the reader's conceptual understanding of the adjustment. We will assume the following data:

Insurance appraisal of buildings and equipment, 12/31/83	$ 5,015
Insurance appraisal of buildings and equipment, 12/31/84	$ 5,570
Appraised value of land, 12/31/83	$ 500
Appraised value of land, 12/31/84	$ 525
New equipment bought on 12/31/84	$ 126

The following data show the increase in specific prices over general prices:

	Building & Equipment	Land	Total
Ending appraised value less acquisitions	$5,444	$525	$5,969
−Accumulated depreciation on appraised value	2,186	—	2,186
Ending net appraised value	$3,258	$525	$3,783
Beginning appraised value	$5,015	$500	$5,515
−Accumulated depreciation on appraised value	1,868	—	1,868
Net appraised value	$3,147	$500	$3,647
Increase in specific prices during the year			$ 136
Effect of increase in general price level	$3,647 × [(315.5/303.5) − 1.0]		$ 144
Increase in specific prices over general price level			$ (8)

These data show that, during 1984, the value of physical assets held by the Williams Convalescent Center did not increase more than the general price level. This may be a positive sign for the center if it is not contemplating a sale. The replacement cost for its assets is increasing less than the general price level. Therefore, revenues could increase less than the general price level and replacement could still be ensured.

Adjusting the Balance Sheet

Monetary Items

None of the monetary items—cash, accounts receivable, prepaid expenses, investments, current liabilities, and long-term debt—requires adjustment. The values of these items already reflect current dollars.

Land

In our discussion of the increase in specific prices over the general price level in the Williams center's income statement, we assumed an appraisal value for land of $525. That value will be used here with the current cost method. With the constant dollar method, we will assume that the land was acquired in 1970 for $200. To restate that amount to purchasing power as of December 31, 1984, the following calculation would be made:

$$\$200 \times 315.5/119.1 = \$530$$

Buildings and Equipment

Values for the center's buildings and equipment and the related accumulated depreciation have already been cited for the current cost method. We will assume those same values here. This produces a value for buildings and equipment of $5,570 (000s omitted) based upon an appraisal. The value for accumulated depreciation was derived as follows:

$$\text{Adjusted accumulated depreciation} =$$
$$\text{Unadjusted accumulated depreciation} \times$$
$$\frac{\text{Appraised value—Current year acquisitions}}{\text{Historical cost—Current year acquisitions}}$$

$$\$2,186 = \$844 \times \frac{(\$5,570 - \$126)}{(\$2,228 - 126)}$$

The constant dollar method values can be derived by using the estimated average age of plant. In earlier discussions relating to depreciation expense, we computed the average age to be 11.4 years and the related price index at acquisition to be 131.8. With this information the following values result:

$$\text{Buildings \& equipment} = \$2,228 \times 315.5/131.8 = \$5,333$$
$$\text{Accumulated depreciation} = \$844 \times 315.5/131.8 = \$2,020$$

Equity

We will not discuss the equity calculations in any detail here. It is enough for our purposes to recognize that equity is a derived figure. Equity must equal total assets less liabilities. In our Williams center example, this generates values of $2,801 for the constant dollar method and $2,867 for the current cost method.

SUMMARY

Financial reporting suffers from its current reliance on the unadjusted historical cost valuation concept. Inflation has made many of the reported values in current financial reports meaningless to decision makers. The example used in this chapter illustrates this point. The total asset investment of Williams Convalescent Center is approximately 100 percent larger when adjusted for inflation under the current cost or constant dollar method. Net income on the other hand decreased. The result is a dramatic deterioration in return on investment—the single most important test of business success.

The following table summarizes return on assets and return on equity for the Williams Convalescent Center:

	Historical Cost	Constant Dollar	Current Cost
Net income/Total assets	5.1%	0.6%	0.4%
Change in equity due to income transactions/Total assets	5.1	1.5	1.1
Net income/Equity	23.4	1.0	0.7
Change in equity due to income transactions/Equity	23.4	2.5	1.9

These reductions are so drastic, they would prompt an investor seriously to question the continuation of the present investment, let alone replacement. More profitable avenues of investment may very likely be available.

To the extent that our Williams Center example is representative of many health care firms—and it probably is—decisions regarding health care business continuation must be seriously evaluated. It is imperative that health care companies, like all other businesses, adjust their financial reports to reflect inflation. Whether the method used is current cost or constant dollar is not the issue. The important point is that ignoring the effects of inflation is unwise at best.

ASSIGNMENTS

Use the data and information presented in Table 5–4 to answer the following questions:

1. What index was used to restate to constant dollars?

2. What method was used to determine current cost values?

3. Is National Medical Enterprises (NME) a net debtor or a net creditor?

4. In 1981, NME showed a minus $24 million value for the increase in specific prices over general prices. What does this mean?

5. Why are NME's net operating revenues in 1984 identical for the historical cost, constant dollar, and current cost methods of reporting?

6. Why is depreciation expense greater in the current cost method than in the constant dollar method?

Table 5–4 Supplementary Financial Information for National Medical Enterprises (NME)

Effects of Changing Prices	The company's financial statements have been prepared in accordance with generally accepted accounting principles and reflect historical cost. The goal of the supplemental information which follows is to reflect the decline in the purchasing power of the dollar resulting from inflation. This information should be viewed only as an indication, however, and not as a specific measure of the inflationary impact.

The constant dollars were calculated by adjusting historical cost amounts by the Consumer Price Index—All Urban Consumers. Current costs, on the other hand, reflect the changes in specific prices of land, buildings, and equipment from the date acquired to the present; they differ from constant dollar amounts to the extent that prices in general have increased more or less rapidly than specific prices. The current cost of buildings and equipment was determined by applying published indexes to the historical cost.

Net income has been adjusted only for the change in depreciation expense. Other operating expenses, which are the result of current transactions, are, in effect, recorded in amounts approximating current purchasing power on the primary financial statements. Depreciation expense was determined by applying primary financial statement depreciation rates to restated building and equipment amounts. Since only historical costs are deductible for income tax purposes, the income tax expense in the primary financial statements was not adjusted.

During a period of inflation, the holding of monetary assets (cash, receivables, etc.) results in a purchasing power loss, while owing monetary liabilities (current liabilities, long-term debt, deferred credits, etc.) results in a gain. Net monetary gains or losses are not included in the adjusted net income amounts reported.

Table 5-4 continued

Consolidated
Statement of
Income
Adjusted
for Changing
Prices

(dollar amounts are expressed in millions)	As Reported in the Primary Statements (Historical Cost)	Adjusted for General Inflation (Constant $)	Adjusted for Changes in Specific Prices (Current Costs)
	For the Year Ended May 31, 1984		
Net operating revenues	$2,065	$2,065	$2,065
Operating and administrative expenses	1,698	1,698	1,698
Depreciation and amortization	84	98	111
Interest	91	91	91
Total costs and expenses	1,873	1,887	1,900
Income from operations	192	178	165
Investment earnings	24	24	24
Income before taxes on income	216	202	189
Taxes on income	95	95	95
Net income	$121	$107	$94
Effective income tax rate	44%	47%	50%

Changing price gains not included in adjusted income:
Increase in specific prices (current cost) of property, plant, and equipment held during the year*		$139
Less effect of increase in general price level		68
Excess of increase in specific prices over increase in the general price level		$ 71

*At May 31, 1984 current cost of property, plant, and equipment, net of accumulated depreciation was $1,915 (historical cost $1,349). "Property, plant, and equipment" in the tables above and below includes land held for expansion.

Selected
Supplementary
Financial
Data
Adjusted
for Effects
of Changing
Prices

(dollar amounts, except per share amounts, are expressed in millions)

For the years ended May 31	1984	1983	1982	1981	1980
Net operating revenues:					
Adjusted for general inflation	$2,065	$1,852	$1,271	$1,070	$832
Net Income:					
Adjusted for general inflation	107	85	73	54	36
Adjusted for changes in specific prices	94	73	64	46	27
Earnings per share:					
Adjusted for general inflation	1.54	1.29	1.18	.95	.82
Adjusted for changes in specific prices	1.35	1.12	1.04	.82	.61

Table 5-4 continued

Purchasing power gain from holding net monetary liabilities during the year	28	15	16	22	32
Increase in specific prices of property, plant and equipment over (under) increases in the general price level	68	85	16	(24)	77
Net assets at year-end (total assets less total liabilities):					
Adjusted for general inflation	1,095	972	756	657	413
Adjusted for changes in specific prices	1,332	1,162	894	809	470
Cash dividends declared per common share:					
Adjusted for general inflation	$0.43	$0.39	$0.34	$0.28	$0.21
Market price per common share at year-end: Adjusted for general inflation	$20.24	$29.41	$12.39	$24.30	$11.66
Average Consumer Price Index—All Urban Consumers	303.9	293.4	280.3	257.5	230.0

Source: National Medical Enterprises (NME) annual report 1984.

SOLUTIONS AND ANSWERS

1. NME used the Consumer Price Index—All Urban Consumers. This index is required by Financial Accounting Standards Board Statement No. 33 to restate historical costs to constant dollars.

2. NME used specific price indexes to restate historical costs to current costs. This method contrasts with the use of appraisals discussed in the chapter example.

3. NME is a net debtor. It has experienced a purchasing power gain in each year from 1980 to 1984. Since prices were increasing during that period, NME must have had a net monetary liability position in each year.

4. In 1981, the specific prices of NME's fixed assets must have increased less than the general price level as determined by using the CPI.

5. NME does not restate revenues or expenses to the fiscal year end, May 31. Instead, they restate to the midpoint of the fiscal year, November 30. Since it is usually assumed that revenues are received equally throughout the year, the midpoint or November 30 would represent the index from which the conversion is made. Since NME is converting to the midpoint index, the adjustment is 1.0. This can be seen in the following equation:

$$\text{Historical revenues} \times \frac{\text{CPI at } 11/30/83}{\text{CPI at } 11/30/83} = \text{Historical revenues}$$

6. Depreciation expense under the current cost method exceeds depreciation expense under the constant dollar method because the current cost value of depreciable assets exceeds the constant dollar value of depreciable assets.

Chapter 6

Analyzing Financial Statements

The major purpose of this chapter is to introduce some analytic tools for evaluating the financial condition of health care entities. Think for a moment how confusing and difficult it would be to reach any decisions on Omega Hospital's financial condition, as presented in Exhibits 4–1 through 4–5, without a key. Unless your training is in business or finance, the statements may look like a mass of endless numbers with little meaning. In short, there may be too much information in most financial statements to be digested easily by a general-purpose user.

An exhaustive list of people who might use general-purpose financial information would be difficult to prepare. Some of the potential users and their reasons for measuring financial condition are listed below:

- *boards of trustees,* to evaluate the solvency of their facilities and establish a framework for various decisions, such as those relating to investment, financing, and pricing

- *creditors,* to determine the amounts and terms of credit to be granted health care facilities and to evaluate the security of presently outstanding credit obligations

- *employee unions,* to evaluate the financial condition of a health care facility and its ability to meet increasing demands for higher wages; also to assess the capability of the facility to meet existing contractual relationships for deferred compensation programs, such as pension plans

- *departmental managers,* to understand better how operations and activities under their direct control contribute to the entity's overall financial position

- *rate regulation agencies,* to assess the adequacy of existing and proposed rates of a health care facility that is subject to rate review

117

- *grant-giving agencies,* (public and private), to determine a grantee's ability to continue to provide services supported by a grant and to assess the need for additional funding
- *public,* to determine a community health care facility's financial condition and assess its need for rate increases and its use of prior funds to enhance and improve the delivery of health care services—as a basis for assessing the need for money in a fund drive.

RATIO ANALYSIS

The technique used to assess financial condition is financial ratio analysis—the examination of the relation of two pieces of financial information to obtain additional information. In this process, the new information is both easier to understand and usually more relevant than the unrelated, freestanding information found in general purpose financial statements. For example, the values of fund balance and total assets may have little meaning when stated independently in a balance sheet. When the ratio of the two is taken, however, it indicates the proportion of assets that have been financed with sources other than debt.

Financial ratios are not another attempt by financial specialists to confuse and confound decision makers. Financial ratios have been empirically tested to determine their value in predicting business failure. The results to date have been quite impressive: financial ratios can, in fact, discern potential problems in financial condition even five years in advance of their emergence.

A sad fact is that much financial information is never really subjected to financial ratio analysis; the mass of figures just seems too voluminous ever to be synthesized. Decision makers tend to assume that, if the entity is breathing at the end of the year and is capable of publishing a financial statement, all must be well. If something goes wrong later, the accountant is blamed for not warning the decision makers. Sometimes the accountant *is* at fault. However, it is often the decision makers' fault for not analyzing and interpreting the financial information given to them in published financial statements.

The accounting profession was bombarded with criticism after the Penn Central collapse in 1970. To many it seemed that reporting standards must be too loose if the imminent financial collapse of a $7 billion business could not be determined from its financial statements. However Paul Dasher, in the March-April 1972 issue of the *Financial Analyst's Journal,* showed that anyone who could apply normal financial ratios to published financial statements could have detected the impending failure. At the conclusion of this chapter, the reader should be able to examine selectively a few specific financial ratios to better assess the financial condition of a health care entity.

Meaningful ratio analysis relies heavily upon the existence of relevant, comparable data. Absolute values of ratios are usually more valuable than the underlying financial information, but they are even more valuable when they can be compared to existing standards. For example, the statement that a hospital earned three percent on its revenues in the previous year is useful, but a statement of the relationship of this three percent to some standard would be far more valuable.

Usually, the analysis of financial ratios involves two types of comparisons. Temporal comparison of ratios, the comparison of year-end ratios to prior year values, gives the analyst some idea of both trend and desirability. A projected financial ratio may similarly be compared to prior, actual values to test the validity of the projection and the desirability of the proposed plan of operation.

A second method of comparison uses industry averages as the relevant standards for comparison. The Financial Analysis Service (FAS), a comparative ratio service of the Healthcare Financial Management Association, provides an excellent set of financial ratio averages for both hospitals and nursing homes.

For some time, the lack of uniformity in financial reporting has inhibited meaningful financial analysis in the health care industry. Specifically, the use of fund accounting has made it difficult to separate the financial effects of operations from the financial effects of other activities of the organization, such as those supported by endowment or grant monies. To some extent, this problem was solved with the publication of the American Institute of Certified Public Accountants' *Hospital Audit Guide* in 1972. This publication, though technically applicable only to audited hospital financial statements, has affected financial reporting of other health care entities. Its major feature is the requirement that funds be separated into restricted and unrestricted categories, as discussed in the last chapter. In most situations, focusing the financial analysis on the unrestricted fund categories provides a better basis for evaluating actual health care operations.

Financial ratios can be classified into five major categories for the purposes of this chapter.

1. liquidity ratios
2. capital structure ratios
3. activity ratios
4. profitability ratios
5. other ratios

In the following discussion, individual ratios within each of these categories are defined with respect to their assessment of financial condition. The specific indicators described are a subset of the 29 ratios used in the FAS. Additional information about FAS can be obtained by contacting the Healthcare Financial Management Association in Oak Brook, Illinois. The financial statements of Willkram Hospital, shown in Exhibits 6–1 and 6–2, illustrate the discussion.

It may seem to some that undue emphasis is being placed on financial reporting and financial analysis in the hospital sector. In terms of coverage in this chapter, this is true. However, ratios are general in nature and are just as relevant in other health care settings. For example, use of a current ratio that measures an entity's liquidity is valid and helpful not only for hospitals but also for nursing homes, HMOs, outpatient clinics, and surgi-centers. Furthermore, understanding the application of financial ratios in the relatively more complex hospital environment makes their application in other settings easier.

LIQUIDITY RATIOS

Liquidity is a term frequently used by business and financial people. It refers to the ability of a firm to meet its short-term maturing obligations. The more liquid a firm, the better it is able to meet its short-term obligations or current liabilities. Liquidity is an important dimension in the assessment of financial condition. Most firms that experience financial problems do so because of a liquidity crisis; they are unable to pay current obligations as they become due. Measuring an entity's liquidity position is central to determining its financial condition. Other long-term factors, such as a poor accounts receivable collection policy, may explain a poor liquidity position, but the worsening of a liquidity position is usually the first clue that something more basic is wrong.

Current Ratio

One of the most widely used measures of liquidity is the current ratio, which equals

$$\frac{\text{Current assets}}{\text{Current liabilities}}$$

For Willkram Hospital, the current ratio values for 1984 and 1983 are as follows:

1984	1983
$\frac{7,326}{2,833} = 2.586$	$\frac{6,201}{2,669} = 2.323$

Exhibit 6-1 Balance Sheet for Willkram Hospital

Willkram Hospital Balance Sheet, Unrestricted Funds, December 30, 1984 (with comparative figures for 1983) (000s omitted)	December 31, 1984	December 31, 1983
Assets		
Current assets		
Cash and marketable securities	$ 119	$ 67
Accounts receivable	$ 6,600	$ 5,900
Less allowances and uncollectibles	868	753
Net accounts receivable	5,732	5,147
Inventories	682	578
Prepaid expenses	397	177
Due from restricted fund	396	232
Total current assets	$ 7,326	$ 6,201
Property, plant, and equipment		
Construction in progress	104	125
Property, plant, and equipment	43,070	40,763
	43,174	40,888
Allowances for depreciation	8,368	6,474
Total property, plant, and equipment	34,806	34,414
Other investments	1,360	1,193
Total assets	$43,492	$41,808
Liabilities and fund balance		
Current liabilities		
Accounts payable	$ 1,472	$ 1,265
Notes payable	0	250
Due to third party	310	188
Accrued expenses	708	611
Due to restricted funds	343	355
Total current liabilities	2,833	2,669
Long-term debt		
Mortgage payable	19,633	18,724
Total liabilities	22,466	21,393
Fund balance	21,026	20,415
Total liabilities and fund balance	$43,492	$41,808

The higher the ratio value, the better the firm's ability to meet its current liabilities. A value commonly used in industry as a standard is 2.00; this means that two dollars of current assets (assets expected to be realized in cash during the year) are available for each one dollar of current liabilities (obligations expected to require cash within the year). The 1984 FAS national

Exhibit 6–2 Statement of Revenue and Expense for Willkram Hospital

	1984	1983
Willkram Hospital Statement of Revenue and Expense Year Ended December 31, 1984 (with comparative figures for 1983) (000s omitted)		
Patient service revenue	$31,824	$27,177
Allowances and uncollectible accounts	1,934	1,411
Net patient service revenue	29,890	25,766
Other operating revenue	1,421	1,150
Total operating revenue	31,311	26,916
Operating expenses		
Nursing services	9,306	7,364
Medical services	7,907	6,523
General services	5,285	5,271
Administrative services	3,683	2,780
Education and research	1,246	1,026
Depreciation	1,944	1,880
Interest	1,403	1,514
Total operating expenses	30,774	26,358
Net operating income	537	558
Nonoperating revenue	60	194
Excess of revenues over expenses	$ 597	$ 752

median was 1.86. On both a trend and a standard-comparison basis, Willkram Hospital is in a favorable position (see Exhibit 6–3).

The current ratio is a basic measure that is widely used. However, if used alone, it does not tell the whole story. Some types of assets—cash and marketable securities for example—are more liquid than accounts receivable or inventory. The current ratio does not account for these differences.

Quick Ratio

Another liquidity ratio, a refinement of the current ratio, is the quick ratio, which equals:

$$\frac{\text{Current assets less inventory}}{\text{Current liabilities}}$$

For Willkram Hospital, the quick ratio values for 1983 and 1984 are:

1984	1983
$\dfrac{7{,}326 - 682}{2{,}833} = 2.345$	$\dfrac{6{,}201 - 578}{2{,}669} = 2.107$

As with the current ratio, the higher the value of this ratio, the better the firm's liquidity position. In industry, a value of 1.0 is often used. However this value is too low for health care facilities because only a small amount of their current asset investment is carried in inventory. The 1984 FAS national median was 1.57. Thus, on both a trend and a standard-comparison basis, Willkram Hospital is in a favorable position with respect to quick ratio values.

In the quick ratio, the numerator is largely composed of cash and marketable securities, plus accounts receivable. These current assets are more liquid and make this a better test of liquidity compared with the current ratio. However, a key assumption is the liquidity of the accounts receivable. If they are not being collected quickly because of poor collection policies or delays in third party payment processing, the quick ratio may not be a good measure of liquidity.

Acid Test Ratio

A refinement of the quick ratio is the acid test ratio, which equals

$$\frac{\text{Cash plus marketable securities}}{\text{Current liabilities}}$$

For Willkram Hospital, the acid test ratios for 1984 and 1983 are:

1984	1983
$\dfrac{119}{2{,}833} = .042$	$\dfrac{67}{2{,}669} = .025$

Higher values again indicate more liquid resources available to meet current liabilities coming due. In this case, the liquid assets are limited to cash and marketable securities. Both these assets could be liquidated with little or no delay to pay maturing current liabilities. In both the quick and current ratios, there are categories of current assets that cannot be converted into cash without significant delays. The 1984 FAS median was .26. Willkram Hospital has a favorable trend but an unfavorable relationship to this standard value. In short, Willkram Hospital appears to be underinvested

Exhibit 6–3 Financial Ratio Analysis of Willkram Hospital

Ratio	1984	1983	FAS Median 1984	Evaluation Trend	Standard
Liquidity					
Current	2.586	2.323	1.86	Favorable	Favorable
Quick	2.345	2.107	1.57	Favorable	Favorable
Acid test	.042	.025	.26	Favorable	Unfavorable
Days in accounts receivable	70.000	72.900	63.70	Favorable	Unfavorable
Days cash on hand	1.510	.999	14.30	Favorable	Unfavorable
Average payment period	35.900	39.800	53.90	Favorable	Favorable
Capital structure					
Equity financing	.483	.488	.48	Unfavorable	Favorable
Long-term debt to equity	.934	.917	.71	Unfavorable	Unfavorable
Fixed asset financing	.564	.544	.62	Unfavorable	Favorable
Times interest earned	1.426	1.497	3.07	Unfavorable	Unfavorable
Debt service coverage	1.750	1.790	3.21	Unfavorable	Unfavorable
Cash flow to debt	.113	.123	.19	Unfavorable	Unfavorable
Activity					
Total asset turnover	.720	.644	.95	Favorable	Unfavorable
Fixed asset turnover	.900	.782	1.74	Favorable	Unfavorable
Current asset turnover	4.274	4.341	3.89	Unfavorable	Favorable
Average age of plant	4.300	3.440	6.87	Unfavorable	Favorable
Inventory turnover	45.910	46.570	69.70	Unfavorable	Unfavorable
Profitability					
Deductible	.061	.052	.183	Unfavorable	Favorable
Markup	1.080	1.067	1.265	Favorable	Unfavorable
Operating margin	.017	.021	.029	Unfavorable	Unfavorable
Operating margin price level adjusted	.001	.004	–.001	Unfavorable	Favorable
Return on total assets	.014	.018	.048	Unfavorable	Unfavorable
Nonoperating revenue	.101	.258	.310	Unfavorable	Unfavorable
Reported income index	.977	.641	.973	Unfavorable	Unfavorable
Other					
Restricted equity	0.000	0.000	.013	Neutral	Unfavorable
Replacement viability	.257	.298	.369	Unfavorable	Unfavorable

in highly liquid assets, like cash and marketable securities, but its trend over the two-year period is favorable.

Days in Patient Accounts Receivable Ratio

All three of the ratios discussed above—current, quick, and acid test—give indexes of the liquidity position of an entity. They do not, however, provide information as to *why* the current liquidity position exists, or what can be done to change it. In contrast, days in patient accounts receivable is a liquidity ratio that indicates the possible cause of a worsening liquidity position. It is simply ending net accounts receivable divided by an average day's revenue. Thus:

$$\frac{\text{Net patient accounts receivable}}{\text{Net patient revenue}/365}$$

For Willkram Hospital, days in accounts receivable for 1984 and 1983 are:

1984	1983
$\dfrac{\dfrac{5{,}732}{29{,}890}}{365} = 70.0$	$\dfrac{\dfrac{5{,}147}{25{,}766}}{365} = 72.9$

Values for this ratio indicate the number of days in the average collection period. For example, Willkram Hospital in 1984 had 70.0 days outstanding in accounts receivable at the year end. This implies that it took the hospital 70.0 days on the average to turn its accounts receivable into cash. High values for this ratio could indicate problems in collection time that may be due to faulty collection policies and billing systems of the entity. However, a high value might also indicate that the underlying quality of the accounts receivable is poor, that is, their collectibility may be in doubt. This might imply that the write-off policy of the entity should be reexamined.

A good way to evaluate the collectibility of accounts receivable is to perform an aging of accounts receivable by payer. For example, let us assume that the following aging of Willkram Hospital's accounts receivable as of December 31, 1984, was performed.

Willkram Hospital
Aging of Accounts Receivable
December 31, 1984
(000s omitted)

	Gross	Self-Pay	Third Party
Less than 30 days	$3,000	$ 800	$2,200
31 – 90 days	1,800	300	1,500
91 – 365 days	500	300	200
Over 365 days	1,300	700	600
Total	$6,600	$2,100	$4,500

The above aging of accounts receivable casts doubt on the collectibility of much of the $700,000 self-pay accounts receivable that is over one year past due. It might also raise a question of why $600,000 of third party payer receivables over one year old are still outstanding. The answer could be a poor collection policy for payment by such third parties as Medicaid, or it may be due to an unresolved dispute between the provider and the payer over the amount actually due.

The 1984 FAS national median for days in patient accounts was 63.7 days. Willkram Hospital thus has a favorable trend in days in accounts receivable but an unfavorable comparison against the standard value. This could be part of the reason that Willkram's acid test ratio is low. For example, if the collection period were sped up by six days, (the difference between Willkram's current collection period and the standard), an additional $491,000 in cash could be collected. If this potential cash balance were added to the present cash value of $119,000, the acid test ratio value would be raised to .215. This represents a 513 percent improvement over its current value.

Care must be exercised in using any of the liquidity ratios if seasonality is a factor. For example, if the dates for financial statement presentation occur during a slack period of the year, certain values of current assets may be understated and others overstated. In particular, the values of accounts receivable and inventory might be at their lowest point of the year, and the corresponding values of cash and marketable securities at their highest, or vice versa, giving a biased view of the liquidity position of the firm. In addition, standards vary by type of health care facility and region of the country. Clinics and HMOs can be expected to have significantly fewer days in accounts receivable than normal hospitals, while long-term care facilities may have significantly longer collection periods than normal hospitals. The collection period also depends heavily upon the composition of payers and their payment practices. Medicaid may pay on a prompt and timely basis in one state and yet be delinquent in another. The same holds true for Blue Cross and other major third party payers.

Average Payment Period Ratio

Another index that provides information about causes of a worsening liquidity position is the average payment period ratio:

$$\frac{\text{Current liabilities}}{(\text{Total operating expenses} - \text{Depreciation})/365}$$

For Willkram Hospital, the values of this ratio for 1984 and 1983 are:

$$\frac{2,833}{(30,774 - 1944)/365} = 35.9 \qquad \frac{2,669}{(26,358 - 1,880)/365} = 39.8$$

From a financial condition standpoint, low values of this ratio are better than higher values. Creditors often use a slight adaptation of this ratio:

$$\frac{\text{Accounts payable}}{\text{Purchases}/365}$$

If the data are available, both of the above average payment period ratios should be calculated. However, in the Willkram Hospital example, a separate listing of purchases for the year is not available.

The average payment period ratio indicates the length of time an entity takes to pay its obligations. The denominator, which is total expenses less depreciation divided by 365, provides an index of average daily cash expenses. (Remember, depreciation is a noncash expense.) The numerator, current liabilities, represents obligations for expenditures during the coming year. Most normal supply items are expensed within the year in which they are purchased. The same is true of payroll expenses, which usually constitute the largest single element of accrued liabilities and expenses. A standard value for this ratio derived from the FAS sample is 53.9. On this basis, Willkram Hospital has both a favorable trend and standard-comparison evaluation.

Day's Cash on Hand Ratio

A final measure of liquidity is day's cash on hand:

$$\frac{\text{Cash} + \text{Marketable securities}}{(\text{Total operating expenses} - \text{Depreciation})/365}$$

For Willkram Hospital, the values of day's cash on hand for 1984 and 1983 are:

$$\frac{119}{(30,774-1,944)/365} = 1.51 \qquad \frac{67}{(26,358-1,880)/365} = .999$$

Higher values of this ratio imply a more liquid position, other factors remaining constant. The ratio measures the number of days an entity could meet its average daily expenditures (as measured by the denominator) with existing liquid assets, namely cash and marketable securities. It is similar to the acid test ratio except that it uses a flow rather than stock concept. It attempts to define a maximum period of safety assuming the worst of all conditions, for example, no conversion of accounts receivable into cash.

The 1984 FAS national median for this ratio was 14.3 days. Using this value as the standard, Willkram Hospital is acutely underinvested in cash and marketable securities, although its trend is favorable. The value of this ratio in conjunction with the value of the acid test ratio strongly implies that Willkram Hospital should seriously consider increasing the amount of cash and marketable securities, especially marketable securities, that it carries. This is the only area where liquidity position is in drastic need of improvement.

It is useful to examine the value of the replacement viability ratio (see page 143) in situations of extremely low day's cash on hand. Sizable values for this ratio indicate the availability of funds that could be used for liquidity purposes. However, Willkram Hospital's values for replacement viability are low when compared with FAS standards, which dramatizes further the need for increases in cash.

CAPITAL STRUCTURE RATIOS

Capital structure ratios are useful in assessing the long-term solvency or liquidity of a firm. While the liquidity ratios just discussed are useful in detection of immediate solvency problems, the capital structure ratios are especially useful in longer-term assessment of financial condition. They are also valuable in detecting some short-term problems. Capital structure ratios are carefully evaluated by long-term creditors and bond-rating agencies to determine an entity's ability to increase its amounts of debt financing. In the last 20 years, the hospital and health care industries have radically increased their percentages of debt financing. This trend makes capital structure ratios vitally important to many individuals. Evaluation of these ratios may well determine the amount of credit available to the industry and thus directly affect its rate of growth.

Equity Financing Ratio

A basic capital structure ratio is the equity financing ratio:

$$\frac{\text{Fund balance}}{\text{Total assets}}$$

For Willkram Hospital the values for this ratio in 1984 and 1983 are:

1984	1983
$\dfrac{21,026}{43,492} = .483$	$\dfrac{20,415}{41,808} = .488$

Higher values for this ratio are regarded as positive indicators of a sound financial condition, all other things being equal. After all, if an entity had zero debt or a fund-balance-to-total-assets ratio of 1.0, there would not be any possible claimants on the entity's assets and thus no fear of bankruptcy or insolvency. The ratio indicates the percentage of total assets that has been financed with sources other than debt. In industry, a value for this ratio of less than 50 percent can cause some alarm. In segments of the health care industry where there is greater stability in earnings, lower ratios may be permitted.

The 1984 FAS national median for the equity financing ratio was .48. Willkram Hospital is very close to this industry norm. Since it has such a high current ratio, we can infer that Willkram Hospital has a greater percentage of long-term debt financing. This will be discussed shortly.

Long-Term Debt to Equity Ratio

Another capital structure ratio used by many analysts is the long-term debt to equity ratio:

$$\frac{\text{Long-term debt}}{\text{Fund balance}}$$

For Willkram Hospital, the values for this ratio in 1984 and 1983 are:

1984	1983
$\dfrac{19,633}{21,026} = .934$	$\dfrac{18,724}{20,415} = .917$

One deficiency of the equity financing ratio is that it includes short-term sources of debt financing, such as current liabilities. When assessing solvency and the ability to increase long-term financing, it is sometimes desirable to focus on "permanent capital." Permanent capital consists of sources of financing that are not temporary, including long-term debt and fund balance. Low values for the long-term debt to equity ratio indicate to creditors an entity's ability to carry additional long-term debt.

A value for this ratio used in general industry is 50 percent; that is, for every one dollar of long-term debt, two dollars should come from equity. In the health care industry this value may be higher, especially for hospitals. A value used by some investment bankers is 2.0. In other words they are willing to allow two dollars of long-term debt for every one dollar of equity. In part, this reflects the stability of the industry. It also reflects the relative difficulty in acquiring equity capital in a largely nonprofit industry.

The 1984 FAS national median for the long-term debt to equity ratio was .705. A comparison of Willkram Hospital's values with this standard yields both an unfavorable trend and standard comparison evaluation. Willkram Hospital has utilized more long-term debt than the average hospital, and its future debt capacity may be limited.

Fixed Asset Financing Ratio

A capital structure ratio of special importance to the health care industry is the fixed asset financing ratio:

$$\frac{\text{Long-term debt}}{\text{Net fixed assets}}$$

For Willkram Hospital, the values for this ratio in 1984 and 1983 are:

1984	1983
$\dfrac{19,633}{34,806} = .564$	$\dfrac{18,724}{34,414} = .544$

The fixed asset financing ratio is of special importance when the payment for capital costs is linked to cost-reimbursement formulas. In most cost payment plans, capital costs are limited to depreciation plus interest expense. The cash payment requirements would, however, consist of interest plus principal retirement. Remember debt principal is an expenditure, not an expense. In this situation, payments for depreciation expense would be needed to meet current and future debt principal payments. If depreciation expense were not of sufficient size to meet debt principal payments, the organization could experience some cash flow problems. In the fixed asset financing ratio, the numerator represents the total future debt principal payments, while the denominator represents a source of payment for debt principal, namely future reimbursable depreciation. As the value for the fixed asset financing ratio increases, the probability of cash flow problems may increase, especially if reimbursement of capital costs on a historical cost basis is a significant factor.

The 1984 FAS national median for the fixed asset financing ratio was .624. Values for Willkram Hospital compare favorably with this standard, but they do exhibit an unfavorable trend upward. Willkram Hospital does have a relatively young physical plant (see average age of plant ratio). This implies that it has probably completed a major renovation recently and will not require significant new long-term debt financing in the immediate future.

Times Interest Earned Ratio

A traditional capital structure ratio that attempts to measure the ability of an entity to meet its interest payment is the times interest earned ratio:

$$\frac{\text{Excess of revenues over expenses + Interest expense}}{\text{Interest expense}}$$

For Willkram Hospital, the values for this ratio in 1984 and 1983 are:

1984	1983
$\dfrac{597 + 1{,}403}{1{,}403} = 1.426$	$\dfrac{752 + 1{,}514}{1{,}514} = 1.497$

Even though a firm has a very low percentage of debt financing, it may not be able to carry additional debt because its profitability cannot meet the increased interest payment. Repayment of interest expense is a very important consideration in long-term financing. Failure to meet interest payment requirements on a timely basis could result in the entire principal value of the loan becoming due. Meeting the fixed annual interest expense obligations is thus highly critical to solvency. The times interest earned ratio measures the extent to which earnings could slip and still not impair the entity's ability to repay its interest obligations. High values for this ratio are obviously preferable. An absolute minimum standard in general industry is 1.5. The 1984 FAS national median for the times interest earned ratio was 3.07. Compared with this standard, Willkram Hospital shows both an unfavorable trend evaluation and an unfavorable standards comparison evaluation. Since this ratio indicates the ability to repay indebtedness, Willkram's low value could seriously impair its ability to acquire additional financing on favorable terms.

Debt Service Coverage Ratio

A commonly used capital structure ratio that measures the ability to pay both components of long-term indebtedness—interest and principal—is the debt service coverage ratio:

$$\frac{\text{Excess of revenues over expenses + Depreciation + Interest}}{\text{Principal payment + Interest expense}}$$

In the financial statements of Willkram Hospital that are available to us, the amount of principal repayments is missing, and thus there are no data to calculate values for this ratio. However, values for debt principal repayments in 1984 and 1983 can be identified in the footnotes to the financial statements (not reprinted here). Using these values, debt service coverage ratios for Willkram Hospital in 1984 and 1983 are:

$$\frac{597 + 1,944 + 1,403}{850 + 1,403} = 1.75 \qquad\qquad \frac{752 + 1,880 + 1,514}{800 + 1,514} = 1.79$$

$$1984 \qquad\qquad\qquad\qquad 1983$$

The debt service coverage ratio is a broader measure of debt repayment ability than the times interest earned ratio because it includes the second component of a debt obligation—the repayment of debt principal. The numerator of the debt service coverage ratio defines the funds available to meet debt service requirements of principal and interest. The ratio indicates the number of times that the debt service requirements can be met from existing funds. Higher ratios indicate that an entity is better able to meet its financing commitments.

A standard minimum debt service coverage ratio value used by investment bankers in the hospital industry is 1.5. The 1984 FAS national median for the debt service coverage ratio was 3.21. With this value as a standard, Willkram Hospital has both an unfavorable trend and an unfavorable standard-comparison evaluation.

Values for Willkram Hospital's debt service coverage ratio corroborate our earlier findings for the times interest earned ratio. The hospital is not in a good position to assume additional long-term debt. In fact, some debt service problems may arise in the future if values for both the times interest earned ratio and the debt service coverage ratio are not increased. Ultimately, increases in these ratios may be linked directly to improvements in profitability, especially operating margins, which are currently depressed.

Cash Flow to Debt

One of the best predictors of financial failure is the cash flow to debt ratio:

$$\frac{\text{Excess of revenues over expenses} + \text{Depreciation}}{\text{Current liabilities} + \text{Long-term debt}}$$

For Willkram Hospital, the values of the cash flow to debt ratio in 1984 and 1983 are:

$$\frac{597 + 1,944}{2,833 + 19,633} = .113 \qquad\qquad \frac{752 + 1,880}{2,669 + 18,724} = .123$$

$$1984 \qquad\qquad\qquad\qquad 1983$$

The cash flow to debt ratio has been found to be an excellent predictor of financial failure, even as much as five years in advance of such failure. The numerator, cash flow, can be thought of as the firm's source of total funds, excluding financing. The denominator, total debt, provides a measure of a major need for future funds, namely, debt retirement. A low value for this ratio often indicates a potential problem in meeting future debt payment requirements.

The 1984 FAS national median for the cash flow to total debt ratio was .192. Again Willkram Hospital demonstrates a potential problem in meeting future debt service requirements. Significant improvements in future profitability are urgently needed at this hospital.

ACTIVITY RATIOS

Activity or turnover ratios measure the relationship between revenue and assets. The numerator is always revenue; it may be thought of as a surrogate measure of output. The denominator is investment in some category of assets; it may be thought of as a measure of input. These ratios are also referred to as efficiency ratios, since efficiency ratios measure output to input. As noted in a later context, activity ratios also have a very important relationship to measures of profitability.

Total Asset Turnover Ratio

The most widely used activity ratio is the total asset turnover ratio:

$$\frac{\text{Total operating revenue}}{\text{Total assets}}$$

For Willkram Hospital, the values of the total asset turnover ratio in 1984 and 1983 are:

1984	1983
$\frac{31,311}{43,492} = .720$	$\frac{26,916}{41,808} = .644$

A high value for this ratio implies that the entity's total investment is being used efficiently, that is, a large number of services is being provided to the community from a limited resource base. However, the ratio can be deceptive. For example, a facility that is relatively old, with most of its plant assets fully depreciated, is quite likely to show a high total asset turnover ratio. Yet it may not be nearly as efficient as a newer facility that has plant and equipment assets that are largely undepreciated.

A measure that may be used to evaluate partially the existence of this problem by detecting the age of a given physical plant is:

$$\frac{\text{Allowance for depreciation}}{\text{Depreciation expense}} = \text{Average age of facility}$$

Using this measure for Willkram Hospital, the values for 1984 and 1983 are:

1984	1983
$\dfrac{8,368}{1,944} = 4.30$	$\dfrac{6,474}{1,880} = 3.44$

The 1984 FAS national median for the average age of plant ratio was 6.87. Willkram Hospital is therefore operating a relatively young physical plant. This means that the costs of their physical assets are much more likely to be close to true current costs. We could therefore expect to see somewhat lower values for both the total asset turnover ratio and the fixed asset turnover ratio and not become too alarmed.

This is in fact the case for the total asset turnover ratio. The 1984 FAS national median for the total asset turnover ratio was .95. Willkram Hospital is significantly below this value, but it does exhibit a favorable trend. This is most likely attributable to the increasing age of the physical plant. As the facility ages, Willkram's total asset turnover will probably approach industry norms.

Fixed Asset Turnover Ratio

Another common turnover ratio is the fixed asset turnover ratio:

$$\frac{\text{Total operating revenue}}{\text{Net fixed assets}}$$

For Willkram Hospital, the values of the fixed assets turnover ratio in 1984 and 1983 are:

1984	1983
$\dfrac{31,311}{34,806} = .900$	$\dfrac{26,916}{34,414} = .782$

The fixed asset turnover ratio is identical to the total asset turnover ratio, except that fixed assets, a specific subset of total assets, is substituted in the denominator. This substitution is an attempt to assess the relative efficiency of an individual category of assets. In fact, all the turnover ratios discussed subsequently are further segregations of various categories of assets.

Fixed assets are the number one investment in most health care entities. The fixed asset ratio can thus be of major importance in assessing the relative efficiency of plant investments. The 1984 FAS national median for the fixed asset turnover ratio was 1.74. Here, Willkram Hospital shows a favorable trend, but an unfavorable standard-comparison evaluation. As the facility becomes older, the value of its fixed asset turnover ratio will probably approach the standard value. In most situations, there are better ways to assess the efficiency of plant investment than by using this very simple ratio; for example, actual measures of utilization may be used. However, an aggregated measure of cost like that used in a fixed asset turnover ratio does provide important information with respect to output per dollar of investment.

Current Asset Turnover Ratio

The complement of the fixed asset turnover ratio is the current asset turnover ratio:

$$\frac{\text{Total operating revenue}}{\text{Current assets}}$$

For Willkram Hospital, the values of this ratio in 1984 and 1983 are:

1984	1983
$\dfrac{31,311}{7,326} = 4.274$	$\dfrac{26,916}{6,201} = 4.341$

The current asset turnover ratio focuses on the relative efficiency of the investment in current assets with respect to the generation of revenue. The valuation of current assets is not subject to the same difficulties encountered in the measurement of fixed assets. The ratio is thus more comparable across facilities. The 1984 FAS national median for the current asset turnover ratio was 3.89. Willkram Hospital thus has a slightly unfavorable trend and a favorable standard-comparison evaluation with respect to this ratio.

Inventory Turnover Ratio

A refinement of the current asset turnover ratio is the inventory turnover ratio:

$$\frac{\text{Total operating revenue}}{\text{Inventory}}$$

For Willkram Hospital, the values of this ratio in 1984 and 1983 are:

1984	1983
$\dfrac{31,311}{682} = 45.91$	$\dfrac{26,916}{578} = 46.57$

The inventory turnover ratio is a very important measure of financial condition in manufacturing and merchandising firms. A low value might imply an overstocking of items that are not selling. Conversely, a high value could indicate that inadequate inventory levels are reducing possible sales because of shortages. In service firms like health care facilities, inventory is of less importance. However, it still is a major category of current asset investment, and its relative efficiency is important. Using the 1984 FAS national median of 69.7, Willkram Hospital produces an unfavorable trend and an unfavorable standard-comparison evaluation. Given this situation, the hospital might do well to investigate its current level of inventory.

Profitability Ratios

To talk of profit in a largely nonprofit industry appears to many to be a contradiction in terms. Yet few, if any, health care facilities can remain liquid and solvent if profits are held to zero. In such a situation, cash flow would not be sufficient to meet normal nonexpense cash flow requirements, such as repayment of debt principal and investment in additional fixed and current assets.

However, recognizing the basic need for profit is not the same thing as determining how much is needed. It is not healthy either for the public or for the health care entity if the entity's profitability is either too great or too small. Discussion of a need for profitability thus centers on a definition of financial requirements. Here we are concerned only with the interpretation of several commonly used financial ratios of profitability.

Deductible Ratio

A common profitability ratio in the health care industry that measures revenue write-offs is the deductible ratio:

$$\frac{\text{Deductions from gross patient revenue}}{\text{Gross patient revenue}}$$

For Willkram Hospital, the values of the deductible ratio in 1984 and 1983 are:

$$\frac{1984}{\underset{31,824}{1,934}} = .061 \qquad\qquad \frac{1983}{\underset{27,177}{1,411}} = .052$$

The deductible ratio measures the proportion of gross patient service revenue that is not expected to be realized in cash. The major categories of deductions are contractual allowances, bad debts, charity care, and courtesy discounts. Ideally, it would be useful to break down the deductible ratio by major payer category. From a profitability perspective, increasing values of the deductible ratio are likely to result in declining profitability, simply because a larger percentage of the total revenue is not being collected. In addition, a large deductible ratio usually results in cross-subsidization between payer categories.

A high deductible ratio does not necessarily imply poor profitability. A hospital may react to high deductibles by raising its rates (high markup ratio) or by increasing its nonoperating sources of funding (high nonoperating revenue ratio or low reported income index ratio). In addition, a hospital should examine the specific causes of the current deductible situation. For example, it may be possible to improve the collection of self-pay accounts by making billing process changes, by instituting a bank financing policy, or by changing the hospital's policy on charity care. Contractual allowances may be reduced by improving reimbursement management. Whatever the ultimate solution(s), it is important to monitor the deductible ratio closely. Small changes in this ratio can have a very profound impact on overall hospital profitability.

The 1984 FAS national median for the deductible ratio was .183. Thus, relatively, Willkram Hospital has an unusually low deductible ratio. The average hospital write-offs are nearly three times the percentage of revenue that Willkram Hospital writes off. At first glance this may appear very positive. However, much of Willkram's low write-off is due to an extremely low markup. An increase in Willkram's rates to reflect its current costs would probably produce significantly higher deductibles, but it would also produce more operating profit which is desperately needed by the hospital to improve its long-term solvency.

Markup Ratio

The markup ratio, used in conjunction with the deductible ratio, determines a firm's operating margin. The markup ratio is defined as:

$$\frac{\text{Gross patient service revenue} + \text{Other operating revenue}}{\text{Operating expenses}}$$

For Willkram Hospital, the values of this ratio in 1984 and 1983 are:

$$1984 \qquad\qquad 1983$$

$$\frac{31,824 + 1,421}{30,774} = 1.080 \qquad\qquad \frac{27,177 + 1,150}{26,538} = 1.067$$

The markup ratio defines the multiple by which rates are set above expenses. The numerator includes both patient service revenue and other operating revenue because the denominator, operating expense, is not usually divided by source of revenue. High values for the markup ratio imply higher rates or prices per dollar of expenses and a greater likelihood of a favorable profitability position. It should be recognized that the objective of most hospitals is not to maximize profit. Therefore, there are upper limits for markups.

As noted earlier, the markup ratio and the deductible ratio interact to determine the hospital's operating margin. High markup ratio values do not guarantee favorable profitability positions if they are associated with unfavorable deductible ratios. Markups are influenced by the age of the plant and the debt principal retirement schedule. Hospitals with relatively old plants and/or high debt service requirements may need to maintain relatively high markup ratios. In such situations, an average markup may not be enough to maintain hospital solvency. Finally, hospitals may also recognize the availability of nonoperating sources of income and choose to keep markups at relatively low values.

The 1984 FAS national median for the markup ratio was 1.265. Willkram Hospital's present rate structure is significantly lower than that of most hospitals. If its costs are not excessive, it should seriously explore the implementation of some sizable rate increases. At the present time, Willkram's poor operating margins are directly traceable to low markups.

Operating Margin Ratio

The most commonly cited measure of profitability is the operating margin ratio:

$$\frac{\text{Net operating income}}{\text{Total operating revenue}}$$

For Willkram Hospital, the values of this ratio in 1984 and 1983 are:

$$1984 \qquad\qquad 1983$$

$$\frac{537}{31,311} = .017 \qquad\qquad \frac{558}{26,916} = .021$$

From the entity's viewpoint, the higher the value of the ratio, the better its financial condition. In most situations, firms that have high profit margins are less likely to experience financial difficulties. A simple way to understand this ratio is to think of it as a measure of profit retained per dollar of sales. For example, in 1984 Willkram Hospital retained 1.7¢ of every revenue dollar as profit. The 1984 FAS national median for the operating margin ratio was .029. Thus, Willkram Hospital shows both an unfavorable trend and an unfavorable standard-comparison evaluation. As discussed earlier, Willkram's rate structure should be reexamined in light of a relatively low operating margin.

Operating Margin Price-Level Adjusted Ratio

It is often useful to adjust the operating margin ratio to reflect replacement cost depreciation. The operating margin price-level adjusted ratio does this:

$$\frac{\text{Total operating revenue} - \text{Operating expenses} + \text{Depreciation} - \text{Price-level depreciation}}{\text{Total operating revenue}}$$

For Willkram Hospital, the values for this ratio in 1984 and 1983 are:

$$\frac{1984}{\frac{31,311 - 30,774 + 1,944 - 2,455}{31,311}} = .001 \qquad \frac{1983}{\frac{26,916 - 26,358 + 1,880 - 2,322}{26,916}} = .004$$

The operating margin price-level adjusted ratio is identical to the operating margin ratio except that it substitutes price-level depreciation for depreciation expense reported on an unadjusted historical cost basis. The ratio defines the proportion of operating revenue net of deductions that is retained as income after deducting price-level adjusted depreciation. Though not totally accurate, this measure of operating profitability attempts to reflect the replacement costs of operating fixed assets in the calculation of the operating margin.

Values for this ratio that are below zero imply that the organization is not currently earning enough operating income to provide funds for the eventual replacement of its fixed assets. Future replacement needs may have to be met from an increased reliance on debt, if available, or from other equity sources, such as grants and contributions, if available. Values for this ratio that exceed zero are not to be interpreted as a guarantee of future fund availability for replacement. To the extent that increased working capital needs are financed with equity, an erosion of the replacement potential of the hospital will occur. Also, it should be remembered that the index used for price-level restatement is the Consumer Price Index for urban wage earners, which may understate the real replacement cost of the hospital.

The 1984 FAS national median for the operating margin price-level adjusted ratio was −.001. Willkram Hospital's ratio compares favorably with this value. Because of the relatively new physical plant at Willkram, operating profitability adjusted for replacement cost is much more favorable than unadjusted operating margins. Willkram is providing for replacement in its current price structure. However, it still needs sizable increases in operating profit to improve its debt service coverage capability.

Nonoperating Revenue Ratio

A profitability ratio that provides a means of analyzing the source of profit is the nonoperating revenue ratio:

$$\frac{\text{Nonoperating revenue}}{\text{Excess of revenues over expenses}}$$

For Willkram Hospital, the values for this ratio in 1984 and 1983 are:

1984	1983
$\dfrac{60}{597} = .101$	$\dfrac{194}{752} = .258$

Depending on the individual situation, a high value for the nonoperating revenue ratio may be good or bad. A high value would indicate that a large percentage of total net income or excess of revenues over expenses was derived from sources other than operations. If the value is stable, it enhances the overall financial condition of the entity and provides a stable source of funding that could be used to meet temporary reversals in operations. However, a high value may also indicate a weak financial condition. For example, there are many health care facilities that are heavily dependent on nonoperating revenue sources to subsidize operations that, by themselves, are incapable of breaking even. If these sources are not guaranteed and exhibit a highly erratic pattern, the financial condition of the entity could be in jeopardy. The 1984 FAS national median for the nonoperating revenue ratio was .31. In the case of Willkram Hospital, comparison with the FAS median indicates significant room for improvement. There was a significant change in the proportion of income contributed by nonoperating revenue sources from 1983 to 1984. During this same period, net operating income was fairly stable. A longer-term trend analysis might reveal the importance of this change in nonoperating revenue. Given Willkram Hospital's low profitability ratio values, the sources of nonoperating revenue and their expected stability should be analyzed.

Return on Total Assets Ratio

A profitability ratio that measures the relationship of profit to investment is the return on total assets ratio:

$$\frac{\text{Excess of revenues over expenses}}{\text{Total assets}}$$

For Willkram Hospital, the values of this ratio in 1984 and 1983 are:

1984	1983
$\dfrac{597}{43,492} = .014$	$\dfrac{752}{41,808} = .018$

The return on total asset ratio defines the amount of net income or excess of revenues over expenses earned per dollar of investment. This profitability measure includes both operating and nonoperating sources of income. It provides a measure of the return on capital invested in operations. Adequate levels of return are essential to the continued viability and replacement of hospital assets. In many situations, the return on total assets ratio is modified by using the excess of revenues over expenses before subtracting interest expense. The rationale for this adaptation is to separate the influence of financing decisions from operating results.

Values for this ratio are affected by the average age of the hospital's plant. A hospital operating with a relatively old and largely depreciated plant may have a very favorable return on assets ratio. However, because of near-term replacement needs, this favorable ratio value may be highly deceiving.

The return on total assets ratio is a function of the product of the total asset turnover ratio, the operating margin ratio, and the nonoperating revenue ratio:

$$\frac{\text{Total asset turnover ratio} \times \text{Operating margin ratio}}{1.0 - \text{Nonoperating revenue ratio}}$$

Return on total assets ratio =

The return on total asset ratio can be increased by improving the total asset turnover ratio, the operating margin ratio, or the nonoperating revenue ratio. It is important to recognize that hospitals with relatively high average age-of-plant ratios should probably try to attain above-average values for the return on total assets ratio.

The 1984 FAS national median for the return on total assets ratio was .048. In light of this standard, Willkram Hospital has both an unfavorable trend and unfavorable standard-comparison evaluation. This is a direct result of its relatively poor position in all three of the ratios that combine to determine the return on total assets ratio—operating margin, total asset turnover, and nonoperating revenue.

Reported Income Index Ratio

Given the peculiar nature of fund accounting in the hospital and health care industry, another valuable profitability ratio is the reported income index ratio:

$$\frac{\text{Excess of revenue over expenses}}{\text{Change in fund balance}}$$

For Willkram Hospital, the values for this ratio in 1984 and 1983 are:

<table>
<tr><td>1984</td><td>1983</td></tr>
<tr><td>$\dfrac{597}{21,026 - 20,415} = .977$</td><td>$\dfrac{752}{20,415 - 19,242} = .641$</td></tr>
</table>

As noted in Chapter 4, there are situations in which funds may be transferred to an unrestricted fund from a restricted fund and not be shown as income to the unrestricted fund. An important example of this is the purchase of fixed assets with dollars from a restricted plant replacement fund. The fixed assets purchased would be transferred to the unrestricted fund and shown as general plant property and equipment; a corresponding direct charge or increase in fund balance of the unrestricted fund would also occur. This increase in fund balance is necessary if the basic accounting equation is to be kept in balance; assets must equal liabilities plus fund balance. If this situation occurs frequently, the financial condition of the entity is far more favorable than its profitability ratios would indicate. The ratio of excess of revenue over expenses to changes in fund balance is designed to determine to what extent such transactions are occurring. Values consistently, and significantly, less than 1.0 indicate that a very important unreported source of income is being used by the entity.

The 1984 FAS national median for the reported income index ratio was .973. In the case of Willkram Hospital, a significant input of unreported income occurred in fiscal year 1983; reported income or the excess of revenues over expenses accounted for only 64.1 percent of the total change in fund balance. A history of such situations could imply a much more favorable financial condition than current profitability ratios might indicate.

OTHER RATIOS

Two ratios do not fit neatly into the four categories discussed above. These ratios are nevertheless useful in providing additional information about the overall assessment of financial position.

Restricted Equity

To assess the availability of capital from third party donor restricted funds, the restricted equity ratio is often used:

$$\frac{\text{Total restricted fund balances}}{\text{Unrestricted fund balance}}$$

Willkram Hospital does not report any restricted funds in their balance sheet. This implies that values for both 1984 and 1983 would be zero.

High values for restricted equity ratios are usually desirable. An underlying assumption about the desirability of high restricted equity ratios is that the entity must already have adequate levels of unrestricted equity. This can be evaluated by analyzing the equity financing ratio. Restricted equity will usually improve hospital profitability in one of two ways. First, if the restricted equity is an endowment, it may provide a very stable flow of investment income that will be reported as nonoperating revenue. Second, if the restricted equity is for plant purposes, there will be future credits to the unrestricted fund balance.

Replacement Viability Ratio

To assess the feasibility of future plant replacement, the replacement viability ratio is frequently used:

$$\frac{\text{Restricted plant fund balance + Unrestricted investments}}{\text{Price-level-adjusted accumulated depreciation} \times 0.50}$$

For Willkram Hospital, the values for replacement viability in 1984 and 1983 are:

1984	1983
$\dfrac{0 + 1,360}{10,569 \times .50} = .257$	$\dfrac{0 + 1,193}{7,995 \times .50} = .298$

The replacement viability ratio is used to measure the adequacy of current investments to meet replacement needs. The numerator, restricted plant fund balance plus unrestricted investments, is a measure of current funds available to meet potential replacement needs. The denominator is a measure of the present need. Price-level-adjusted accumulated depreciation is a measure of the current cost of fixed assets that has been written off as depreciation. It is not a perfect measure of a hospital's replacement need, but it gives a far better estimate than that produced by simply using unadjusted historical cost accumulated depreciation. Its value is multiplied by 0.50 to recognize that debt financing may be used; the assumption being that 50 percent of replacement needs will be financed with debt.

A standard value for the replacement viability ratio is 1.0. This implies a situation in which exactly enough funds are available for replacement needs. Values greater than 1.0 may indicate more than adequate levels of investment, while values less than 1.0 indicate deficiencies. Hospitals may adjust this ratio to reflect their own desired future financing patterns. This is done by multiplying the calculated replacement viability ratio as follows:

$$\text{Adjusted replacement viability} =$$

$$\text{Replacement viability} \times \frac{0.50}{\text{Expected proportion of equity financing}}$$

Willkram Hospital is significantly underinvested in relation to its potential replacement needs. Again, low profitability would appear to be the major cause for this problem. Unless Willkram adds significantly to its replacement reserves, it will be forced either to borrow a very large percentage of its future replacement cost or to reduce the size and scope of any renovation and replacement program. Either course would seriously jeopardize the hospital's long-term solvency.

SOME CAVEATS

In this chapter, we have demonstrated, through an examination of 26 separate financial ratios, the use of financial ratio analysis in the assessment of the financial condition of health care facilities. At this point, it is appropriate to add some general limitations that should be recognized when evaluating financial condition through financial ratio analysis.

Validity of Standards

The standards used in this chapter should be helpful in many health care settings. They are, however, of special importance in the hospital industry, since that is where they were derived. These ratios will vary by region of the country and time period. This implies that standards should be updated frequently. It also implies the importance of using adequate trend data.

Financial ratios should be calculated over a minimum of five years if meaningful trends are to be discovered. The two-year comparisons developed in this chapter were used only to discuss basic methodology and are clearly inadequate. In this connection, participation in a financial service like the Healthcare Financial Management Association's Financial Analysis Service (FAS) is strongly encouraged.

Cost Valuation

The values reported in a balance sheet are usually stated at unadjusted historical cost. Though this valuation does have some advantages in terms of objectivity of reporting, it limits the utility of comparisons across facilities when inflation is a predominant factor. The need for adjustment of ratios that use balance sheet values, especially fixed asset values, cannot be overstated.

Projections

Financial ratio analysis uses historical data. It provides a picture of where the entity has been; it does not necessarily tell where it is going. Budgetary data are required for this purpose. The value of financial ratio analysis as a predictor rests on the assumption that past behavior validly indicates future behavior.

Accounting Alternatives

It should be recognized that there are available a number of acceptable accounting alternatives for measuring the financial effects of various transactions. The use of different accounting methods can create significantly different values for financial ratios, even when the underlying financial events are identical. There may even be situations in which differences in accounting methods impair the comparability of financial ratios across health care facilities or over time. Consistent use of a given set of accounting methods can help a health care facility avoid such comparability problems and should be encouraged.

ASSIGNMENTS

1. Operating margins in your hospital have been consistently below national norms for the past three years. Discuss the factors that might have created this situation and the ways in which you might determine specific causes.

2. Exhibit 6–4 contains financial statements and some key financial ratios for Multiplan, an HMO corporation. Analyze the data and describe areas of strength and weakness.

Exhibit 6–4 Financial Statements and Ratios for Multiplan, Inc.

Multiplan Inc., and Subsidiaries
Financial Statements and Financial Ratios
(Amounts in thousands except per share data)

A. Consolidated Statements of Income

Revenue

Premiums	$188,018	$113,482
Hospital services	4,786	3,936
Pharmacy sales	1,022	1,014
Other income	2,898	3,118
Total revenue	196,724	121,550

Costs and expenses

Medical services	74,838	45,963
Hospital services	72,378	42,905
Outpatient services	11,761	8,159
Other health care expense	7,386	6,161
Salary expense	9,174	5,766
Marketing, general and administrative	7,981	5,281
Depreciation and amortization	1,689	1,237
Interest	1,597	1,519
Total costs and expenses	186,804	116,991
	9,920	4,559
Minority interests	523	588
Income before income taxes	10,443	5,147
Provision for income taxes	5,057	2,640
Net income	$ 5,386	$ 2,507
Net income per common share	$ .35	$ .17

B. Consolidated Balance Sheets

Assets

Current assets

Cash and cash equivalents	$34,264	$15,996
Accounts receivable (net of allowance for doubtful accounts 1987, $1,367 and 1986, $173)	14,069	9,664
Inventory	715	529
Prepaid expenses	2,435	814
Total current assets	51,483	27,003

Exhibit 6-4 continued

| | Years Ended December 31 | |
	1987	1986
Property and equipment		
Land	1,725	1,682
Building and leasehold improvements	7,350	4,847
Furniture and equipment	6,822	5,044
	15,897	11,573
Less accumulated depreciation and amortization	2,947	1,718
Total property and equipment	12,950	9,855
Other assets		
Intangible assets	12,183	12,985
Long-term receivable	1,494	1,747
Other assets	508	570
Total Other Assets	14,185	15,302
Total Assets	$78,618	$52,160
Liabilities and Shareholders' Equity		
Current liabilities		
Estimated claims payable	$16,977	$12,275
Accounts payable	1,306	2,068
Accrued income taxes	2,740	2,470
Current portion of long-term debt	940	961
Accrued hospital incentive	2,370	511
Accrued salary expense	1,627	1,293
Other current liabilities	1,969	1,640
Total current liabilities	27,929	21,218
Long-term debt	11,475	12,567
Deferred income taxes	352	293
Other long-term liabilities	807	1,292
Total liabilities	40,563	35,370
Shareholders' equity		
Preferred stock; 6,000,000 shares authorized, none issued		
Common stock, no stated value; authorized 60,000,000 shares; 1987, 16,186,000 shares, and 1986, 15,000,000 shares, and outstanding	18,581	2,702
Additional paid-in capital	11,581	11,581
Retained earnings	7,893	2,507
Total shareholders' equity	38,055	16,790
Total liabilities and shareholders' equity	$78,618	$52,160

Exhibit 6–4 continued

	Years Ended December 31	
	1987	1986
C. Financial ratios		
Liquidity		
Current	1.843	1.273
Quick	1.818	1.248
Acid test	1.227	0.754
Days in patient receivable	26.494	29.784
Average payment period	53.752	65.740
Days' cash on hand	65.945	49.561
Capital structure		
Equity financing	0.484	0.322
Cash flow to debt	0.176	0.107
Long-term debt to equity	0.323	0.825
Fixed asset financing	0.948	1.406
Times interest earned	4.373	2.650
Debt service coverage	3.390	2.140
Activity		
Total asset turnover	2.502	2.330
Fixed asset turnover	15.191	12.334
Current asset turnover	3.821	4.501
Inventory	275.138	229.773
Profitability		
Operating margin	0.027	0.021
Reported income index	0.253	0.165
Return on total assets	0.069	0.048
Return on equity	0.142	0.149
Other		
Average age of plant	1.745	1.389

3. An income index ratio of 1.5 is reported by a health care entity. What could account for this value?

4. How could a firm have a negative times interest earned ratio and a positive debt service coverage ratio?

5. Your firm's current ratio is 1.2. Is your liquidity position poor? What other factors would you check?

6. Your total asset turnover ratio has been declining over the past few years. How might you determine the cause for this decline?

7. Your firm has a replacement viability ratio of .20. If you were to replace your fixed assets today, what percentage of debt financing would you use?

8. Howard Ruhl has just been selected as the new chief executive officer of Suburban Hospital, a well-known, 600-bed teaching hospital located in the suburb of a stable Western city of approximately 1.5 million population. Howard is concerned about the future of the hospital. He fears that, over the years, it has relied too much on its good location and excellent medical staff. Although all the operating indicators point to a good future—for example, outpatient and inpatient volumes are up—Howard is specifically concerned about the financial welfare of the hospital.

   The man whom Howard is replacing is well-respected and was unquestionably a good manager. He personally brought the hospital through a significant growth period and is probably the major cause of its current success. He was, however, was not well-versed in finance and did not recruit competent fiscal help. The present chief fiscal officer is an old friend of the outgoing CEO and has no financial background; he received an MHA more than 20 years ago from the same school as the outgoing CEO.

   Suburban Hospital has borrowed very little in the past. Most of its present plant was financed with county general obligation bonds. That financing vehicle is no longer available.

   At the present time, Suburban has a fairly active outpatient clinic operation. It does not have an attached medical office building. Howard believes that major growth in a number of areas is essential if Suburban is to remain strong. However, he is not certain which areas of growth to suggest to his fiscally conservative board, or how to suggest them. As a first step, Howard has asked for and received the two most recent financial statements. His present fiscal officer has calculated some key financial ratios for him to consider in his review. These statements and ratios are shown in Exhibit 6–5.

   a. Define key areas of concern for Suburban Hospital and state the rationales for your concern.

   b. Propose a set of possible actions that may correct the problems in these key areas.

Exhibit 6-5 Financial Statements and Ratios for Suburban Hospital

Suburban Hospital
Financial Statement and Financial Ratios
(amounts in thousands)

A. Income Statement

Operating revenues

Routine services	$28,453	$22,914
Ancillary services	33,376	27,133
Total patient revenues	$61,829	$50,047

Deductions from revenue

Charity and bad debts	$ 2,160	$ 1,549
Contractual adjustments	3,263	2,388
Other	229	63
Total deduction from revenue	5,652	4,000
Net patient revenue	56,177	46,047
Other operating revenues	2,547	48
Total operating revenues	$58,724	$46,095

Operating expenses

Salaries	$30,620	$24,670
Supplies and other	27,026	20,723
Total operating expenses	57,646	45,393
Net operating gain	1,078	702
Nonoperating revenues—Net	1,363	497
excess of revenues over expenses	2,441	1,199
before changes in method of accounting	671	—
Excess of revenues over expenses	$ 3,112	$ 1,199

B. Balance Sheet

1. Unrestricted Funds
Assets

Current assets

Cash and cash equivalents	$ 974	$ 2,606
Accounts receivable	8,734	6,398
Other current assets	988	1,829
Current assets	10,696	10,833

Other assets

Replacement funds	4,668	7,215
Other funds	2,256	1,182

Exhibit 6–5 continued

	1987	1986
Other assets	6,924	8,397
Property, plant, and equipment	36,579	31,508
Total assets	54,199	50,738
Liabilities and current liabilities		
Accounts payable	1,948	2,644
Accrued expenses	3,005	2,174
Current maturities of long-term debt	1,031	837
Other	85	792
Current liabilities	6,069	6,447
Long-term debt	13,658	13,213
State equity	1,408	1,372
Fund balance	33,064	29,706
Total liabilities and fund balance	54,199	50,738

2. Restricted funds		
Total restricted funds	773	665
Fund balance	$ 773	$ 665

C. Financial ratios

	1987	1986
Liquidity		
Current	1.760	1.680
Quick	1.600	1.400
Acid test	.160	.400
Days in accounts receivable	56.700	50.700
Average payment period	40.100	54.200
Days' cash on hand	6.400	21.900
Capital structure		
Equity financing	.610	.590
Long-term debt to equity	.420	.450
Fixed asset financing	.370	.420
Times interest earned	4.430	4.350
Debt service coverage	3.660	2.880
Cash flow to total debt	.260	.150
Activity		
Total asset turnover	1.080	.910
Fixed asset turnover	1.610	1.460
Current asset turnover	5.490	4.260
Inventory turnover	76.900	85.000

Exhibit 6–5 continued

	1987	1986
Profitability		
Deductible	.091	.080
Markup	1.117	1.104
Operating margin	.018	.015
Nonoperating revenue	.440	.410
Reported income index	.970	.270
Return on total assets	.057	.024
Return on equity	.094	.040
Other		
Average age of plant	8.500	9.090
Operating margin (PLA)	−.029	−.029
Restricted equity	.023	.022
Replacement viability	.212	.394

SOLUTIONS AND ANSWERS

1. Operating margins are related to the values of markup and deductible ratios. A low operating margin ratio could result from a low markup ratio, a high deductible ratio, or some combination of the two. Low markup ratios in turn result from low prices or high expenses. A high deductible ratio results from large write-offs of revenue to third party payers for contractual allowances or from large bad debt and charity care write-offs. Ideally, operating margins should be broken down by major product lines, such as pediatrics, obstetrics, ambulatory surgery, and so on.

2. An examination of Multiplan's financial data yields the following conclusions:

   • Multiplan has experienced a sizable growth in equity during the last two years, as evidenced by the reported income index. The funds involved resulted from the issuance of stock.

   • Multiplan has a low days in accounts receivable ratio, but this is based upon a comparison with hospital norms. HMOs usually have a low days in accounts receivable ratio due to the prepayment nature of their business. However, the trend is still favorable.

   • Multiplan has a relatively good total asset turnover compared with hospital norms. Again, HMOs usually have far less investment in fixed assets than hospitals. This can be seen from an analysis of the fixed asset turnover ratio.

   • Multiplan has shown significant improvement in its operating margin. The 1987 value of 2.7 percent is comparable with hospitals, but it probably should be higher to finance future growth needs. No deductible or markup ratios are calculated because Multiplan does not have significant contractual allowances and provides only net revenue measures.

   • Multiplan appears to have significant additional debt capacity available, as can be seen from an examination of its capital structure ratios. This additional debt capacity is, however, contingent upon the maintenance and improvement of existing operating margins.

3. A transfer of funds out of the entity may have taken place. This is often the case in investor-owned companies, due to the payment of dividends. It may also occur in a voluntary entity because of a corporate restructuring. A positive reported income index can result if there is a positive transfer of funds into the firm when a loss occurs. For example, a firm may have a loss of $15 million and transfer of $5 million into the firm. The resulting reported income index would be 1.5 (–15.0/–10.0).

4. The firm may have an extensive amount of depreciation and very low debt principal payments. This is often the case in the early years immediately following a major construction program.

5. A low current ratio is not always an indication of a poor liquidity position. If significant cash reserves are available, as measured by a high acid test ratio or a high replacement viability ratio, a liquidity problem may not exist. Alternatively, a high current ratio that results from a high days in accounts receivable position may not indicate good liquidity.

6. A declining total asset turnover can usually be traced to a declining fixed asset turnover ratio or a declining current asset turnover ratio. A declining fixed asset turnover ratio often results from declining utilization or from new plant investment, which should be associated with a declining average age of plant ratio. A declining current asset turnover ratio can be traced to an increasing days in accounts receivable, an increasing days cash on hand, or a declining inventory turnover ratio.

7. The required percentage of debt financing for the firm would be 90 percent, or, alternatively, 10 percent equity financing. The following formulas can be used:

Requiring debt financing %
$$\begin{aligned} &= [1.0 - .5 \times \text{Replacement viability ratio}] \times 100.0\% \\ &= [1.0 - .5 \times .20] \times 100.0\% \\ &= 90.0\% \end{aligned}$$

8. a. The major areas of concern for Suburban Hospital are:

- relatively low operating profitability
- a relatively old physical plant
- a dramatic decline in liquid assets, as evidenced by days cash on hand

b. Possible courses of action to be considered are:

- Improve markup position through an increase in rates or curtailment of operating expenses. Suburban's markups have been historically low.
- Investigate the reasons for the build-up of accounts receivable. The increase appears to have required Suburban to expend more of its cash reserves to meet operating expenses.
- Consider additional debt financing to meet physical asset replacement and expansion needs. Suburban appears to have additional debt capacity at the present time. However, a successful financing package is highly contingent upon an improvement in operating profitability.

Chapter 7

Strategic Financial Planning

Is there a need to define corporate financial policy in a health care firm? If so, who should be responsible—the board of trustees, the chief executive officer, the chief financial officer, or some combination of these? How should the definition of financial policy be accomplished? What are the steps required?

These kinds of questions are only now beginning to surface in the health care industry. Finance and financial management have long been areas of concern, but their orientation has recently shifted. Reimbursement and payment system management have given way to financial planning. Survival tomorrow is no longer a guaranteed option. Health care firms must establish realistic and achievable financial plans that are consistent with their strategic plans. The primary purpose of this chapter is to help provide a basis for the very crucial task of financial policy formation in health care firms.

THE STRATEGIC PLANNING PROCESS

Most observers would probably agree that financial policy and financial planning should be closely integrated within the strategic planning process. Understanding the strategic planning process is thus a first step in defining and developing financial policy and financial planning. It would be ideal if there was agreement among leading experts regarding the definition of strategic planning. But such is not the case. The literature on strategic planning is fairly recent; most of it has appeared since 1965. And the application of strategic planning principles to the health care industry is even more recent; the bulk of the literature on such applications has been published since 1980.

One trend in health care strategic planning does appear clear, however: There is a definite movement away from "facilities planning" to a more market-oriented approach. Health care firms can no longer decide which services they want to deliver without assessing need or market. This requirement appears consistent with the concept of strategic planning as it is used in general industry. Indeed, as the business environments of the health care industry and general industry become more alike, strategic planning in the two areas should become increasingly similar.

Much of the literature that deals with the strategic planning process in business organizations appears to be concerned with two basic decision outcomes: First, a statement of mission and/or goals is required to provide guidance to the organization. Second, a set of programs or activities to which the organization will commit resources during the planning period is defined.

Figure 7–1 shows the integration of the financial planning process with the strategic planning process. Financial planning is fashioned by the definition of programs and services and then assesses the financial feasibility of those programs and services. In many cases, a desired set of programs and services may not be financially feasible. This may cause a redefinition of the organization's mission and its desired programs and services. For example, a hospital may decide to change from a full-service hospital to a specialty hospital, or it may decide to drop specific clinical programs, such as pediatrics or obstetrics.

Three points concerning the integration of strategic and financial planning should be emphasized. First, both strategic planning and financial planning are the primary responsibility of the board of trustees. This does not exclude top management from the process, since they should be active and participative members of the board. Second, strategic planning should precede financial planning. In some situations, the board may make strategic decisions based upon the availability of funding. While this may be fiscally conservative, it can often inhibit creative thinking. Third, the board should play an active, not a passive, role in the financial planning process. The board should not await word concerning the financial feasibility of its desired programs and services; it should actively provide guidelines for management and/or its consultants to use in developing the financial plan. Specifically, the board should establish key financial policy targets in three major areas:

1. growth rate
2. debt capacity
3. profitability objective (return on equity)

Figure 7–1 Integration of Strategic and Financial Planning

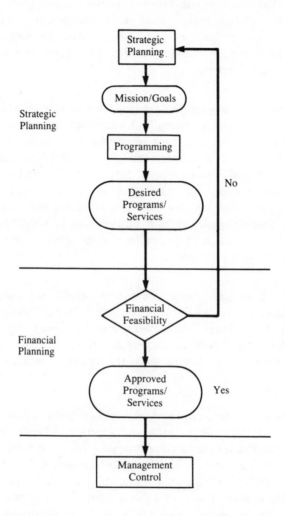

Financial Policy Targets

The term *financial feasibility* is often associated with an expensive study performed by a consulting firm in conjunction with the issue of debt. In such cases, the financial projections are so incredibly complex that few people profess to understand them, and even fewer actually do. In many people's minds, financial planning consists of a large number of mathematical relationships that can simulate future financial results, given certain key inputs. The validity of the projections is dependent upon the reliability of the mathematical relationships, or model, and upon the accuracy of the assumptions. Most financial feasibility studies developed in this way are never reviewed and never updated.

But conditions are changing, and changing very rapidly. A large number of health care firms are now beginning to develop formal strategic plans. They are beginning to redefine, or at least reconsider, their basic mission and to identify future market areas. It is increasingly clear that their financial plans and financial strategies must be integral parts of their overall strategic plan. With the elimination of cost reimbursement and increased competition among health care providers, board members are beginning to insist on a greater role in financial policy making. Future financial viability is no longer a virtual certainty; some analysts predict that as many as one out of four existing hospitals will not survive.

Granted that health care board members and health care executives have an urgent need to understand financial policy and financial planning, can the requisite body of knowledge be conveyed in a manner that is capable of being understood? Must board members and executives remain passive observers in financial planning, or can they be given the means to establish key policy directives?

The simplest way to categorize and describe key financial relationships in a financial plan is through a balance sheet presentation. A financial plan can be thought of as a bridge between a current balance sheet and a balance sheet at some future date (see Figure 7–2). The bridge consists of three spans: First, the plan must specify what the *growth rate* and level of investment in assets should be at future dates. This span is directly linked to the strategic planning outcome that defines desired programs. Second, the plan must specify the *profitability rate* or the amount of equity financing that will be available. This span is dependent upon the definition and profit rates of the desired programs. The third and final span involves the definition of *debt capacity*. Having defined required investment and available equity, the amount of debt is predetermined. However, the plan must assess both the desirability and the feasibility of the required debt levels. In short, does the organization want to assume that level of indebtedness, and can they meet the associated debt service requirements?

Figure 7–2 The Bridge Spans in Effective Financial Planning

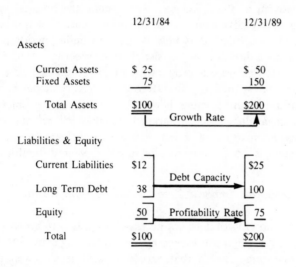

	12/31/84		12/31/89
Assets			
Current Assets	$ 25		$ 50
Fixed Assets	75		150
Total Assets	$100		$200
		Growth Rate	
Liabilities & Equity			
Current Liabilities	$12		$25
		Debt Capacity	
Long Term Debt	38		100
Equity	50	Profitability Rate	75
Total	$100		$200

Requirements for Effective Financial Policy Making

The preceding discussion of the elements of financial planning and the three major target areas of financial policy suggests certain requirements for effective financial planning and policy making. The following ten requirements are of special importance.

The Accounting System Should Be Capable of Providing Data on Cost, Revenue, and Investment along Program Lines

Programs or "strategic business units" are the basic building blocks of any strategic plan. The financial plan must be developed on a basis consistent with the strategic plan. Unfortunately, present accounting systems are geared to provide data along responsibility center or departmental lines. For example, psychiatry may represent a program in the strategic plan, but the financial data on costs, investments, and revenues for the program may be intertwined with many departments, such as dietary, housekeeping, occupational therapy, and pharmacy. Still, this problem is not unique to the hospital and health care industry. Many organizations have programs that cut across departmental lines. In such cases, the financial data can be accumulated along programmatic lines, but some adjustments in cost and revenue assignments are necessary.

With the advent of the DRG payment system, the hospital industry has been making major advancements in the accumulation of financial data in terms of DRG categories. It is now possible to define major programs or product lines in a hospital as consisting of a specific set of DRGs. For example, if obstetrics were a program, it might be defined as DRG #370 (Caesarian section with C.C.) to DRG #391 (Normal newborns).

The important point to note here is that, although problems exist in obtaining financial data along program lines, they are not insurmountable. The health care industry is of course different from the automotive industry, but the differences do not necessarily imply greater difficulties.

No Growth Does Not Imply a Zero Growth Rate in Assets

The fact that no growth does not necessarily imply zero growth in assets is so obvious that it is often overlooked by many planning committees. Inflation will create investment needs that exceed present levels, even though the organization's strategic plan may call for program stabilization or an actual retrenchment. An annual rate of inflation equal to 7 percent means a doubling of investment values every ten years. For example, a hospital with assets of $25 million today should plan on being a $50-million-asset firm ten years from now. Just because the investment involved may not represent a real increase in value does not negate the need for a plan of finance that will generate $25 million in new equity and debt financing over the next ten years.

Over time, of course, expectations about future rates of inflation may change. The financial plan should reflect the best current thinking in this area. This may necessitate periodic changes in the financial plan (examined below). It is also important to recognize that there may be differences in investment inflation rates across programs. In some programs, such as oncology, where dramatic technology changes are likely to occur, a greater relative inflation rate may have to be assigned.

Working Capital Is a Major Element in Computing Total Future Asset Needs

In computing future investment needs, it is not uncommon to omit the working capital category. The majority of investment in any strategic plan is usually in bricks and mortar and equipment. However, working capital can still be a rather sizable component, accounting for 20 to 30 percent of total investment in many health care firms.

The term *net working capital* is often used to describe the amount of permanent financing required to finance working capital or current assets. Net working capital is defined as current assets less current liabilities. It is important to remember this, since some current liability financing is automatic or unnegotiated. Just as inflation increases the dollar value of outstanding accounts receivable, it also increases wages or salaries payable and accounts payable. It is the net amount that must be financed. In the Figure 7–2 example, the increase in net working capital was $12 ($25 – $13).

Working capital requirements vary by program. New programs usually have significant working capital requirements, whereas existing programs may experience only modest increases resulting from inflation. One of the primary causes for failure in new business ventures is often an inadequate amount of available working capital. New programs also may have significantly different working capital requirements. For example, a home health program may require little fixed investment in plant and equipment, but significant amounts of working capital may be required to finance a long collection cycle and initial development costs. Many firms who rushed into the development of home health agency (HHA) programs have become acutely aware of this problem.

If inadequate amounts of working capital are included in the financial plan, the entire plan may be jeopardized. For example, an unanticipated $2 million increase in receivables requires an immediate source of finance, such as the liquidation of investments. If those investments are essential to provide needed equity in a larger financing program, certain key investments may be delayed or cancelled in the future. A number of firms have had to reduce the scope of their strategic plans because of unanticipated demands for working capital.

Some Accumulation of Funds for Future Investment Is Critical to Long-Term Solvency

Saving for a rainy day has not been a policy practiced by many health care firms to any significant degree. As of 1984, the average hospital had approximately 37 percent of its replacement needs available in investments assuming 50 percent debt financing. This implies that the average hospital would need to borrow approximately 80 percent of its replacement needs. This level of debt financing may no longer be feasible in the hospital industry as lenders reassess the relative degree of risk involved.

It is critical that health care boards and management establish formal policies for retention of funds for future investment. Health care firms can no longer expect to finance all of their investment needs with debt. They must set aside funds for investment to meet future needs in the same manner that pension plans are funded. An actuarially determined pension funding requirement is analogous to a board policy of replacement reserve funding. Yet, very few hospitals have seriously undertaken to set aside funds for future investment needs, which partially explains the dramatic growth in debt in the hospital industry.

A Formally Defined Debt Capacity Ceiling Should Be Established

Few health care firms have formally defined their firm's debt capacity or debt policy. This is in sharp contrast to most other industries. Without such a formally established debt policy, one of two unfavorable outcomes may result. First, debt may be viewed as the balancing variable in the financial plan. If a firm expects a $25 million increase in its investment and a $5 million increase in equity, $20 million of debt is required to make the strategic plan financially feasible. The firm will then try to arrange for $20 million of new debt financing. This is the situation in which many hospitals have found themselves. In such cases, additional debt could usually be obtained and adequate debt service could be demonstrated to lenders. Cost reimbursement had its advantages in that it could be used to provide payment for debt service costs. The strategic plan could remain unchanged, but a potential problem was that the debt to equity ratio might increase significantly.

Second, the balancing variable in the financial plan may shift to the investment side, but on an ex post facto basis. An approved financial plan may be unrealistic because the level of indebtedness required to finance the strategic plan exposes the hospital to excessive risks. Management may not realize this until the actual financing is needed. At that point, a scaling down of the programs specified in the strategic plan may be required. If a realistic debt capacity ceiling had been established earlier, existing funded programs might have been cancelled or cut back to make funds available for more desirable programs.

Debt capacity can be defined in a number of ways. It may be expressed as a ratio, such as a long-term debt to equity ratio. Or it could be defined in terms of demonstrated debt service coverage. Whatever the method used, some limit on debt financing should be established. That limit should represent a balance between the organization's desire to avoid financial risk exposure and the investment needs of its strategic plan. Debt policy should be clearly and concisely established before the fact; it should not be an ad hoc result.

Return on Investment by Program Area Should Be an Important Criterion in Program Selection

The principle that return on investment by program area should govern program selection is related to the need for accounting data along product lines, as discussed above. In order to calculate return on investment along program lines, financial data on revenues, expenses, and investment must be available along program lines. Return on investment should be used as part of an overall system of program evaluation and selection.

Portfolio analysis is a buzz word that has been used lately to categorize programs in terms of market share and growth rate. Health care writers have applied the concept in the literature on health care planning and marketing. However, one difficulty with the application of portfolio analysis in the health care industry is in the selection of the dimensions for developing the portfolio matrix. In most portfolio matrixes, the dimensions used are market share and growth. Market share and growth are assumed to have an explicit relationship to cash flow. High market share is associated with high profitability and thus with good cash flow. High market growth is assumed to require cash flow for investment. For example, a program with a high market share and low growth is regarded as a "cash cow." It produces high cash flow but requires little cash flow for reinvestment, due to its low growth needs.

Here, we will employ a slight modification of the portfolio analysis paradigm, incorporating the dimension of profitability. Figure 7–3 illustrates the revised portfolio analysis matrix. Its two dimensions are (1) return on investment and (2) community need. Return on investment is used as the measure of profitability because it has the most direct tie to strategic and financial planning. Profit is merely new equity that can be used to finance new investment. Absolute levels of profit or cash flow mean little unless they are related to the underlying investment. For example, if Program A has profit of $100,000 and an investment of $2,000,000 while Program B has profit of $50,000 and an investment of $100,000, which program is a better cash cow if both programs have low community need?

In our revised portfolio analysis matrix, community need replaces the traditional marketing dimensions of growth and market share. Community need may be difficult to measure quantitatively, but the concept appears closely aligned to the missions of most voluntary health care firms—firms that were usually formed to provide health services to some reasonably well-defined market.

Figure 7–3 categorizes programs as "dogs," "cash cows," "stars," and "samaritans." With the exception of samaritans, these terms are identical to those used in the existing literature. An example of a samaritan program is one with a small or negative return on investment but a high community

Figure 7–3 Revised Portfolio Analysis Matrix

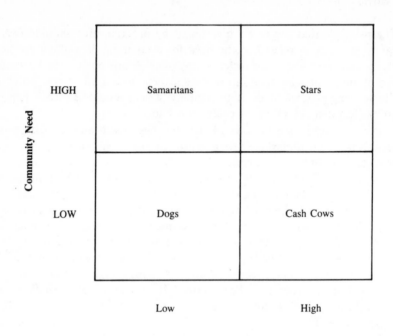

need. Thus, a hospital may provide a drug abuse program that loses money but meets a community need not met by any other health care provider. The program can continue if, and only if, the hospital has some stars or cash cows to subsidize the program's poor profitability. Dogs, that is, programs with low community need and low profit, should be considered in light of the resources they draw from potential samaritans. The new payment environment makes this kind of analysis mandatory.

Nonoperating Sources of Equity Should Be Included in the Financial Plan

In the preceding discussion of return on investment, we were concerned primarily with operating profitability. However, in most voluntary health care firms, nonoperating income can also be extremely important. In fact, in 1984, nonoperating revenue accounted for 30 percent of total reported net income in the hospital industry. If nonoperating income can be improved, a significant new source of funding will be available to help finance the strategic plan. This could mean either that a greater percentage of desired programs can be undertaken or that reduced levels of indebtedness are possible.

The investment portfolio of many health care firms is quite large. Funds are available for retirement plans, professional liability self-insurance plans, funded depreciation, bond funds, endowments, and other purposes. Thus, small increases in investment yields can create sizable increases in income. For example, a one percent improvement in the yield on invested pension funds may reduce annual pension expense by as much as ten percent. Clearly, hospital management should formally establish and incorporate target investment yields in its financial plans.

It should be noted that new equity can come from sources other than operating and nonoperating income. Corporate restructuring arrangements can create proprietary subsidiaries that can issue stock. Joint venture relationships with medical staff and others can be used to finance plant assets. It is important that both board members and executives have a clear understanding of the possible alternatives available for raising new equity to finance the strategic plan. Raising new equity through stock or partnerships is no longer the exclusive domain of proprietary entities.

The Financial Plan Must Be Integrated with the Management Control System

The integration of the financial plan with the management control system is an obvious requirement, but it is often overlooked. Frequently, a large fee is paid to a consultant or enormous amounts of internal staff time are used to develop a financial plan that is never used.

Ideally, the financial plan is the basis for the annual budget. The key link between the budget and the financial plan should be the return on investment (ROI) targets specified in the financial plan. These ROI targets are critical to the long-run fulfillment of the strategic plan. Failure to achieve the targeted levels of profit will require revisions in the strategic plan.

Health care boards would not have to be involved in pricing debates if approved financial plans were available. In such situations, the profitability targets by program would already have been approved in the plans. The primary issues in the budgeting process should be the translation of profit targets by program lines to departmental lines via pricing allocations and the assessment of departmental operating efficiencies. Long, involved discussions about whether budgeted profit is too much or not enough should not be necessary.

The Financial Plan Should Be Updated at Least Annually

Management should have the most recent financial road map available at all times. Few people would plan a drive to San Francisco from Boston with a five-year-old road map, yet many organizations operate either with no long-range financial plan or with an outdated one. This can be especially dangerous for health care firms at the present time, as the business environment continues to change rapidly. Today, financial plans based on cost reimbursement and minimal competition may be useless, or even misleading. In all financial plans, a careful reassessment of relative program profitability is periodically required, possibly prompting major revisions of the strategic plan. Knowing both where you are going and how you expect to get there is critical to survival in a competitive environment.

The Financial Plan Is a Board Document and Should Be Formally Approved by the Board

In many firms the financial plan, if it exists, is regarded as a management document. The board may be only mildly interested in reviewing it, and not interested at all in relating it to a strategic plan. This is rather strange behavior. Most boards would never dream of letting management operate without a board-approved annual budget for fear of failing to fulfill their board responsibilities. Yet planning for periods of time greater than one year is not regarded as important.

A recent hospital board meeting that followed a two-day strategic planning retreat illustrates this traditional perspective. During the retreat, strategic discussions about the future were held. The board and management agreed on a plan for the future that called for significant expansion into new market areas, such as long-term care. At the subsequent board meeting the CEO and the chief finance officer presented the strategic plan and the related financial plan. The board members regarded approval of the financial plan as a waste of time. They did approve it, but in body only—not in spirit. Their rationale for apathy was clear. They could not foresee any problem with the financing. Most of them had been board members for a long time. Whenever money was needed in the past, they raised rates or borrowed. And they could not see any reason to change this policy in the future. Behavior today would hopefully be different.

Fortunately, this kind of reaction is becoming less common. Board members today are beginning to realize that the financial plan and the strategic plan are integrally related. It is impossible to develop one without the other. And both are ultimately the responsibility of the board.

DEVELOPING THE FINANCIAL PLAN

In this section, we describe in some detail the steps involved in preparing a financial plan, using an actual case example. For our purposes, a financial plan may be defined as the bridge between two balance sheets. Here, we limit our attention to the financial plan as a projection of the balance sheet; discussion of methods used to project other financial statements, such as those involving income or cash flow, is beyond the scope of this chapter.

The Developmental Process

Four steps are involved in the development of a financial plan:

1. Assess financial position and prior growth patterns.
2. Define growth needs in total assets for the planning period.
3. Define acceptable level of debt, for both current and long-term categories.
4. Assess reasonableness of required growth rate in equity.

Assessment of Present Financial Position

The first step in the development of a financial plan is the assessment of present financial position. It is extremely important to determine the present financial health and position of the firm. Without such information, projections about future growth can be dangerous at best. In most situations, past performance is usually a good basis for projecting future performance. For example, a financial plan may call for a future growth rate in equity of 15 percent per year. If, however, the prior five-year period showed an average annual growth rate in equity of only 5 percent, there may be some doubt about the validity of the 15 percent assumption and thus about the reasonableness of the financial plan.

Three categories of financial information need to be assembled to assess present financial position:

1. prior financial statements for the past three to five years
2. compounded growth rates in individual balance sheet accounts
3. financial evaluation of the firm, using ratio analysis

To illustrate the application of this information in financial planning, the balance sheets presented in Exhibit 7–1 will be used. These balance sheets provide information for ABC Medical Center for the years 1982 and 1987. The column at the far right identifies the average five-year compounded growth rate. This average rate of growth can be determined by using financial mathematics tables (see Chapter 11), by using a calculator with financial functions, or by solving the following equation:

$$(1+i)^5 = \frac{1987\ \text{Value}}{1982\ \text{Value}}$$

where i equals the average annual compounded rate of growth

The Exhibit 7–1 balance sheets are somewhat abbreviated but they provide sufficient information to illustrate the mechanics of financial planning. The

Exhibit 7–1 Balance Sheets for ABC Medical Center

ABC Medical Center
Balance Sheets
(000s omitted)

	1982	*1987*	*5-Year Growth Rate (percent)*
Assets			
Cash	$ 161	$ 568	29
Accounts receivable	1,605	3,714	18
Inventories	211	102	–14
Other current assets	177	709	32
Total current assets	$ 2,154	$ 5,093	19
Replacement funds	4,981	7,705	9
Net fixed assets	9,789	12,245	5
Other	569	1,375	19
Total assets	$17,493	$26,418	9
Liabilities and Fund Balance			
Current liabilities	$ 1,079	$ 2,957	22
Long-term debt	10,070	7,330	–6
Deferred Medicare liability	456	1,285	23
Fund balance	5,888	14,846	20
Total liabilities and fund balance	$17,493	$26,418	9

data reveal some very interesting information about ABC's growth rate patterns. First, current assets have been growing at a much higher rate than other individual asset categories. During the past five years, the average rate of growth has been approximately 19 percent per year. This, of course, explains the very large increase in current assets. This finding is typical of most health care firms over the past decade. Current assets in general, and accounts receivable in particular, have experienced relatively high rates of growth; in projecting future growth rates, this should be kept in mind. Second, the growth rate in current liabilities is approximately equal to the growth rate in current assets. This finding is also very common and should be incorporated into the assumptions utilized in the financial plan. Third, the ABC Center has experienced a very large rate of growth in equity during the past five years. This is a very positive finding and lends support for the continuation of significant equity growth in the future.

Financial ratios for ABC Medical Center are presented in Exhibit 7–2. A review of these data provides us with a good assessment of both the firm's present financial position and its past financial trends. Among the significant findings that are likely to have a direct effect upon the firm's financial plan are the following:

- There was a large increase in days in accounts receivable over the past five years. This might cause us to assume that little real growth in days in accounts receivable will occur during the planning period. There might even be a slight reduction in days in accounts receivable during the period.

- The present average payment period has increased significantly during the last year. Future growth in current liability financing may not be as feasible, given the center's present position.

- The center's ability to assume additional long-term debt appears to be confirmed. Debt service coverage and times interest earned ratios indicate good coverage of existing debt, and the present capital structure does not appear to be heavily leveraged relative to industry norms.

- The center's need for additional capital expenditures to renovate and replace its existing plant does not appear to be excessive. The center's present average age of plant ratio is only 6.35 years, which compares favorably with industry norms.

- The center's present replacement viability ratio is excellent. It has an unusually large amount of existing replacement funds that can be used to finance future capital needs.

Exhibit 7–2 Financial Ratios for ABC Medical Center

	ABC Medical Center					
	Financial Ratios (1982 – 1987)					
Liquidity	1982	1983	1984	1985	1986	1987
Current	1.996	2.091	2.067	2.037	2.398	1.722
Quick	1.636	1.758	1.775	1.775	2.137	1.448
Acid test	.149	.378	.159	.229	.229	.192
Days' in patient receivable	54.335	48.849	50.832	55.615	61.979	63.207
Average payment period	40.092	38.624	33.671	38.145	35.012	53.901
Days' cash on hand	5.979	14.599	5.360	8.743	7.812	10.376
Capital structure						
Equity financing	.337	.392	.433	.472	.522	.561
Cash flow to debt	.127	.165	.191	.209	.227	.395
Long-term debt to equity ·	1.710	1.311	1.094	.893	.740	.493
Fixed asset financing	.982	.818	.805	.767	.752	.598
Times interest earned	3.255	2.888	2.688	2.937	3.577	5.027
Debt service coverage	2.508	3.343	3.275	3.574	4.284	5.573
Activity						
Total asset turnover	.629	.723	.829	.897	.909	.844
Fixed asset turnover	1.123	1.150	1.410	1.634	1.769	1.822
Current asset turnover	5.105	5.054	5.757	5.149	4.881	4.381
Inventory	52.106	55.146	68.646	70.208	75.006	78.932
Profitability						
Deductible	.121	.144	.122	.150	.142	.168
Markup	1.208	1.233	1.180	1.220	1.231	1.254
Operating margin	.060	.056	.038	.040	.058	.047
Nonoperating revenue	.222	.326	.482	.430	.319	.285
Reported income index	.892	.710	.749	.778	.647	.587
Return on total assets	.049	.060	.061	.063	.077	.107
Return on equity	.145	.152	.142	.133	.148	.191
Other						
Average age plant	6.361	5.798	5.632	5.952	6.064	6.350
Price level depreciation	1.710	1.640	1.675	1.672	1.638	1.605
Operating margin price-level adjusted	.028	.024	.004	.008	.025	.014
Reserve equity	.128	.079	.058	.030	.024	.000
Viability	1.036	.925	.939	.881	.628	.836
Replacement viability	.471	.943	1.042	1.051	1.079	1.236

• The center's operating profitability has been consistently above average. Its unusually high growth rate in equity is largely attributable to this factor.

Definition of Growth Rate of Assets

The preceding discussion of ABC's financial position and prior growth patterns gives us a good basis for defining future growth rates for individual asset categories. These growth rates must in turn be related to the center's strategic plan. Specifically, we must know what new programs and services the firm anticipates developing over the planning period, which is usually three to five years. These broad policy projections must be translated into specific financial requirements for future investment. Because of space constraints, we are not able to pursue this phase of the financial plan's development in the present context. It should be noted, however, that the projection of financial requirements for future investment is the key to successful financial plan development, in that it provides the link between strategic planning and financial planning.

In our case example, we assume a status quo model. In other words, the ABC Medical Center will attempt to maintain its present market share and position over the next five years with very little additional real growth into new market areas. This simplifies its projections and provides a basis for future plan modifications to take into account the impact of growth in new market areas.

One of the most important aspects of financial plan development is the assumption of a rate of inflation. In our economy, inflation is almost a given. It is assumed that assets will be replaced at values greater than original cost and that additional working capital will be required to meet operating needs. Financial projections are extremely sensitive to the assumed rate of inflation. In our example, we assume that the projected rate of inflation over the next five years (1987 to 1992) will be ten percent. This gives us a benchmark for the definition of specific growth rates in individual asset categories. These growth rates are summarized in the financial projections in Exhibit 7–3.

The following comments may be made on the individual growth rate projections in Exhibit 7–3:

• *Cash.* Cash was projected forward using an 11 percent growth rate, which is slightly higher than the assumed 10 percent inflation rate. This small increment above inflation was made because of the current weakness in operating cash position. The present days cash on hand is slightly below the national average.

Exhibit 7–3 Projected Balance Sheet for ABC Medical Center

ABC Medical Center

Projected Balance Sheet
(000s omitted)

	Historical 1987	Projected 1992	Model Assumption
Assets			
Cash	$ 568	$ 957	11% Growth rate
Accounts receivable	3,714	5,981	10% Growth rate
Inventories	102	205	15% Growth rate
Other current assets	709	1,142	10% Growth rate
Total current assets	$ 5,093	$ 8,285	Summation
Replacement funds	7,705	9,834	5% Growth rate
Net fixed assets	12,245	20,634	11% Growth rate
Other	1,375	1,755	5% Growth rate
Total assets	$26,418	$40,508	Summation
Liabilities and Fund Balance			
Current liabilities	$ 2,957	$ 4,143	2:1 Current ratio
Long-term debt	7,330	12,380	60% of net fixed asets
Deferred Medicare liability	1,285	0	Elimination
Fund balance	14,846	23,985	Residual
Total liabilities and fund balance	$26,418	$40,508	Summation

- *Accounts receivable.* The inflationary rate of ten percent was used to project accounts receivable. No increment above this rate was made because the current days in accounts receivable appear to be close to national norms. Therefore, the financial plan assumed that the present position would be maintained into the future. If ABC's days in accounts receivable were much higher, for example 90 days, an argument might be made for using a rate lower than the inflationary rate.

- *Inventories.* Inventories were increased substantially above the current inflationary rate, to 15%. Present levels of inventory appear to be slightly below national norms as measured by the inventory ratio. This, coupled with the decline in inventory values during the past five-year historical period, led us to increase our inventory levels. Note that the financial plan will not be very sensitive to alternative inventory projections because inventory accounts for such a small percentage of total investment.

- *Other current assets.* Other current assets were projected to increase at the inflationary rate. This estimate may be understated if the rate of increase in the future parallels prior growth rates. Note that the past five-year period showed a 32 percent annual growth rate.

- *Current assets.* The value for current assets represents the summation of the individual elements that constitute current assets. The 1992 value of current assets represents a 10.2 percent compounded yearly growth rate.

- *Replacement funds.* A five percent rate was used to project replacement funds for the next five years. The rationale for using a rate that is significantly below the inflationary rate is based upon the present value of the replacement viability ratio. It is assumed that ABC will begin to use some of these funds for replacement purposes and not expand its replacement reserves at the same rate it has in the past. The absolute level of funds will increase by approximately $2.1 million, but the relative level in terms of replacement needs will fall.

- *Net fixed assets.* A slight increment above the inflationary rate was used to project net fixed assets. Even though the current average age of plant ratio is slightly below the national norm, we are providing a small cushion for the hospital to expand into some areas that might require new investment.

- *Other assets.* A rate of five percent was used to project other assets. Much of the investment in this category will be amortized over the coming five-year period. Therefore, we have provided for only marginal real future growth.

- *Total assets.* Total assets, like current assets, are the result of summing the individual elements. The projected value of total assets ($40,508) represents an annual growth rate of 8.9 percent, which is slightly below the inflationary rate. This is the result of the low growth rates used to project replacement funds and, to a lesser degree, of the lower rate used to project other assets.

Definition of Acceptable Levels of Debt

The third step in the development of the financial plan is the definition of an acceptable debt policy. Debt should not be viewed as the balancing variable in a financial plan. That is, the financial plan should not project assets and equity and then balance the equation with debt. Sound financial policy requires that the board and management define in advance what their position is regarding the assumption of debt. Exhibit 7–3 projects the various categories of debt to 1992 and defines the assumption underlying the projections. The relevant projections and assumptions are delineated below:

- *Current liabilities.* Current liabilities are projected forward using a desired current ratio of 2 to 1. Since the projected current assets in 1992 are $8,285, the projected value for current liabilities would be one-half of that value, or $4,143. The current ratio of 2.000 represents a change from the present current (1987) ratio of 1.722. The assumption underlying the change is that the center will be relying upon current liability financing to a lesser degree than they are now. This means that the center will have to increase its equity financing in the planning period to replace the portion of current assets that is presently financed with current liabilities. If the center had used its present current ratio of 1.722 to project current liabilities in 1992, the projected value would have been $4,811 (rather than $4,143 as projected with a current ratio of 2.000). This means that the ABC Medical Center will have to generate approximately $670,000 in additional equity over the five-year planning period to replace the amount of current liability financing presently implied in its current ratio of 1.722.

- *Long-term debt.* ABC Medical Center is assumed to have a stated long-term debt policy of 60 percent debt financing of net fixed assets. This policy is consistent with its present fixed asset financing ratio of .598. To generate the 1992 long-term debt value, we simply multiply net fixed assets in 1992 by .60. The projected value for long-term debt in 1992 would therefore be $12,380. It is important to note that long-term debt does not usually change by constant increments each year. In most situations, a major financing will take place every five years or so. In our example, ABC Medical Center may do no long-term debt financing for the first three years of the financial plan and then borrow heavily in 1991. The target of 60 percent fixed asset financing simply provides it with an objective that it would like to see attained in the year 1992.

- *Deferred Medicare liability.* The deferred Medicare liability is projected to be zero in 1992. In other words, the balance will disappear as the method of payment for capital costs changes under the Medicare program. The present liability resulted from the use of accelerated depreciation and a gain on an advance bond refunding.

Assessment of the Reasonableness of the Required Equity Growth Rate

Determining whether the equity growth rate is reasonable is perhaps the most crucial step in the financial planning process. Defining the actual amount of required equity capital in the financial plan is relatively simple: Once the actual level of total assets has been projected and the entity's debt policy has been defined, the level of required equity is the residual figure. In our example of ABC Medical Center, we can determine that it needs to have $23,985 in equity in 1992. That is the amount of equity needed to keep the balance sheet equation in balance. Anything less than that amount and the center will be forced either to reduce its level of total assets or to increase its level of debt.

The question of reasonableness in equity growth still remains, however. In our example, increasing ABC's equity to $23,985 in 1992 translates into a 10.1 percent annual growth rate. Is this level of growth actually attainable?

The best way to assess the reasonableness of equity growth is to factor the growth rate into a number of specific areas that can be analyzed in terms of reasonableness. The following equation defines equity growth as a product of five factors:

$$\text{Equity growth rate} = \text{OM} \times \text{TAT} \times \frac{1}{\text{EF}} \times \frac{1}{\text{RII}} \times \frac{1}{\text{1-NOR}}$$

where:

OM = Operating margin ratio
TAT = Total asset turnover ratio
EF   = Equity financing ratio
RII   = Reported income index ratio
NOR = Nonoperating revenue ratio

By stating equity growth as a product of the five factors cited above, the analyst is better able to assess whether a required growth rate in equity is actually attainable. The best starting point is to examine the historical pattern of values for these five factors. Exhibit 7–4 provides the relevant data for ABC Medical Center.

Historically, ABC Medical Center has demonstrated a growth rate in equity that is far above the required growth rate of 10.1 percent called for in the financial plan. It has averaged approximately 20 percent per year in equity growth. The specific values for each of the five factors that determine equity growth show how this growth rate was accomplished. These data also serve as a basis for projecting into the future. The last column of Exhibit 7–4 provides details about ABC Medical Center's projected or targeted equity growth rate. The rationale for projecting the specific ratio values in this forecast is presented below:

Exhibit 7–4 Equity Growth Rates for ABC Medical Center

	Historical Values					Target 1987 – 1992
	1983	1984	1985	1986	1987	
Equity growth rate	21.7%	19.0%	17.2%	22.9%	16.8%	10.1%
Operating margin ratio	.056	.038	.040	.058	.047	.050
Total asset turnover ratio	.72	.82	.90	.91	.84	.76
Equity financing ratio	.39	.43	.47	.52	.56	.59
Nonoperating revenue ratio	.33	.48	.43	.32	.29	.25
Reported income index ratio	.71	.75	.78	.65	.59	.85

- *Operating margin ratio.* The plan calls for an operating margin of 5.0 percent per year during the five-year planning period. This value is fairly consistent with prior values and represents a reasonable estimate of future levels of operating profitability. If the center had information to indicate that levels of competition might increase in the future, it might wish to reduce its operating margin projection. In this regard, it is useful to undertake a sensitivity analysis. For example, the effect of reducing the operating margin to 4.0 percent over the planning period would be to reduce the growth rate in equity to approximately 8.1 percent. Other scenarios could be tested to determine the effects upon the attainability of the targeted equity growth rate and thus the feasibility of the center's financial plan.

- *Total asset turnover ratio.* A small reduction in the value of the total asset turnover ratio from prior values is reflected in the forecast. The assumption for the reduction is based upon the prior trend, which has been declining over the last three years. The forecast calls for the total asset turnover ratio to be .76 in the five-year planning period, which is below the 1987 value of .84. Again, a sensitivity analysis could be performed to test the effects of possible changes upon equity growth. In situations calling for major capital replacement or renovation, total asset turnover ratios usually decline substantially. However, since ABC Medical Center does not anticipate major capital expenditures during the planning period, the lowered total asset turnover forecast appears to be reasonable, given prior trends.

- *Equity financing ratio.* Over the past five years, ABC Medical Center has shown a substantial increase in its level of equity financing. The percentage of assets financed with equity in 1987 was 56 percent, compared with only 39 percent in 1983. The projection calls for an equity financing ratio of .59 during the planning period. This value is consistent with the percentage of equity financing shown in the 1992 projected balance sheet in Exhibit 7–3. It reflects the slower rate of equity growth assumed in the initial financial plan for the ABC Medical Center.

- *Nonoperating revenue ratio.* The ratio of nonoperating revenue to net income has declined over the past four years for ABC Medical Center, to a value of .29 in 1987. A value of .25 is projected during the planning period. This projection appears reasonable given the small increase in operating margin forecasted for the planning period. Note that the targeted operating margin is 5.0 percent, compared with 4.7 percent in 1987. Nonoperating revenue usually represents a smaller percentage of total net income when operating profits are increasing. In addition, investment income or replacement funds may decrease relatively, due to the lower growth rate used to project replacement funds.

- *Reported income index ratio.* The value projected for the reported income index ratio during the planning period is greater than in any period during the past five years. This is based on the conservative assumption that ABC Medical Center will be relying less on unreported income during the next five years than it has in the past. The rationale for this assumption is related to information that is not available in the data presented here, namely, that ABC Medical Center has benefited in the past from sizable levels of donor-restricted monies. The relative importance of these funds is decreasing, however, and ABC is rapidly drawing on them for operating purposes. Though these funds will continue to exist in the planning period, the center believes that there will be a significant reduction in fund transfers during the next five years. This reduction is reflected in the increased value assumed for the reported income index ratio.

The individual values assumed for the five ratios that determine equity growth rate yield the projected rate of 10.1 percent

$$\text{Equity growth rate} = .05 \times .76 + \frac{1}{.59} \times \frac{1}{(1-.25)} \times \frac{1}{.85} = .101 \times 100 = 10.1\%$$

Comments and Conclusions

At this juncture in the planning process, alternative plans could be developed that would reflect different assumptions. For example, the ABC Medical Center might decide to expand its operations, embark upon a major renovation program, or change its debt policy. Each of these changes would require new sets of financial projections and new tests to determine if the required growth rate in equity is reasonable.

One final point should be made before we begin our discussion of the next stage, integrating the financial plan with the management control process. In most financial feasibility studies, the projection of funds flow and net income is extremely important; financial officers need to have very precise estimates of the flow of funds by period to plan their financing patterns. However, the financial planning process described here does not provide a basis for the projection of funds flow or net income. Our perspective has been more global; in this context, we have not concerned ourselves with the detail required for projecting funds flow. This does not mean, however, that our approach is inconsistent with a more detailed funds flow projection. In fact, the assumptions made in the ABC Center's projected balance sheet would provide the basis for more detailed funds projections. The assumptions we have made concerning the factors that determine equity growth would also be integral to funds flow projections.

Finally, even though we have not projected revenues and expenses for the ABC Medical Center, we have specified, through our definition of the operating margin, the percentage of revenues that will be realized as income from operations. In this regard, it is useful to remember that a statement of revenues and expenses or net income provides detail about how a given change in equity was accomplished. The values specified in an equity growth model collectively provide the same data, but the approach described in this chapter is easier to understand and utilize. This is especially important as a basis for presentation to board members and executives who are interested in broad policy formulation and goal setting rather than the details of specific transactions.

INTEGRATION OF THE FINANCIAL PLAN WITH MANAGEMENT CONTROL

The development of a financial plan is a useless exercise unless that plan is integrated into the management control process. Management needs to know if the plan is being realized and, if it is not, what corrective action can be taken. In some cases, there is little that management can do. For example, assume that the entity has experienced an unusually large reduction in its operating margins, due to increased competition. In this case, perhaps the only course of action open to management is to revise its plan to reflect more accurately the current situation. Indeed it is important for management to assess the accuracy of its financial plan annually and to make appropriate changes in it as needed.

To integrate the financial plan with the management control process, some structure is needed. Financial ratios provide that structure. The chart in Figure 7–4 depicts detailed targets for the ABC Medical Center, reflecting its financial plan. In the chart, specific ratio values are delineated. The primary targets involve the five major ratios that together determine the center's equity growth rate. The secondary targets are concerned with additional data that can be used to monitor actual performance and detect possible problems.

To see how the Figure 7–4 chart might be used in management control, let us assume that 1988 has just ended and the financial data essential to the calculation of the ratios are now available. ABC Medical Center's actual growth rate in equity for 1988 is assumed to be 8.7 percent, which represents an unfavorable variance from the required value of 10.1 percent. Actual values for the primary indicators are:

	1988 Values
Operating margin ratio	.040
Total asset turnover ratio	.810
Equity financing ratio	.570
Nonoperating revenue ratio	.300
Reported income index ratio	.930

The major cause of the unfavorable variance in equity growth rate during 1988 is an unfavorable operating margin (.040 versus the .050 target) and an unfavorable reported income index (.930 versus the .850 target). The improvement in the nonoperating revenue ratio is the result of the reduction in operating profit.

We could also identify the cause of the unfavorable operating margin ratio by examining the values of the deductible ratio and the markup ratio. Let us assume that the markup ratio in 1988 was 1.20 and the deductible ratio was .17. This would narrow our attention to the markup ratio as the source of the problem. Upon examination, we might learn that the primary reason for the unfavorable variation in the markup ratio was an unexpected increase in expenses. This situation may be correctable in future periods, putting the center back on track in terms of realizing its financial plan projections. However, it should be noted that because it did not realize a 10.1 percent growth rate in equity in the current year, it will need to plan on larger increases in the remaining four years. If it fails to realize growth rates in

Figure 7–4 Financial Ratio Targets for ABC Medical Center

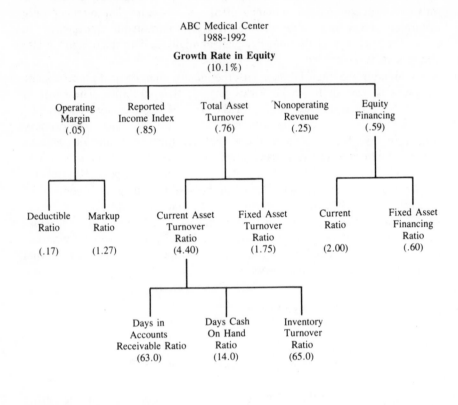

excess of 10.1 percent in future years, its financial projections will not be realized.

The reported income index value was also significantly above the projected value. This means that the center did not derive as much new equity from unreported sources as it had originally planned. If this trend continues, the center might be forced to change its initial assumptions and redefine its financial plan to reflect current circumstances.

The preceding framework for integrating management control and financial planning is reasonably concise and simple. It can be used by board members to assess more accurately the financial situation of their organization, and it provides a useful tool for communication by management. Finally, it relates directly to established financial planning targets and thus provides a structure for the delineation of secondary and tertiary targets, which may be particularly useful for lower levels of management.

SUMMARY

In the process of identifying the requirements for effective financial policy formulation in health care firms, it is especially important to relate the strategic plan to the financial plan. The financial plan should not be developed in isolation from strategic planning, nor should the strategic plan be developed in isolation from the financial plan. Both need to be developed together, reflecting in that context their individual requirements and assumptions. A strategic plan is not valid if it is not financially feasible, and a financial plan is of little value if it does not reflect the strategic decisions reached by management and the board.

A financial plan should be updated at least annually, projecting a forecast period of three to five years. Financial plans that are not updated stand a good chance of becoming invalid. The environment of health care delivery is changing, and a health care entity's financial plan must reflect the changes. In fact, a failure to update its financial plan can have disastrous consequences for an entity, leading perhaps to market share retrenchment or even financial failure.

Finally, financial plans should be integrated into the management control process. Financial ratios can be very useful in this regard. In particular, specific ratios can be usefully related to the key financial planning target of growth rate in equity.

ASSIGNMENTS

1. A financial plan may be thought of as a bridge between two balance sheets. What are the major categories of assumptions that must be specified to project a future balance sheet, given a current balance sheet?

2. What problems result from the present responsibility-center orientation of most accounting systems in providing data for financial planning?

3. Your director of marketing is urging you to develop a new drug abuse program. She has argued that there is no capital investment involved in the development of the new service. Do you believe this is an accurate statement?

4. Your hospital has a current replacement viability ratio of .20. What are the implications of this indicator for your hospital's financial planning?

5. Your controller has just provided you with return on investment (ROI) figures for your firm's major product lines. You have noticed that obstetrics has a very low ROI. What factors should be considered before you drop this service?

6. You are in the process of developing your firm's financial plan for the next five years. As an initial step, you are analyzing financial ratios for the last five years. You notice that, over the

five-year period, the average age of plant ratio has increased from 8.5 years to 12.2 years. What are the implications of this for your financial plan?

7. If current assets are expected to increase by $4 million over the next five years and you wish to increase your current ratio from 1.5 to 2.0, what additional amount of new equity must be generated to finance the increase in the current ratio?

8. Beginning equity is $50 million and equity in five years is projected to be $100 million. What is the annual rate of growth implied by these values?

9. You are assessing the financial plan developed for you by a prestigious "Big-8" accounting firm. You are especially interested in the attainability of the projected growth rate in equity. You know that, if that growth rate is not realistic, the financial plan is not valid and you may have to scale back your projected increase in assets. The following schedule summarizes your findings:

	Historical Average	5-Year Projected
Reported income index ratio	1.000	.900
Operating margin ratio	.025	.027
Total asset turnover ratio	1.100	1.200
Nonoperating revenue ratio	.300	.300
Equity financing ratio	.500	.500
Equity growth rate	7.86%	10.29%

Does the accounting firm's plan appear to be reasonable?

10. During the next five years, Meredith Hospital must spend $2 million to renovate its plant. Data for the most recent two years are presented in the hospital's financial statements in Exhibits 7–5 through 7–8. Based on these data, develop a projected balance sheet for 1992. Assume that Meredith Hospital will be experiencing a general inflationary rate of 8 percent over the next five years. Does it appear that the hospital can realistically finance its asset needs?

Exhibit 7–5 Balance Sheets for Meredith Hospital

Meredith Hospital

Balance Sheets, December 31, 1986 and 1987

Assets

Unrestricted Funds

	1987	1986
Current assets		
Cash		
Demand deposits	$ 4,855	$ 49,953
Savings	22,948	79,849
Certificates of deposit	9,187	103,362
Accounts receivable:		
Patient accounts	910,596	634,867
Less allowance for uncollectible accounts and contractual allowance	52,000	75,000
	858,596	559,867
Other	83,845	40,445
	942,441	600,312
Inventory	115,356	101,542
Prepaid expenses	24,128	42,369
Total current assets	1,118,915	977,387
Other assets		
Other	69,085	71,501
Property, plant, and equipment less accumulated depreciation of $1,474,395 in 1987 and $1,473,063 in 1986	2,008,589	1,850,819
	$3,196,589	$2,899,707

Restricted Funds

	1987	1986
Special purpose funds		
Investments	$ 169	$ 169
Endowment funds		
Cash and investments	$155,302	$155,302

Exhibit 7–6 Statements of Liabilities and Fund Balances for Meredith Hospital

---

Meredith Hospital

Liabilities and Fund Balances
Years Ended December 31, 1987 and 1986

Unrestricted Funds

	1987	1986
Current liabilities		
Current maturities of long-term debt	$ 20,282	$ 0
Trade accounts payable	299,607	138,655
Accrued expenses		
Salaries and wages	61,618	119,709
Other	270,327	175,769
Amounts due Blue Cross, Blue Shield, Medicare, and Medicaid from adjustments of interim payments	144,402	77,851
Total current liabilities	796,236	511,984
Long-term debt, less current maturities	121,415	0
Fund balance	2,278,938	2,387,723
	$3,196,589	$2,899,707

Restricted Funds

Special purpose funds		
Fund balance	$ 169	$ 169
Endowment funds		
Fund balance	$155,302	$155,302

Exhibit 7–7 Statements of Revenue and Expense and Changes in
Unrestricted Fund Balances for Meredith Hospital

Meredith Hospital

Statements of Revenue and Expense and
Changes in Unrestricted Fund Balances
Years Ended December 31, 1987 and 1986

	1987	1986
Operating revenue		
Patient revenue	$6,116,268	$4,476,208
Revenue deductions	785,465	430,380
Net patient revenue	5,330,803	4,045,828
Other operating revenue	138,179	103,259
Total operating revenue	5,468,982	4,149,087
Operating expenses		
Nursing service	1,572,884	1,106,979
Emergency service	354,441	268,728
Ancillary service	1,100,823	793,752
Medical administration	129,259	114,344
General service	799,767	674,755
Administrative and fiscal services	811,718	620,180
Interest	3,151	0
Depreciation	190,583	165,896
Other operating expense	497,920	453,847
Total operating expense	5,460,546	4,198,481
Income (loss) from operations	8,436	(49,394)
Net nonoperating income (expense)	(133,913)	124,385
Excess of revenues over expenses (expenses over revenues)	(125,477)	74,991
Fund balance		
Beginning	2,387,723	2,298,255
Transfer from restricted fund	16,692	14,477
Ending	$2,278,938	$2,387,723

Exhibit 7–8 Statement of Changes in Fund Balances, Restricted Funds, for Meredith Hospital

	Special Purpose Funds		Endowment Funds	
	1987	1986	1987	1986
Balance, beginning	$169	$169	$155,302	$155,302
Additions (deductions)				
Interest income	20	20	16,019	13,940
Contributions	653	517	0	0
Transfer to unrestricted funds	(673)	(537)	(16,019)	(13,940)
Balance, ending	$169	$169	$155,302	$155,302

Meredith Hospital
Statement of Changes in Fund Balances
Restricted Funds
Years Ended December 31, 1987 and 1986

SOLUTIONS AND ANSWERS

1. Projection of a future balance sheet requires assumptions in three categories:

    1. rates of growth for individual asset accounts

    2. debt financing policy for both current and long-term debt

    3. realizable rate of growth in equity that is factored into five ratio areas: operating margins, nonoperating revenue, equity financing, total asset turnover, and reported income index

2. Strategic financial planning is usually done along program or product lines, not responsibility centers. This requires the financial planner to transfer revenue, cost, and investment assignments from responsibility centers to product lines. This can be a very difficult and inexact process.

3. Although there may be a little new investment in fixed assets required to start a drug abuse program, the investment in working capital may be sizable. Some projection of the investment should be made to assess the potential return on investment that is likely to result.

4. A replacement viability ratio of .20 implies that your hospital will need to borrow 90 percent of its replacement needs in the future. The percentage of debt financing is derived by the following formula:

$$\text{Debt Financing} = 100\% - .5 \times \text{Replacement Viability Ratio}$$

This directly affects the debt policy assumptions that will be used in the financial plan. It will also impact the firm's operating margins because of the potentially large increase in debt and the resulting increase in interest expense.

5. Eliminating a product line solely on the basis of an inadequate return on investment may not be consistent with the firm's goals and objectives. Specifically, obstetrics may meet an unmet community need and may be essential to the firm's mission; it may in fact be classified as a samaritan (see Figure 7–3). Alternatively, a low return on investment can sometimes be deceiving. The product line may have important externalities. For example, obstetrics may lose money, but gynecology may be very profitable. Removing obstetrics may mean that the firm's gynecology line, and its profits, would be reduced.

6. The current average age of plant ratio implies that the firm has a very old plant relative to industry norms. This will almost certainly mean that significant new investment will be required in the planning period.

7. Use of a current ratio of 2.0 implies that the incremental investment of $4.00 million in current assets would be financed with $2.00 million of current liabilities. Use of a current ratio of 1.5 would imply current liability financing of $2.67 million. Therefore, the change in the current ratio implies that an additional equity requirement of $670,000 would be required.

8. The implied annual rate of growth is 14.86 percent.

9. The accounting firm's plan specifies a 30 percent increase in the annual growth rate in equity, compared with the historical five-year average (7.86 percent versus 10.29 percent). The major changes are in the reported income index and total asset turnover ratios. In the past five years, the firm has had no unreported income, since the value for the reported income index is 1.0. It is very important to find out what the source of the new equity is expected to be. The increase in total asset turnover, though not large, does play an important role in the higher projected growth rate in equity. Reasons for this increase should be verified.

10. The data in Table 7–1 are the results of a financial ratio analysis conducted for Meredith Hospital. The ratios indicate that the hospital's cash position is presently very weak. A significant build-up in cash may be required to meet liquidity concerns. There is very little long-term debt, but profitably is very weak, which means that debt service coverage is marginal. Virtually no replacement funds are present to finance future asset growth. Table 7–2 shows data for the projected balance sheet for Meredith Hospital with supporting assumptions. From these data, it can be seen that the projected growth rate in equity is fairly modest, 2.32 percent per annum. This rate appears feasible, provided the hospital can increase its operating margin and not lose money from nonoperating sources. A key concern is the ability of the hospital to borrow long-term debt. Its present levels of income may not justify additional long-term debt in the amount required in the plan.

Table 7–1 Financial Ratios for Meredith Hospital

Ratios	1986	1987
Liquidity		
Current	1.909	1.405
Quick	1.549	1.125
Acid test	.455	.046
Days in patient receivable	50.509	58.788
Average payment period	46.341	55.148
Days' cash on hand	21.104	2.562

Ratios	1986	1987
Capital structure		
Equity financing	.823	.713
Cash flow to debt	.470	.071
Long-term debt to equity	.000	.053
Fixed asset financing	.000	.060
Times interest earned	NA	− 38.821
Debt service coverage	NA	20.662
Activity		
Total asset turnover	1.431	1.711
Fixed asset turnover	2.242	2.723
Current asset turnover	4.245	4.888
Inventory	40.861	47.410
Profitability		
Deductible	.096	.128
Markup	1.091	1.145
Operating margin	− .012	.002
Nonoperating revenue	1.659	1.067
Reported income index	.838	1.153
Return on total assets	.026	− .039
Return on equity	.031	− .055
Other		
Average age plant	8.879	7.736
Price level depreciation	2.091	1.982
Operating margin price-level adjusted	− .056	− .033
Restricted equity	.065	.068
Viability	.388	.812
Replacement viability	.046	.047

Table 7–2 Projected Balance Sheet for Meredith Hospital (000s Omitted)

	1987	1992
Current Assets		
Cash and certificates of deposit	$ 37	$ 217[a]
Accounts receivable	942	1,384[b]
Inventory	115	169[c]
Prepaid expenses	24	35[d]
Total Current Assets	$1,118	$1,805
Other	69	852[e]
Property, plant, and equipment	2,009	2,456[f]
Total Assets	$3,196	$5,113

	1987	1992
Current liabilities	$796	1,002[g]
Long-term debt	121	1,555[h]
Fund balance	2,279	2,556[i]
Total	$3,196	$5,113

Assumptions

[a]Present cash should be around $148 to yield a 10.5 days' cash on hand position. Inflating that value forward at 8 percent yields $217.

[b]Present days in accounts receivable is acceptable. Present receivables inflated at 8 percent.

[c]Present inventory may be excessive, but this is not significant. Current value inflated at 8 percent.

[d]Inflated at 8 percent.

[e]Other assets represent replacement funds. Their present position is inadequate, given their low replacement viability ratio. To be near normal, the present level of investments should be near $580. Inflating $580 at 8 percent yields the 1992 projected value.

[f]The hospital expects to add $2,000,000 in new investment over the five-year period. This would yield $4,009,000 in 1992 before subtracting depreciation. Present depreciation expense is $190,583. The assumption that the new assets will be put in operation in Year 3 and have an average ten-year life means $200,000 of additional depreciation expense in Years 3, 4, and 5. Total depreciation expense would be $1,552,915 ((5 × $190,583) + (3 × $200,000)). This means net plant would be $2,456,085 in 1992.

[g]The current ratio will be 1.8 in 1992.

[h]It is assumed that the hospital desires an equity financing ratio of .5. Therefore, current liabilities plus long-term debt cannot exceed $2,557 (50 percent of $5,113). Long-term debt is therefore $1,555.

[i]Equity is a residue figure (5113-1002-1555).

Chapter 8

Cost Concepts and Decision Making

In the last five chapters, we have focused on understanding and interpreting the financial information prepared by the financial accounting system and presented in general-purpose financial statements. This chapter is directed more narrowly at the utilization of cost information in decision making. Cost information is produced by the cost accounting system of an entity. In most situations, it is shaped by the financial accounting system and the generally accepted principles of financial accounting. However, it is flexible, since it usually provides information for identifiable and specific decision-making groups, such as budgetary cost variance reports to department managers, cost reports to third party payers, and forecasted project cost reports to planning agencies.

Cost is a noun that never really stands alone. In most situations, two additional pieces of information are added that enhance the meaning and relevance of the cost statistic.

First, the object being costed is defined. For example, we might say that the cost of routine nursing care in Willkram Hospital is $200. Objects of costing are usually of two types:

1. products (outputs or services)
2. responsibility centers (departments or larger units)

Quite often, we oversimplify this classification system and refer to cost information about products as *planning information* and cost information about responsibility centers as *control information*.

Second, usually an adjective is added to modify cost. For example, we might say that the *direct* cost of routine nursing care in Willkram Hospital is $100. A number of major categories of adjective modifiers refine the concept of cost; they are all used to improve the decision-making process by precisely defining cost to make it more relevant to decisions.

This chapter discusses some of the basic concepts of cost used in cost analysis. It is important to explain this jargon if decision makers are to use cost information correctly. Different concepts of cost are required for different decision purposes. In most situations, these concepts require specific, unique methodologies for cost measurement.

CONCEPTS OF COST

Cost may be categorized in a variety of ways to meet decision makers' specific needs. However, in most situations, the total value of cost is the same. Using one cost concept in place of another simply slices the total cost pie differently. For example, in Table 8–1, the total cost of a laboratory for June, 1986, was $21,360. Of that amount, $20,000 could be classified as direct cost and $1,360 as indirect cost. However, classifying costs by controllability might determine that $15,000 of the laboratory cost was controllable and $6,360 was not controllable. The total cost, however, is the same in both cases.

This brings us to another important point. Since, in most cases, different concepts of cost simply slice total cost in different ways, there may be underlying relationships between the various concepts of costs. For example, direct costs and controllable costs may be related. In many situations, there are standard rules of thumb that may be used to relate cost measures.

The difference between cost and expense is another crucial definitional point. Accountants have traditionally defined cost in a way that leads one to think of cost as an expenditure. However, in most reported cost statistics, the definition is usually one of expense, not necessarily expenditure. For example, in Table 8–1, depreciation is listed as a cost. However, depreciation is not an actual expenditure of cash but an amortization of prior cost. In the present context, unless otherwise indicated, when we are discussing cost statistics, the term costs and expenses may be used interchangeably.

For purposes of discussion, we examine below the four major categories within which costs can be classified:

1. traceability to the object being costed
2. behavior of cost to output or activity
3. management responsibility for control
4. future vs. historical

Table 8–1 Cost Report, Laboratory, June, 1986

DIRECT COSTS	
Salaries	$10,000
Supplies	5,000
Other	5,000
TOTAL	$20,000
DEPRECIATION	
Building and Fixed Equipment	100
Major Movable Equipment	60
TOTAL	160
ALLOCATED COSTS	
Employee Benefits	150
Administration	500
Maintenance	250
Housekeeping	200
Laundry	100
TOTAL	1,200
TOTAL COSTS	$21,360
RELATIVE VALUE UNITS (RVU) PRODUCED	10,000
AVERAGE COST PER RVU	$ 2,136

Traceability

Of all cost classifications, traceability is the most basic. Two major categories of costs classified by traceability are (1) direct costs and (2) indirect costs. A direct cost is specifically traceable to a given cost objective. For example, the salaries, supplies, and other costs of Table 8–1 are classified as direct costs of the laboratory. Indirect costs cannot be traced to a given cost objective without resorting to some arbitrary method of assignment. In Table 8–1, depreciation, employee benefits, and costs of other departments would be classified as indirect costs.

Not all costs classified as indirect may actually be indirect, however. In some situations, they could be redefined as direct costs. For example, it might be possible to calculate employee benefits for specific employees; these costs could then be charged to the departments where the employees worked and thus become direct costs. However, the actual costs of performing these calculations might be prohibitive.

The classification of a cost as either direct or indirect depends on the given cost objective. This is a simple observation, but one that is forgotten by many users of cost information. For example, the $20,000 of direct cost identified in Table 8–1 is a direct cost only with respect to the laboratory department. If another cost objective is specified, the cost may no longer be direct. For example, dividing the $20,000 of direct costs by the number of relative value units (RVUs) yields a direct cost per RVU of $2.00. But, this is not really true. The direct cost of any given RVU may be higher or lower than the $2.00 calculated, which is the average value for all RVUs and not necessarily the cost for any specific unit.

Incorrect classification is a common problem in cost accounting. Costs are accumulated on a department or responsibility-center basis and may be direct or indirect with respect to that department. However, it can be misleading to say that the same set of direct costs is also direct with respect to the outputs of that department.

The major direct cost categories of most departments would include the following three:

- salaries
- supplies
- other (usually fees and purchased services, such as utilities, dues, travel, and rents)

Indirect cost categories usually include:

- depreciation
- employee benefits
- allocated costs of other departments

The concept of direct versus indirect cost may not appear to have much specific relevance to decision makers. To some extent this is true, however, the concept of direct versus indirect costs is pervasive. It influences both the definition and measurement of other alternative cost concepts that do have specific relevance.

Cost Behavior

Cost is also classified by the degree of variability in relation to output. The actual measurement of cost behavior is influenced by a department's classifications of cost, which provides the basis for categorizing costs as direct or indirect.

For our purposes, we can identify four major categories of costs that are classified according to their relationship to output:

1. variable
2. fixed
3. semifixed
4. semivariable

Variable costs change as output or volume changes in a constant, proportional manner. That is, if output increases by 10 percent, costs should also increase by 10 percent, that is, there is some constant cost increment per unit of output. Figure 8–1 illustrates, graphically and mathematically, the concept of variable cost for the laboratory example of Table 8–1. It is assumed that all supply costs in this case are variable. For each unit increase in RVUs, supply costs will increase by $.50.

Fixed costs do not change in response to changes in volume. They are a function of the passage of time, not output. Figure 8–2 illustrates fixed cost behavior patterns for the depreciation costs of the laboratory example. Each month, irrespective of output levels, depreciation cost will be $160.

Semifixed, or step, costs do change with respect to changes in output, but they are not proportional. A semifixed cost might be considered variable or fixed—depending on the size of the steps relative to the range of volume under consideration. For example, in Figure 8–3, it is assumed that the

---

Figure 8–1 Cost Behavior of Supplies Cost, Variable

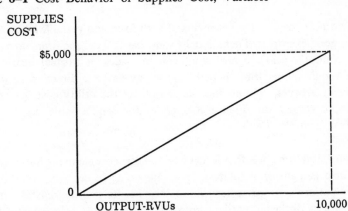

Note: Supplies cost = $.50 × number of RVUs.

Figure 8-2 Cost Behavior of Depreciation, Fixed

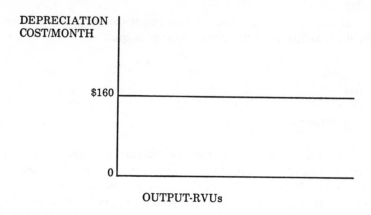

DEPRECIATION
COST/MONTH

$160

0

OUTPUT-RVUs

Note: Depreciation cost = $160 per month.

salaries cost of the laboratory is semifixed. If the volume of output under consideration for a specific decision were between 6,000 and 8,000 RVUs, salary costs could be considered fixed at $9,000. Some semifixed costs may be considered variable for cost analysis purposes. For example, if smaller units of people could be employed instead of full-time equivalents (FTEs), such as on the basis of hours generated by an available part-time pool, the size of the steps might be significantly smaller than 2,000 RVUs in our laboratory example. At the present, it is assumed that one additional FTE must be employed for every increment of 2,000 RVUs. Treating salary costs as variable in this situation might not be a bad procedure (see Figure 8-3).

Semivariable costs include elements of both fixed and variable costs. Utility costs are good examples. There may be some basic, fixed requirement per unit of time, (month, year) regardless of volume—such as normal heating and lighting requirements. But there is also likely to be a direct, proportional relationship between volume and the amount of the utility cost. As volume increases, costs go up. Figure 8-4 illustrates semivariable costs in our laboratory example.

In many situations, we do not focus on specific cost elements but aggregate several cost categories of interest. It is interesting to see what type of cost behavior pattern emerges when we do this. Figure 8-5 aggregates the four cost categories discussed earlier—supplies, depreciation, salaries, and other. A semivariable cost behavior pattern closely approximates the actual

Figure 8–3 Cost Behavior of Salary Costs, Semifixed

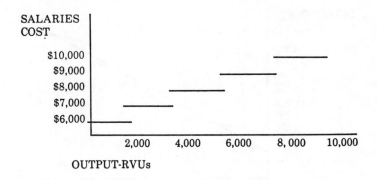

Note: Salary costs = $6,000 if RVUs are less than 2,000, $7,000 if RVUs are between 2,001 and 4,000, $8,000 if RVUs are between 4,001 and 6,000, $9,000 if RVUs are between 6,001 and 8,000, and $10,000 if RVUs are between 8,001 and 10,000.

aggregated cost behavior pattern; this is true for many types of operations. In the next section, we discuss some very simple but useful methods for approximating this cost function.

Figure 8–4 Cost Behavior of Other Costs, Semivariable

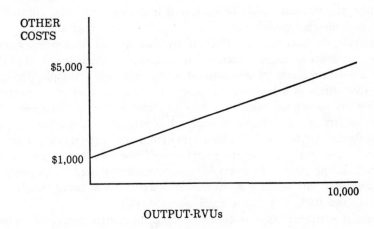

Note: Other costs = $1,000 per month + $.40 × RVUs.

Figure 8–5 Cost Behavior of Aggregated Costs, Direct Cost and Depreciation

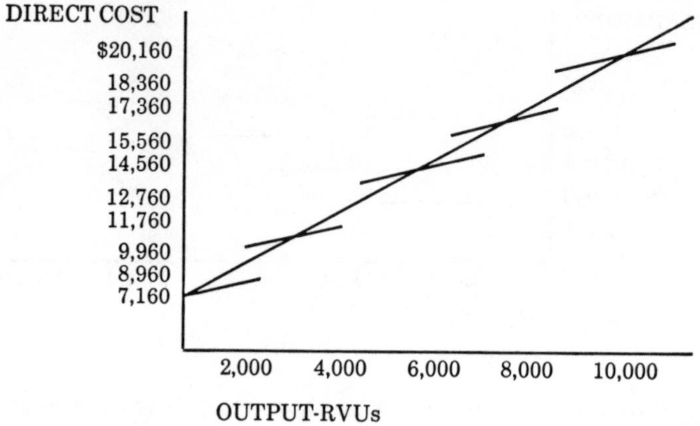

Note: Direct cost and depreciation = $7,160 per month + $1.30 × RVUs (approximation).

Controllability

One of the primary purposes of gathering cost information is to aid the management control process. To facilitate evaluation of the management control process, costs must be assigned to individual responsibility centers, usually departments, where a designated manager is responsible for cost control. A natural question that arises is, what proportion of the total costs charged to a department is the manager responsible for? The answer to this question requires that costs be separated into two categories: controllable costs and noncontrollable costs.

Controllable costs can be influenced by a designated responsibility center or departmental manager within a defined control period. It is said that all costs are controllable by someone at some time. For example, the chief executive officer of a health care facility, through the authority granted to him by his governing board, is ultimately responsible for all costs.

The matrix of costs shown in Figure 8–6 categorizes the laboratory cost report data of Table 8–1. All costs must fall into one of the six cells, however it may be possible to categorize an aggregated cost category into more than one cell. In the laboratory example, other cost was viewed as semivariable, implying that part of the cost would be described as a direct variable cost ($4,000) and part as a direct fixed cost ($1,000).

There is a tendency in developing management control programs, especially in the health care industry, to use one of three approaches in designating controllable costs. First, controllable costs may be defined to be the total

Figure 8–6 Laboratory Cost Behavior Categorization

Traceability	Variable		Fixed		Semifixed		Total
Direct	Other Supplies	$4,000 5,000	Other	$1,000	Salaries	$10,000	
		$9,000		$1,000		$10,000	$20,000
Indirect	Employee Benefits Housekeeping	$150 $100	Depreciation Administration Housekeeping	$160 $500 $100	Maintenance Laundry	$250 $100	
		$250		$760		$350	$1,360
Totals		$9,250		$1,760		$10,350	$21,360

costs charged to the department; the department manager would view all costs in the above six categories as controllable. In our example, all $21,360 of cost would be viewed as controllable by the laboratory manager. In most normal situations, however, this grossly overstates the amount of cost actually controllable by a given departmental manager. The result of this overstatement has been negative in many situations. Departmental managers have rightfully viewed this basis of control as highly inequitable.

Second, controllable costs may be limited to those costs classified as direct. This system is also not without fault: specifically, there may be fixed costs attributed directly to the department that should not be considered controllable. Rents on pieces of equipment for example, may not be under the departmental manager's control. There may also be indirect costs, especially costs that are variable, that the department manager can control. For example, employee benefits may legitimately be the department manager's responsibility.

Third, in some situations, controllable costs may be defined as only those costs that are direct/variable. This limits costs that are controllable by the department manager to their lowest level. However, it excludes what could be a relatively large amount of cost influenced by the department manager. Failure to include the latter cost in the manager's control sphere may weaken management control.

Future Costs

Decision making involves selection among alternatives; it is a forward-looking process. Actual historical cost may be useful as a basis for projecting future costs, but it should not be used without adjustment unless it can be assumed that future conditions will be identical to past conditions.

A variety of concepts and definitions have been used in current discussion of costs for decision making purposes. The following four types of costs appear to be basic to the process of selecting among alternative decisions.

1. avoidable costs
2. sunk costs
3. incremental costs
4. opportunity costs

Avoidable Costs

Avoidable costs will be affected by the decision under consideration. Specifically, they are costs that can be eliminated or saved if an activity is discontinued; they will continue only if the activity is left unchanged. For example, if a hospital were considering curtailing its volume by 50 percent in response to cost-containment pressures, what would it save? The answer is those costs that are avoidable. In most situations, multiplication of current, average, and total cost per unit of output (patient days or admissions) by the projected change in output would overstate avoidable costs; a considerable proportion of the cost may be classified as sunk.

Sunk Costs

Sunk costs are unaffected by the decision under consideration. In the example above, large portions of cost—depreciation, administrative salaries, insurance and others—are sunk or not avoidable in the proposed 50 percent reduction in volume.

The distinction between fixed and variable costs, on the one hand, and sunk and avoidable costs, on the other, is not perfect. Many costs classified as fixed may also be thought of as sunk, but some are not. For example, malpractice insurance premiums may be generally considered fixed cost, given an expected normal level of activity. However, if the institution is considering a drastic reduction in volume, malpractice premiums may not be entirely fixed.

Incremental Costs

Incremental costs are the changes in total cost resulting from various alternative courses of action. Avoidable costs may be thought of as a subset of incremental costs, but most people regard avoidable costs as the result of a comparison of cost in which one alternative is reduction in volume or discontinuation of some activity. Incremental costs usually arise in situations in which an alternative is an expansion of volume or the initiation of a new activity. For decisions involving only modest changes in output, incremental costs and variable costs may be used interchangeably. In most situations, however, incremental costs are more comprehensive. A decision to construct a surgi-center adjacent to a hospital would involve fixed and variable costs. Depreciation on the facility would be a fixed cost but it would be incremental to the decision to construct the surgi-center.

Opportunity Costs

Opportunity cost is the value foregone by using a resource in a particular way instead of in its next best alternative way. Assume that a nursing home is considering expanding its facility and would use land acquired 20 years ago. If the land had a historical cost of $1 million but a present market value of $10 million, what is the opportunity cost of the land? Practically everyone would agree that if sale of the land constituted the next best alternative, the opportunity cost would be $10 million, not $1 million. Alternatively, a hospital might consider converting part of its acute care facility into a skilled nursing facility because of a reduction in demand or obsolescence in the facility. The question arises, what is the value, or what would be the cost of the facility, to the skilled nursing facility operation? If there is no way that the facility can be renovated or if the facility is not needed for the provision of acute care, its opportunity cost may be zero. This could contrast sharply to the recorded historical cost of the facility.

COST MEASUREMENT

In this section, we examine the methods of cost measurement for two cost categories: (1) direct and indirect full cost, and (2) variable and fixed cost. Both of these cost categories are useful in financial decisions, but the cost accounting system does not directly provide estimates for them.

Direct and Indirect Full Cost

In most cost accounting systems, costs are classified by department or responsibility center or by the object of expenditure. When costs are classified primarily along departmental lines, individual cost items are charged to the departments to which they are traceable. When costs are classified by object of expenditure, they may be identified as relating to supplies, salaries, rent, insurance, or some other category.

Departments in a health care facility can be classified generally as direct or indirect departments, depending on whether they provide services directly to the patient or not. Sometimes the terms *revenue* and *nonrevenue* are substituted for direct and indirect. In the hospital industry, the following breakdown is used in general-purpose financial statements.

Operating Expense Area	Type of Department
Nursing services area	Direct/revenue
Other professional services	Direct/revenue
General services	Indirect/nonrevenue
Fiscal services	Indirect/nonrevenue
Administrative services	Indirect/nonrevenue

Whatever the nomenclature used to describe the classification of departments, cost allocation is a fundamental need. The costs of the indirect, nonrevenue departments need to be allocated to the direct revenue departments for many decision-making purposes. For example, some payers reimburse on the basis of the full costs of direct departments and are interested in the cost of indirect departments only insofar as it affects the calculation of the direct departments' full costs. Pricing decisions need to be based on full costs, not just direct costs, if the costs of the indirect departments are to be covered equitably.

Equity is a key concept in allocating indirect department costs to direct departments. Ideally, the allocation should reflect as nearly as possible the actual cost incurred by the indirect department to provide services for a direct department. Department managers who receive cost reports showing indirect allocations are vitally interested in this equity principle, and for good reason. Even if indirect costs are not regarded as controllable by the department manager, the allocation of costs to a given direct department can have an important effect on a variety of management decisions. Pricing, expansion or contraction of a department, the purchase of new equipment, and the salaries of departmental managers are all affected by the allocation of indirect costs.

Costs of indirect departments are in most cases not traceable to direct departments. If they were, they could be reassigned. In such cases, they must

Table 8–2 Cost Allocation Example

Department	Direct Costs	Pounds of Laundry Used	Square Feet	Hours of Housekeeping Used
Laundry/Linen	$ 15,000	$ —	$ 50,000	$ 150
Housekeeping	30,000	5,000	—	—
Radiology	135,000	5,000	10,000	900
Nursing	270,000	90,000	140,000	1,950
Totals	$450,000	$100,000	$200,000	$3,000

be allocated to the direct departments in some systematic and rational manner. In general, two allocation decisions must be made: (1) selection of the allocation basis and (2) selection of the method of cost apportionment.

Table 8–2 provides sample data for a cost allocation. In this example, there are four departments: two are indirect—laundry/linen and housekeeping—and two are direct—radiology and nursing. Pounds of laundry is the only allocation basis under consideration for the laundry and linen department. The housekeeping department can use one of two allocation bases, either square feet of area served or hours of service actually worked.

In general, there are only three acceptable methods of cost allocation:

1. step-down
2. double-distribution
3. simultaneous-equations

Most health care facilities still use the step-down method of cost allocation. In this method, the indirect department that receives the least amount of service from other indirect departments and provides the most service to other departments allocates its cost first. A similar analysis follows to determine the order of cost allocation for each of the remaining indirect departments. This determination can be subjective to allow some flexibility, as we shall see shortly.

In the step-down allocation process illustrated below, laundry/linen allocates its cost first. Then, housekeeping allocates its direct cost, plus the allocated cost of laundry and linen, to the direct departments of radiology and nursing, based on the ratio of services provided to those departments. The allocation proportions are given in parentheses.

	Direct Costs	Laundry/Linen	Housekeeping	Total
Laundry/Linen	$ 15,000	$15,000		
Housekeeping	30,000	750 (.05)	$30,750	
Radiology	135,000	750 (.05)	9,711 (.3158)	$145,461
Nursing	270,000	13,500 (.90)	21,039 (.6842)	304,539
Totals	$450,000	$15,000	$30,750	$450,000

The order of departmental allocation can be an important variable in a step-down method of cost allocation. Shown below is an alternative step-down cost allocation in which housekeeping allocates its cost first and precedes laundry/linen.

	Direct Costs	Housekeeping	Laundry/Linen	Total
Housekeeping	$ 30,000	$30,000		
Laundry/Linen	15,000	1,500 (.05)	$16,500	
Radiology	135,000	9,000 (.30)	868 (.053)	$144,868
Nursing	270,000	19,500 (.65)	15,632 (.947)	305,132
Totals	$450,000	$30,000	$16,500	$450,000

The double-distribution method of cost allocation is just a refinement of the step-down method. Instead of closing the individual department after allocating its costs, it is kept open and receives the costs of other indirect departments. After one complete allocation sequence, the former departments are then closed, using the normal step-down method. The simultaneous-equations method of cost allocation is used in an attempt to be exact about the cost allocation amounts. A system of equations is established and mathematically correct allocations are computed. In the above example, if simultaneous equations had been used, the cost of radiology would be $145,075 and the cost of nursing would be $304,925.

Finally, it should be noted that using a different allocation base can create differences in cost allocation. For example, the use of square footage for housekeeping, instead of hours served, produces the following pattern of cost allocation when housekeeping allocates its cost first, using the step-down method:

	Direct Cost	Housekeeping	Laundry/Linen	Total
Housekeeping	$ 30,000	$30,000		
Laundry/Linen	15,000	7,500 (.25)	$22,500	
Radiology	135,000	1,500 (.05)	1,125 (.05)	$137,625
Nursing	270,000	21,000 (.70)	21,375 (.95)	312,375
Totals	$450,000	$30,000	$22,500	$450,000

The important point in this discussion is that full cost is not as objective and exact a figure as one might normally think. Indirect costs can be allocated in a variety of ways that can create significant differences in full costs for given departments. This flexibility should be remembered when examining and interpreting full-cost data.

Variable and Fixed Cost

A very important and widely used cost concept is variability with respect to output. It is involved in determining for decision-making purposes such costs as avoidable, sunk, incremental, and controllable. However, accounting records do not directly yield this type of cost information. Instead, the costs are classified by department and by object of expenditure. Thus, in order to develop estimates of variable and fixed costs, the relevant data must be analyzed in some way.

Our discussion of cost concepts classified by variability with respect to output indicated that a semivariable cost pattern may be a good representation of many types of costs. A semivariable cost function is one that has both a fixed and variable element in it. A semivariable cost function often results when various types of costs are aggregated together.

Estimating Methods

Estimation of a semivariable cost function requires separation of the cost into variable and fixed components. A variety of methods, varying in complexity and accuracy, may be used. Three of the simplest methods are (1) visual-fit, (2) high-low, and (3) semi-averages.

To illustrate each of these methods, assume that we are trying to determine the labor cost function for the radiology department and we have the following six biweekly payroll data points:

Pay Period	Number of Films	Hours Worked
1	300	180 (low)
2	240	140 (low)
3	400	230 (high)
4	340	190 (high)
5	180	110 (lowest)
6	600	320 (highest)

In the visual-fit method of cost estimation, the above individual data points are plotted on graph paper. A straight line is then drawn through the points

Figure 8–7 Visual Fitting of Radiology Data

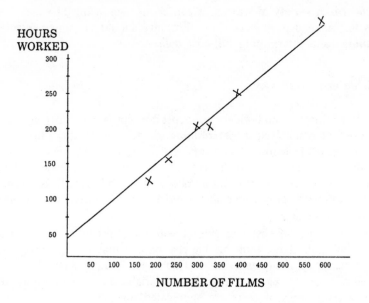

to provide the best fit. Visual fitting of data is a good first step in any method of cost estimation. Figure 8–7 shows a visual fitting of the above radiology data.

The high-low method is a simple technique that can be used to estimate the variable and fixed-cost coefficients of a semivariable cost function. The variable cost parameter is solved first. It equals the change in cost from the highest to the lowest data point, divided by the change in output. In the above radiology example, the variable *hours worked* would be calculated as follows:

$$\frac{\text{Variable labor hours}}{\text{Film}} = \frac{320 - 110}{600 - 180} = \frac{210}{420} = .50$$

The fixed-cost parameter may then be solved by subtracting the estimated variable cost (determined by multiplying the variable cost parameter estimate by output at the high level) from total cost. In our radiology example, fixed cost would equal

Fixed labor hours/

Biweekly pay period $= 320 - (.50 \times 600) = 320 - 300 = 20$

Alternatively, it is possible to plot the high and low points and then draw a straight line through them.

The semi-averages method is very similar to the high-low method in terms of its mathematical solution. To derive the estimate of variable cost, the difference between the mean of the high-cost points and the mean of the low-cost points is divided by the change in output from the mean of the high-cost points to the mean of the low-cost points. In the radiology example, variable cost would be calculated as follows:

$$\text{Variable Labor Hours/Film} = \frac{\dfrac{320 + 230 + 190}{3} - \dfrac{180 + 140 + 110}{3}}{\dfrac{600 + 400 + 340}{3} - \dfrac{300 + 240 + 180}{3}} = \frac{246.67 - 143.33}{446.67 - 240.00} = .50$$

Fixed cost is solved in a manner identical to that used in the high-low method. In the radiology example, fixed cost would equal

Fixed labor hours/
Biweekly pay period $= 246.67 - (.50 \times 446.67) = 23.34$

These three methods of estimating variable and fixed cost are highly simplistic. They are useful only in limited ways to provide a basis for further discussing and analyzing what the true cost behavioral pattern might be. However, in most situations a limited attempt, based on simplistic methods, to discover the underlying fixed/variable cost patterns, is better than no effort.

Data Checks

When any of the above methods are used, several data checks should be performed. First, the cost data being used to estimate the cost behavior pattern should be stated in a common dollar. If the wages paid for employees have changed dramatically from one year to the next, the use of unadjusted wage and salary data from the two years can create measurement problems. In our radiology example, we used a physical quantity measure of cost, namely, hours worked. A physical measure of cost should be used whenever possible.

Second, cost and output data should be matched; the figures for reported cost should relate to the activity of the period. In most situations, accounting records provide this type of relationship, based on the accrual principle of accounting. However, in some situations this may not happen; supply costs may be charged to a department when the items are purchased, not when they are used.

Third, the period of time during which a cost function is being estimated should be one of a stable technology and case mix. If the technology under consideration has changed dramatically during that period, there will be measurement problems.

BREAK-EVEN ANALYSIS

Certain techniques can be applied in analyzing the relationship between cost, volume, and profit. These techniques rely on categorizing costs as fixed and variable. They can serve as powerful management decision aids and may be valuable in a wide range of decisions. An understanding of these techniques is crucial for decision makers whose choices affect the financial results of health care facilities.

Profit in a health care facility is influenced by various factors, including:

- rates
- volume
- variable cost
- fixed cost
- payer mix
- bad debts

The primary value of break-even analysis, or, as it is sometimes called, cost-volume-profit analysis, is its ability to quantify the relationships between the above factors and profit.

Traditional Applications

Break-even analysis has been used in industry for decades with a high degree of satisfaction. Its name comes from the solution to an equation that sets profit equal to zero and revenue equal to costs. To illustrate, assume that a hospital has the following financial information:

Variable cost per case	$1,000.00
Fixed cost per period	$100,000.00
Rate per case	$2,400.00

The break-even volume may be solved by dividing fixed costs by the contribution margin, which is the difference between rate and variable cost:

$$\text{Break-even volume in units} = \frac{\text{Fixed Cost}}{\text{Rate} - \text{Variable cost}}$$

Thus, in our hospital example, break-even volume would be

$$\text{Break-even volume in units} = \frac{\$100,000}{\$2,400 - \$1,000} = 71.4 \text{ Cases}$$

If volume exceeds 72 cases, the hospital will make a profit; but if volume goes below 71 cases it will incur a loss. Sometimes, a revenue-and-cost relationship is put into graphic form to illustrate profit at various levels. Such a presentation is referred to as a break-even chart. For our hospital example, a break-even chart is shown in Figure 8–8.

In many cases, some targeted level of net income or profit is desired. The break-even model is easily adapted to this purpose; the new break-even point would become

$$\text{Break-even volume in units} = \frac{\text{Fixed cost} + \text{Targeted net income}}{\text{Rate} - \text{Variable cost}}$$

In our example, assuming that a desired profit of $6,000 were required, the new break-even point would be

$$\text{Break-even volume in units} = \frac{\$100,000 + \$6,000}{\$1,400} = 75.7 \text{ Cases}$$

Figure 8–8 Break-Even Chart

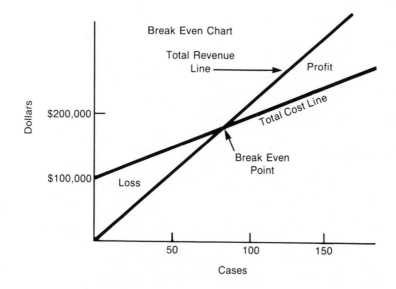

Multiple-Payer Model

Although break-even analysis is a powerful management tool, it cannot be employed in the health care industry without adaptation. The major revision required relates to the revenue function. The preceding discussion of break-even analysis assumed that there was only one payer or purchaser of services. That payer was assumed to pay a fixed price per unit of product. However, this situation does not exist in the health care industry, where there may be three or more major categories of payers. For our purposes, we will assume that there are three categories of payers:

1. cost payers (paying average cost of services provided)
2. fixed-price payers (paying an established fee per unit of service, for example, a fixed price per DRG)
3. charge payers (paying on the basis of internally set prices)

The break-even formula in these three payer situations can be generalized as follows:

$$\text{Break-even volume in units} = \frac{(1 - CO)\ F + NI}{CHxP_I + FPxP_E - (1 - CO)V}$$

This formula may look complex at first glance, but it is really very similar to the previous one-payer break-even formula. In fact, the above equation can be used in the one-payer situation and provides an identical result. To aid in our understanding of the formula, we should first define the individual variables:

V = Variable cost per unit of output
F = Fixed cost per period
NI = Targeted net income
P_I = Internally set price that is paid by charge payers
P_E = Externally set price paid by fixed-price payers
CO = Proportion of cost payers
CH = Proportion of charge payers
FP = Proportion of fixed-price payers

Let us now examine each term in the equation:

- $(1 - CO)\ F$—This term represents the proportion of fixed cost (F) that is not paid by cost payers (CO). Cost payers are assumed to pay their proportionate share of fixed costs. This leaves the residual portion $(1 - CO)$ unpaid; it is included in the numerator as a financial requirement that must be covered before break-even takes place. If there were no cost payers, $(1 - CO)$ would be 1, and all of the fixed costs would be included. This is the case in traditional break-even analysis.

- NI—This term, targeted net income, is included as a financial requirement as in the traditional break-even formula. NI is not reduced by the
cost payer portion because it is assumed that cost payers are not
contributing toward meeting the net income requirement. Cost payers
pay cost, nothing less and nothing more.

- $CHxP_I$—This term represents the weighted price paid by charge payers.
When added to the next term ($FPxP_E$), we have a measure of the price
paid by the two price-paying categories of customers—charge payers and
fixed-price payers. It should be emphasized that P_I represents the price
received, not the charge made. For example, if 10 percent of the patients
paid established charges of $2,400 per case and 20 percent paid 90
percent of established charges of $2,400 per case, the following values
would result:

CH = .10 + .20 = .30
P_I = (1.0 × $2,400) × 1/3 + (.90 × $2,400) × 2/3 = $2,240

- $FPxP_E$—This term represents the weighted price paid by fixed price
payers. The addition of this term to $CHxP_I$ yields a measure of the price
received for price-paying patients. The summation of the two terms can
be compared to the rate term used in the traditional break-even formula.
Again, there may be circumstances in which a subweighting may be
necessary. For example, assume that Medicare pays $2,000 per case and
that 40 percent of the cases are Medicare. Also assume that 10 percent of
the cases are from an HMO that pays $2,200 per case. The following
values would result:

FP = .40 + .10 = .50
P_E = .8 × $2,000 + .2 × $2,200 = $2,040

- (1 − CO)V—This term represents the net variable cost that remains after
reflecting the proportion paid by cost payers. Cost payers pay their share
of both fixed and variable cost. If there were no cost payers, the entire
value of the variable cost per unit would be subtracted to yield the
contribution margin per unit.

To see that the traditional break-even formula is actually derived from our
more general three-payer model, let us compute the break-even point using
the data from the case example developed in our discussion of traditional
break-even analysis:

$$\text{Break-even volume in units} = \frac{(1-0) \times \$100,000 + \$6,000}{1.0 \times \$2,400 + 0 \times \$0 - (1-0) \times \$1,000} = 75.7 \text{ cases}$$

Now, having tested the accuracy of the three-payer break-even formula in a one-payer situation, let us expand out initial case example to a more realistic multiple-payer situation. The following data are assumed:

Payer Proportion	Payment Method
.20	pay average cost
.40	pay $2,000 per case (fixed price payer)
.10	pay $2,200 per case (fixed price payer)
.10	pay 100% of charges, $2,400 per case
.20	pay 90% of charges, $2,160 per case

Also assume that the variable cost is $1,000 per case and fixed costs are $100,000 per period. In addition the firm needs a profit of $6,000 to meet other financial requirements. The use of these data in our break-down model would produce the following result:

$$\text{Break-even volume in cases} = \frac{(.8 \times \$100{,}000) + \$6{,}000}{(.3 \times \$2{,}240) + (.5 \times \$2{,}040) - (.8 \times \$1{,}000)}$$

$$= \frac{\$86{,}000}{\$892} = 96.413$$

To demonstrate the accuracy of the break-even formula, we can derive the following income statement for our case example, assuming 96.4 cases as the break-even volume:

Patient revenue	
.20 × 96.4 × $2,037.34[a]	$ 39,279.92
.40 × 96.4 × $2,000.00	77,120.00
.10 × 96.4 × $2,200.00	21,208.00
.10 × 96.4 × $2,400.00	23,136.00
.20 × 96.4 × $2,160.00	41,644.80
Net patient revenue	$202,388.72
Fixed cost	100,000.00
Variable cost (96.4 × $1,000)	96,400.00
Net income	$ 5,988.72

[a] Average cost × ($100,000 + $96,400)/96.4 × $2,037.34

This income statement demonstrates that, at a volume of 96.4 patients, the firm's net income would be $5,988.72. This value does not exactly match the targeted net income level of $6,000.00 because of a small rounding error; the actual break-even volume was 96.413, not 96.4.

Special Applications

The break-even formula has many applications other than that of computing break-even points. Two specific applications are in (1) the computation of marginal profit of volume changes and (2) rate-setting analysis.

Computation of Marginal Profit of Volume Changes

In most business situations, executives are very concerned about the impact of volume changes upon operating profitability. At the beginning of a budget period, management may not be sure what its actual volumes will be, but it still needs to know how sensitive profit will be to possible swings in volume. If the payer mix is expected to remain constant, the following simple formula can be used to calculate the marginal changes in profit associated with volume swings:

Change in profit = Change in units $\times$ Profitability index
where:
Profitability index = CH $(P_I - V)$ + FP $(P_E - V)$

The profitability index remains constant and is simply multiplied by projected volume change to determine the profit change. Using our earlier case example, the profitability index would be

Profitability index = .3($2,240 - $1,000) + .5($2,040 - $1,000) = $892

The value for the profitability index is really the weighted contribution margin per unit of output. This fact is easily seen by comparing the value calculated above with that from our three-payer break-even example. The values are the same, $892 in each case. This means that, for every one unit change in output, the profit increases by $892. An increase of one unit will raise profit by $892, and a decrease of one unit will lower profit by $892. A useful question to raise at this point is, How large a reduction in volume can the firm experience before its profit falls to $2,000? Using the preceding formula, the answer would be:

Change in profit   = Volume change $\times$ Profitability index
($6,000 - $2,000)   = Volume change $\times$ $892
Volume change   = 4.48 cases

If volume falls by 4.48 cases, the firm's profit will fall to $2,000. Further analysis could be used to portray other scenarios or to answer other what-if type questions. In each case, the resulting data could be displayed in a table or graph.

Rate-Setting Analysis

Rate setting is an extremely important activity for most health care organizations. Usually the objective is not profit maximization but rather fulfillment of financial requirements. In general, pricing services can be stated in the following conceptual terms:

Price = Average cost + Profit requirement + Loss on fixed-price patients

If Q represents total budgeted volume in units, we can use our earlier break-even model to develop the following pricing formula:

$$P_I = AC + \frac{NI}{CHxQ} + \frac{(AC - P_E) \times FP \times Q}{CHxQ}$$

where:

$$AC = \text{Average cost per unit} = \frac{F}{Q} + V$$

Again, it is useful to examine the individual terms in order to understand their conceptual relationships:

- AC—This term represents the average cost per unit. Average cost is the basis on which the firm marks up to establish a price that can meet its financial requirements.

- NI/(CHxQ)—This term divides the target net income (NI) by the number of charge paying units (CHxQ). This payment source generates the firm's profit. Internally set prices will not affect the amount of payment received from cost payers or fixed price payers.

- $(AC-P_E) \times (FPxQ)/(CHxQ)$—This term is complex but has a simple interpretation. The difference between average cost (AC) and the fixed price (P_E) represents an additional requirement that must be covered by the firm's charge paying units. This difference per unit is then multiplied by total fixed-price payer units (FPxQ) to generate the total loss resulting from selling services to fixed price payers. Dividing by the number of charge payers (CHxQ) translates this loss into an additional pricing increment that must be recovered from the charge payers. It is important to note that, if the fixed price paid by fixed price payers exceeds average cost, this term will be negative. Prices to the charge payers could then be reduced because the fixed price payers would be making a positive contribution to the firm's profit requirement.

To test the validity of the pricing formula, let us apply it to the data in our earlier three-payer break-even example. Assume that the volume is 96.4 cases:

$$P_I = \$2,037.34 + \frac{\$6,000}{.3 \times 96.4} + \frac{(\$2,037.34 - 2,040) \times .5 \times 96.4}{.3 \times 96.4}$$

$$= \$2,037.34 + \$207.47 - 4.43 = \$2,240.38$$

The required price as determined above, $2,240.38, is approximately equal to the price established for charge payers, $2,240. Again, a small discrepancy exists because of rounding errors.

It should be noted that $2,240 is not the actual charge or price set per case. The actual posted charge is $2,400. P_I represents the net amount actually received. Because the firm had one category of payers who paid 90 percent of charges, the effective price realized was only $2,240. When using this pricing formula to define hospital charges, the defined price must be increased to reflect write-offs due to discounts, bad debts, or charity care. The following general formula represents the markup requirement:

$$\text{Price} = P_I/(1 - \text{write-off proportion})$$

The write-off proportion is not based upon total revenue; it is based only on the revenue from charge payers. For example, in our case example, the charge payers represented 30 percent of total cases. Of that 30 percent, 10 percent paid 100 percent of charges and 20 percent paid 90 percent of charges. The write-off percentage is thus:

$$(1/3) \times (1.0 - 1.0) + (2/3) \times (1.0 - .9) = .0667$$

Using this value to mark up the required net price of $2,240 would yield $2,400 ($2,240/[1 - .0667] = $2,400), which is the firm's established charge.

An important issue for many health care organizations concerns the maximization of profit per dollar of rate increase. In a number of states and regions, rate regulations impose restraints upon a firm's ability to raise its rates. In addition, boards may wish to minimize rate increases in any given budgetary cycle.

The percentage of any price increase that will be realized as profit can be expressed as follows:

% Price increase realized as profit = (% Charge payers) $\times$ (1 - Write-off proportion)

Let us assume that a nursing home is interested in learning what effect a $5 increase in its per diem would have on its profitability. Its present payer mix and write-off proportions are:

Payer Percentage	Payer Mode	Write-off Proportion
10%	Medicare — pays cost	.00
50%	Private payer — pays charges	.10
40%	Medicaid — pays fixed charge per diem	.00

Thus, a $5.00 per diem increase would generate a 45 percent increase in profit, or $2.25 per day:

$$50\% \times (1 - .10) = 45\%$$

SUMMARY

Cost accounting systems can be designed to provide different measures of cost for different decision-making purposes. This is a desirable characteristic, not an exercise in numbers playing. To understand what measure of cost is needed for a specific purpose, the decision maker must have some knowledge of the variety of alternative concepts of cost. The terms covered in this chapter should be useful in helping decision makers define their needs more precisely.

Break-even analysis presents management with a set of simple analytical tools to provide information about the effects of costs, volume, and prices upon profitability. In this chapter, we examined the application of several break-even models for health care providers with three categories of payers. Utilization of these models should help analysts understand the conceptual framework for improving profitability in their health care organization.

ASSIGNMENTS

1. What are the two major categories of decisions that utilize cost information?

2. What does it mean to say that a cost is direct?

3. Define the terms *variable costs* and *fixed costs*. Give some examples of each.

4. Is it true that indirect costs should never be included in the determination of controllable costs?

5. A hospital is considering using a vacant wing to set up a skilled nursing facility. What is the cost of the space?

6. A free-standing ambulatory care center averages $60 in charges per patient. Variable costs are approximately $10 per patient, and fixed costs are about $1.2 million per year. Using this data, how many patients must be seen each day, assuming a 365-day operation, to reach the break-even point?

Table 8–3 Budgeted Clinical Service Volumes for Harding Hospital

	Medicare	Medicaid	Charge	Total
Cardiology				
DRG 127—Heart failure	20	5	15	40
DRG 140—Angina	15	2	3	20
Pulmonary				
DRG 88—Chronic obstruction	20	2	8	30
Surgery				
DRG 115—Pacemaker implant	15	3	12	30
DRG 210—Major joint	20	3	17	40

7. Howard Hamilton, administrator of Harding Hospital, is assessing the adequacy of the hospital's rate structure for fiscal year 1985. Harding has three primary clinical service lines with abbreviated budgeted volumes as indicated in Table 8–3.

   The hospital's projected gross revenue, using last year's prices and this year's projected volume, is depicted in Table 8–4.

   Harding's budgeted costs by department are shown in Table 8–5.

   Harding Hospital's Medicaid patients are reimbursed on a ratio of charges-to-charges formula, applied departmentally. Assume that indirect costs are allocated proportionately to nursing, surgery, and ancillary. Medicare patients use the following rates for payment:

DRG No.	Price
127	$2,520
140	1,800
88	2,500
115	9,360
210	5,520

   Charge payers have an average 10 percent write-off.

   Given the above background and data:

   a. Project Harding Hospital's operating income at last year's prices.

   b. Develop a rate increase proposal that will generate $50,000 of income. Prices must exceed cost in each area. Minimize the total value of the revenue increase above the present $694,000.

8. Your hospital's board of trustees has just determined that the maximum revenue increase it will permit next year is five percent. It has also specified maximum and minimum rate increases by department. Data for the hospital's five departments are:

Table 8–4 Projected Gross Revenue for Harding Hospital

	Nursing ($300/PD)	Surgery ($1,000/Hr.)	Ancillary ($20/Unit)	Total
DRG 127				
Medicare	$ 48,000	$ 0	$ 6,000	$ 54,000
Medicaid	10,500	0	1,500	12,000
Other	31,500	0	4,500	36,000
DRG 140				
Medicare	27,000	0	3,000	30,000
Medicaid	3,000	0	400	3,400
Other	4,500	0	600	5,100
DRG 88				
Medicare	42,000	0	8,000	50,000
Medicaid	4,200	0	800	5,000
Other	16,800	0	3,200	20,000
DRG 115				
Medicare	67,500	67,500	6,000	141,000
Medicaid	10,800	13,500	1,200	25,500
Other	43,200	54,000	4,800	102,000
DRG 210				
Medicare	108,000	10,000	2,000	120,000
Medicaid	11,700	1,500	300	13,500
Other	66,300	8,500	1,700	76,500
	$495,000	$155,000	$44,000	$694,000

Table 8–5 Budgeted Costs for Harding Hospital, by Department

	Activity Unit	Projected Volume	Projected Cost	Variable Cost/Unit	Fixed Cost
Nursing	Patient day	1,650	$325,000	$100	$160,000
Surgery	Hours	155	100,000	300	53,500
Ancillary	Unit	2,200	30,000	6	16,800
Dietary and housekeeping	Patient day	1,650	150,000	50	67,500
Business office	Cases	160	20,000	60	10,400
Overhead	None	—	80,000	0	80,000
			$705,000		$388,200

	Current Charges	Budgeted Cost	Payer Composition%			Bad Debt	Physi-cian Fee	Rate Change%	
			Cost	Fixed Price	Charge			Min.	Max.
Nursing	$2,000	$2,200	30	30%	40%	10%	0%	5	20%
Emergency room	200	190	70	10	20	10	0	0	10
Operating room	300	330	35	40	25	20	0	10	25
Laboratory	1,000	750	50	30	20	15	10	−10	20
Anesthesiology	360	300	40	30	30	10	30	0	10
	$3,860	$3,770							

Given the above information, develop a rate-change plan that will maximize the hospital's net income yet still adhere to the board's guidelines.

9. Develop an estimate of fixed and variable costs for labor expenses, based on the following data. Develop your estimates using the high-low and the semi-averages methods:

Period	Output in Units	Hours Worked
1	16,156	3,525
2	19,160	4,151
3	17,846	3,829
4	20,238	4,454
5	21,198	4,657
6	14,640	3,406

10. An interdepartmental service structure and its direct costs are as follows:

Department	Direct Costs	% of Service Consumed by					
		S_1	S_2	S_3	R_1	R_2	R_3
Service Center 1	$10,000	—	10	10	40	20	20
Service Center 2	12,000	10	—	10	20	40	20
Service Center 3	10,000	10	10	—	20	20	40
Revenue Center 1	30,000						
Revenue Center 2	25,000						
Revenue Center 3	50,000						

Compute the total costs, direct and allocated, for each of the three revenue centers, using the direct and step-down methods of cost apportionment.

SOLUTIONS AND ANSWERS

1. The two major categories of decisions that use cost data are planning and control. Planning decisions usually require costs that are accumulated by program or product line, whereas control decisions usually require costs that are accumulated by responsibility centers or departments.

2. A direct cost is one that can be traced or associated with a specific cost objective, usually related to a department or responsibility center.

3. A variable cost is one that changes proportionately with volume. Common examples are materials and supplies. A fixed cost does not change with volume but remains constant. Common examples are rent, depreciation, and interest. Fixed costs are usually constant only for some "relevant range" of volume. For example, depreciation will probably increase if a facility experiences volume increases that exceed existing capacity.

4. It is not invariably true that indirect costs should never be included in the determination of controllable costs. There are some costs that may be classified as indirect but could be controlled by a manager. For example, housekeeping costs may be classified as an indirect cost to the physical therapy department. However, the actual amount of housekeeping services required by the physical therapy department may be affected by the actions of the physical therapy department manager.

5. The opportunity cost of the space—that is, its value in the next best alternative use—should be measured. Possible alternative uses might be use as physician offices or as sleeping accommodations for patient families.

6. The number of patients that must be seen is 65.75 patients per day, based on the following calculation:

$$\text{Annual break-even volume} = \frac{1,200,000}{\$50} = 24,000 \text{ patient per year}$$

$$\text{Daily Break-even volume} = \frac{24,000}{365} = 65.75 \text{ patient per day}$$

7. a. The projection of Harding Hospital's operating income at last year's prices is developed in the following financial statements:

• Cost allocation

	Initial	Overhead	Business Office	Dietary and Housekeeping	Total
Overhead	$ 80,000	—	—	—	—
Business office	20,000	—	—	—	—
Dietary and housekeeping	150,000	—	—	—	—
Ancillary	30,000	5,275	1,319	9,893	46,487
Surgery	100,000	17,582	4,396	32,970	154,948
Nursing	325,000	57,143	14,285	107,137	503,565
	$705,000	$80,000	$20,000	$150,000	$705,000

● Medicaid net patient revenue

	Medicaid Revenue	Medicaid Proportion (Medicaid Revenue/ Total Revenue)	Medicaid Cost Share (Medicaid Proportion × Total Cost)
Nursing	$40,200	.08121	$40,896
Surgery	15,000	.09677	14,995
Ancillary	4,200	.09545	4,437
	$59,400		$60,328

● Charge payer net patient revenue

	Collected revenue Charge revenue	.9 × Charge Revenue
Nursing	$162,300	$146,070
Surgery	62,500	56,250
Ancillary	14,800	13,320
		$215,640

● Medicare net patient revenue

DRG #	Price	Volume	Revenue
127	$2,520	20	$ 50,400
140	1,800	15	27,000
88	2,500	20	50,000
115	9,360	15	140,400
210	5,520	20	110,400
			$378,200

● Projected income

Gross patient revenue	$694,000
Less deductions	39,832
Net patient revenue	654,168
Less cost	705,000
Loss	($ 50,832)

b. The rate increase proposal could be developed as shown in the following calculations:

● Percentage of price realized as profit

Nursing $= (162,300/495,000) \times (1-.10) = .29509 = 29.509\%$
Surgery $= (62,500/155,000) \times (1-.10) = .362903 = 36.2903\%$
Ancillary $= (14,800/44,000) \times (1-.10) = .30273 = 30.273\%$

- Initial rate increases/Set rate equal costs

	Cost	Present Revenue	Increase	New Rate Per Unit
Nursing	$503,565	$495,000	$ 8,565	$ 305.19
Surgery	154,948	155,000	0	$1000.00
Ancillary	46,487	44,000	2,487	21.13
	$705,000	$694,000	$11,052	

- Required profit increment

$$\text{Increase} = 50,832 + 50,000 = \$100,832$$

- Profit generated from initial rate increase

Nursing	$8,565 × .29509 = $2,527
Ancillary	2,487 × .30273 = 753
	$3,280

- Remaining profit required

$$
\begin{array}{r}
\$100,832 \\
- \ 3,280 \\
\hline
\$ \ 97,552
\end{array}
$$

- Price Strategy

  Load into Surgery because surgery has the highest profit potential:

.362903 × Price increase	= $97,552
Price increase	= $268,809 or $1,734 per hour
New surgery price	= $2,734 per hour

- Charge revenue

$$\text{Nursing} \quad \$305.19 \times \frac{162,300}{300} \times .9 = \$148,597$$

$$\text{Surgery} \quad \$2,734 \times \frac{62,500}{1,000} \times .9 = \$153,788$$

$$\text{Ancillary} \ \$21.13 \times \frac{14,800}{20} \times .9 = \underline{14,073}$$
$$\$316,458$$

- Projected income with new price structure

Net Medicaid revenue	$ 60,328
Net Medicare revenue	378,200
Net charge revenue	316,458
Net patient revenue	754,986
Less cost	705,000
Net operating income	$ 49,986

8. The rate change plan could be developed in the following manner:

- Percentage of price realized as profit

Department	% Price Realized As Profit
Nursing	40.0% × .9 = 36.0%
Emergency room	20.0% × .9 = 18.0%
Operating room	25.0% × .8 = 20.0%
Laboratory	(20.0% − 10%) × .85 = 8.5%
Anesthesiology	(30% − 30%) × .9 = 0%

- Results of loading as much of the rate increase as possible into nursing

Department	Current Charges	Required Minimum	Additional Charge	Final Charges
Nursing	$2,000	$100	163	$2,263
Emergency room	200	0	0	200
Operating room	300	30	0	330
Laboratory	1,000	−100	0	900
Anesthesiology	360	0	0	360
	$3,860	$ 30	$163	$4,053

9. The following estimates of fixed and variable costs for labor expenses could be developed:

	Variable Hours Per Unit	Fixed Hours
High-low method	.1908	613
Semi-averages method	.2093	193

10. The total costs for the three revenue centers would be as follows:

	Cost Apportionment Method	
	Direct	Step-Down
Revenue Center 1	$ 40,500	$ 40,000
Revenue Center 2	36,000	35,889
Revenue Center 3	60,500	61,111
	$137,000	$137,000

Chapter 9

Product Costing

Since the implementation of the prospective payment system, there has been a rapidly growing interest in cost accounting. The increased interest in developing sophisticated cost accounting systems is not limited to the hospital industry; it has infected all health care industry sectors. Most, if not all, of this interest is due to the establishment of fixed prices for services and to the increasing economic competition among health care providers.

A variety of terms have been used to describe the new methodology in cost accounting. Some refer to it as costing by DRGs, others call it standard costing, and still others refer to it as costing by product line or as product costing. For the purposes of this chapter, we shall use the term *product costing*. A product or product line is more generic, compared with the terms used in the other definitions. Also the concept of product costing can be related to costing in other industries; most of the principles of product costing have been examined and debated for many years in the manufacturing sector. Thus, we do not have to reinvent the wheel in order to develop costing principles for the health care industry.

RELATIONSHIP TO PLANNING, BUDGETING, AND CONTROL

Cost information is of value only as it aids in the management decision-making process. Figure 9–1 presents a schematic that summarizes the planning-budgeting-control process in a business. Of special interest is the decision output of the planning process. The planning process should detail the products or product lines that the business will produce during the planning horizon.

Figure 9–1 The Planning-Budgeting-Control Process

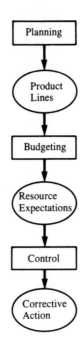

Products and Product Lines

The terms *product* and *product line* seem fairly simple and easy to understand in most businesses. For example, a finished car is the product of the automobile company; individual types of cars may then be grouped to form product lines, such as the Chevrolet product line of General Motors.

Can this definition of a product be transposed to the health care sector? Many individuals feel very strongly that products cannot be defined so easily in health care firms. The major dilemma seems to arise in the area of patients versus products. In short, is the product the patient, or is it the individual services provided, such as lab tests, nursing care, and meals? In most situations, we believe that the patient is the basic product of a health care firm. This means that the wide range of services provided to patients—such as nursing, prescriptions, and tests—are to be viewed as intermediate products, not final products. There is in fact little difference between this interpretation and that applied in most manufacturing settings. For example, automobile fenders are, on one hand, a final product; on the other, they are only an intermediate product in preparation of the final product, the completed automobile. Ultimately, it is the automobile that is sold to the public, not the fenders. In the same vein, it is the treated patient that generates revenue, not the individual service provided in isolation. Indeed, a hospital that provided only lab tests would not be a hospital but rather a laboratory. In short, it takes patients to be a health care provider.

Product lines represent an amalgamation of patients in a way that makes business sense. Sometimes people use the term *strategic business units* to refer to areas of activity that may stand alone. For our purpose, a product line is a unit of business activity that requires a go or no-go decision. For example, eliminating one DRG is probably not possible, because that DRG may be linked to other DRGs within a clinical specialty area; it may be impossible to stop producing DRG # 36 (Retinal Procedures) without also eliminating other DRGs, such as DRG # 39 (Lens Procedure). Thus, in many cases, it is the clinical specialty, for example, ophthalmology, that defines the product line.

Budgeting and Resource Expectations

The budgeting phase of operations involves a translation of the product-line decisions reached earlier into a set of resource expectations. The primary purpose of this is twofold. First, management must assure itself that there will be sufficient funds flow to maintain financial solvency. Just as you and I must live within our financial means, so must any health care business entity. Second, the resulting budget serves as a basis for management control. If budget expectations are not realized, management must discover why not and take corrective actions. A budget or set of resource expectations can be thought of as a standard costing system. The budget represents management's expectations of how costs should behave, given a certain set of volume assumptions.

The key aspect of budgeting is the translation of product-line decisions into precise and specific sets of resource expectations. This involves five basic steps:

1. Define the volume of patients by case type to be treated in the budget period.

2. Define the standard treatment protocol by case type.
3. Define the required departmental volumes.
4. Define the standard cost profiles for departmental outputs.
5. Define the prices to be paid for resources.

The primary output of the budgeting process is a series of departmental budgets that spell out what costs should be during the coming budget period. Three separate sets of standards are involved in the development of these budgets (the three sets of standards are described later in the chapter).

Control and Corrective Action

The control phase of business operations monitors actual cost experience and compares it with budgetary expectations. If there are deviations from expectations, management analyzes the causes of the deviation. If the deviation is favorable, management may seek to make whatever created the variance a permanent part of operations. If the variance is unfavorable, action will be taken in an attempt to prevent a recurrence. Much of the control phase centers around the topic of variance analysis, which is explored in depth in Chapter 11.

THE COSTING PROCESS

Most firms, whether they are hospitals, nursing homes or steel manufacturers, have fairly similar costing systems. In fact, in most cases, the similarities outweigh the differences. Figure 9–2 presents a schematic of the cost measurement process that exists in most businesses.

Valuation

Valuation has always been a thorny issue for accountants, one that has not been satisfactorily resolved even today. We need only to look at the current controversy over replacement costs versus historical costs to see the problem in full bloom. Here, for discussion purposes, we have chosen to split the valuation process into two areas: (1) basis and (2) assignment over time. These two areas are not mutually exclusive; to some degree they overlap with one another. However, both determine the total value of a resource that is used to cost a final product.

Figure 9–2 The Cost Measurement Process

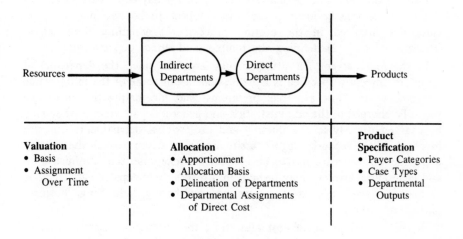

The valuation basis is the process by which a value is assigned to each and every resource transaction occurring between the entity being accounted for and another entity. In most situations this value is historical cost.

Having established a basis value for the resource transaction, there are two major types of situations in which that value will have to be assigned over time: First, the value may be expended prior to the actual reporting of expense. The best example of this is depreciation. Second, the expense may be recognized prior to an actual expenditure. Normal accruals such as wages and salaries are examples of this situation.

Allocation

The end result of the cost allocation process is to assign to direct departments all costs or values determined in the valuation phase of costing. Two phases of activity are involved in this assignment: First, all resource values to be recorded as expense in a given period are assigned or allocated to the direct and indirect departments as direct expenses. Second, once the initial cost assignment to individual departments has been made, a further allocation is required. In this phase the expenses of the indirect departments are assigned to the direct departments.

Using this framework for analysis, costing issues may be subcategorized. In the initial cost assignment phase, there appear to be two major action categories involved in the costing process: (1) assigning the cost to departments and (2) defining the indirect and direct departments.

In the first category, a situation may arise in which the departmental structure currently specified is not questioned, but some of the initial value assignments are. For example, premiums paid for malpractice insurance might be charged to the administration and general department, or they may be charged directly to the nursing and professional departments that are involved. In the second category, a situation may arise in which the existing departmental structure has to be revised. For example, the administration and general department may be split into several new departments, such as nonpatient telephones, data processing, purchasing, admitting, business office, and other.

In the second phase of cost allocation, the reassignment from indirect departments to direct departments, there are also two primary categories of action involved: (1) selection of the cost apportionment method and (2) selection of the appropriate allocation basis. With respect to the first category, cost apportionment methods—such as step-down, double-distribution or simultaneous-equations—are simply mathematical algorithms that redistribute cost from existing indirect departments to direct departments, given defined allocation bases. An example of the second action category is the selection of square feet or hours worked for housekeeping as an appropriate allocation basis for an indirect department.

Product Specification

In most health care firms, there are two phases in the production (or treatment) process. The schematic in Figure 9–3 illustrates this process and also introduces a few new terms.

In Stage 1 of the production process, resources are acquired and consumed within departments to produce a product, defined as a service unit. Here, two points need to be emphasized. First, all departments have service units, but not all departments have the same number of service units. For example, nursing may provide four levels of care: Acuity Levels 1, 2, 3, and 4. Laboratory in contrast, may have a hundred or more separate service units that relate to the provision of specific tests. Second, not all service units can

Figure 9–3 The Production Process for Health Care Firms

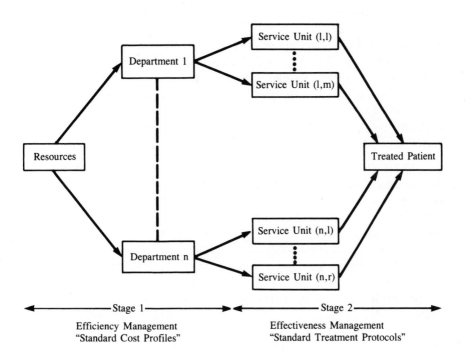

be directly associated with the delivery of patient care; some of the service units may be only indirectly associated with patient treatment. For example, housekeeping cleans laboratory areas, but there is no direct association between this function and patient treatment. However, the cleaning of a patient's room could be regarded as a service that is directly associated with a patient.

Stage 2 of the production process relates to the actual consumption of specific service units in the treatment of a patient. Much of the production process is managed by the physician. This is true regardless of the setting, (hospital, nursing home, home health care firm, or clinic). The physician prescribes the specific service units that will be required to treat a given patient effectively.

The lack of management authority in this area complicates management's efforts to budget and control its costs. This is not meant to be a negative criticism of current health care delivery systems; all of us would prefer to have a qualified physician rather than a lay health care executive direct our care. Yet this is perhaps the area of greatest difference between health care firms and other business entities. Management at General Motors can decide which automobiles will have factory-installed air conditioning and tinted glass and which will not. In contrast, a hospital manager will have great difficulty in attempting to direct a physician to either prescribe or not prescribe a given procedure in the treatment of a patient.

Health care products to be costed may vary depending upon the specific decision under consideration. At one level, management may be interested in the cost of a specific service unit or departmental output. Prices for some service units, for example, for x-ray procedures, may have to be established, and to do that management must know their costs. In other situations, the cost of an individual treated patient or a grouping of treated patients may be desired. For example, management may wish to bid on a contract to provide home health services to an HMO. In this case, it is important for them to understand what the costs of treating HMO patients are likely to be. If the contract is signed, management then needs to determine the actual costs of treating the patients from the HMO in order to measure the overall profitability from that segment of the business. Alternatively, a grouping of patients by specialty may be necessary. A hospital may wish to know if it is losing money from treating a particular DRG entity or some grouping of DRGs, such as obstetrics.

STANDARD DEVELOPMENT

The key to successful product costing is management's ability to develop and maintain two systems: (1) a system of standard cost profiles and (2) a system of standard treatment protocols. The relationship between these two systems is shown in Figure 9–3. The link pin between them is the service unit (SU) concept. Specifically, management must know what it costs to produce an SU, and it must know what particular SUs are needed to treat a given patient.

Standard Cost Profiles

The standard cost profile (SCP) is not a new concept; it has been used in manufacturing cost accounting systems for many years. For our purposes, there are two key elements in an SCP: (1) the definition of the SU being costed and (2) the profile of resources required to produce the SU.

As noted earlier, the number of SUs in a given department may vary; some departments may have one, while others may have a hundred or more. If the number of SUs is very large, however, there may be an unacceptable level of costing detail involved to make the system feasible. In these situations, it may be useful to aggregate some of the SUs. For example, the laboratory may perform a thousand or more tests. In this situation, it may make sense to develop cost profiles for only the most commonly performed tests and to employ some arbitrary assignment method for the remaining noncommon tests.

The SU does not have to be a product or service that is directly performed for a patient. Many indirect departments do not provide services or products to the patient; instead, their products or services are consumed by other departments, both direct and indirect. However, many indirect departments have SUs that are directly provided to the patient. For example, dietary, often regarded as an indirect department, may not have revenue billed for its product to the patient. However, a meal furnished by it to a patient is an SU that is just as direct as a lab test or a chest x-ray. In a similar vein, housekeeping may provide cleaning for a patient's room that is, in effect, a direct service consumed by the patient.

Thus, SUs may be categorized as either direct or indirect. A direct SU is one that is associated with a given patient. An indirect SU is one provided to another department of the hospital, as opposed to a patient. The differentiation between direct and indirect SUs is important, not only in the development of standard cost profiles but also in the development of standard treatment protocols. Direct SUs must be identified when standard treatment protocols are defined, whereas indirect SUs need not be specifically identified, although some estimate of allocated cost is often required.

In the development of a SCP for a given SU, the following resource expense categories are listed: (1) direct expenses (labor, materials, and departmental overhead) and (2) allocated overhead. Ideally, the expense should also be categorized as variable or fixed. This distinction is particularly important in certain areas of management decision making, as pointed out in Chapter 8. Specifically, the differentiation between variable and fixed cost is critical to many incremental pricing and volume decisions. It is also important in flexible budgeting systems and management control. These topics are explored in greater depth in Chapters 10 and 11.

Table 9–1 Standard Cost Profile for a Dietary/Regular Patient Meal SU #181

Cost Category	Quantity Required Variable	Quantity Required Fixed	Unit Cost	Variable Cost	Average Fixed Cost	Average Total Cost
Direct labor	.05	.05	$6.00	$ .30	$ .30	$ .60
Direct materials	1.00	.00	1.00	1.00	.00	1.00
Department overhead	.00	1.00	.50	.00	.50	.50
Allocated costs						
Housekeeping	.00	.10	1.00	.00	.10	.10
Plant operation	.00	1.00	.10	.00	.10	.10
Administration	.00	.02	10.00	.00	.20	.20
Total				$1.30	$1.20	$2.50

Table 9–1 presents a SCP for a regular patient meal in a dietary department. The total cost of providing one regular patient meal, or SU #181, is $2.50. The variable cost per meal is $1.30, and the average fixed cost per meal is $1.20.

In most situations, direct labor is the largest single expense category. In our dietary meal example, this is not true because the direct material cost, mostly raw food, is larger. It is possible, and in many cases desirable, to define direct labor costs by labor category. Thus, in our dietary meal example, we might provide separate listings for cooks, dietary aides, and dishwashers.

An important point here is the division of cost into fixed and variable quantities. Table 9–1 indicates that .05 units of variable labor time are required per meal and .05 units of fixed labor are required per meal. (In Chapter 8 we discussed several methods for splitting costs into fixed and variable elements.) The fixed cost assignment is an average based upon some expected level of volume. This is an important point to remember when developing SCPs; a decline in volume below expected levels will raise the average cost of production.

The third column of Table 9–1 unit cost. This represents management's best guess as to the cost or price of the resources to be used in the production process. Our dietary meal SCP indicates a price of $6 per unit of direct labor. This value reflects the expected wage per hour to be paid for direct labor in the dietary department. Again, it might be possible and desirable to further break out direct labor into specific job classifications. This usually permits better costing, but it does require more effort.

Any fringe benefit cost associated with labor should be included in the unit cost. For example, the average direct hourly wage in our dietary meal example might be $5 per hour, but fringe benefits may average 20 percent. In this case, the effective wage would be $6 per hour.

Departmental overhead consists of expenses that are directly charged to a department and do not represent either labor or materials. Common examples are equipment costs, travel allowances, expenses for outside purchased services, and cost of publications. Usually these items do not vary with level of activity or volume but remain fixed for the budgetary period. If this is the case, assignment to a SCP can be based on a simple average. For example, assume that our dietary department expects to provide 200,000 regular patient meals next year. Assume further that the department has been authorized to spend $100,000 in discretionary areas that constitute departmental overhead. The average cost per meal for these discretionary costs would be $.50 and would be fixed.

Allocated costs are probably the most difficult to assign in most situations. In our dietary example, we include only three allocated cost areas. This is probably a low figure; a number of other departments would most likely provide service to dietary and should properly be included in the SCP.

There are two major alternatives to the use of estimates of allocated costs in a SCP. First, individual costing studies could be performed, and services from one department to another could be recorded. This process may be expensive, however, and not worth the effort. For example, if separate meters were installed, utility costs could be associated with each user department. However, the installation of such meters is probably not an effective expenditure of funds; costing accuracy would not be improved enough to justify the extra expenditure.

The second alternative would be a simple averaging method. All overhead costs might be aggregated and apportioned to other departments on the basis of direct expenses, FTEs, or some other criterion. This method is relatively simple, but its accuracy would be suspect if significant variation in departmental utilization exists.

We believe that the best approach to costing is to identify all possible direct SUs. These SUs, which can be directly associated with a patient, are far more numerous than one would suspect. For example, a meal provided to a patient is a direct SU but is currently treated as an indirect product in most costing systems. Laundry and linen have certain SUs that are directly associated with a patient, such as clean sheets and gowns. Housekeeping provides direct services to patients when its personnel clean rooms. Administration and medical records also provide specific direct services to patients in the form of processed paperwork and insurance forms. If such costs, currently regarded as indirect, were reclassified as direct, there would be a substantially lower level of indirect costs that would require allocation. This would improve the costing of patients, the health care product, and make the allocation of indirect costs less critical. Currently, indirect costs in many health care settings are in excess of 50 percent of total cost. With better identification of services or SUs, we believe that level could be reduced to 25 percent or lower.

Standard Treatment Protocols

There is an analogy between a standard treatment protocol (STP) and a job order cost sheet used in industrial cost accounting. In a job order cost system, a separate cost sheet is completed for each specific job. This is necessary because each job is different from jobs performed in the past and jobs to be performed in the future. Automobile repairs are an excellent example of a job order cost system. A separate cost sheet is prepared for each job. That cost sheet then serves as the bill or invoice to the customer.

Health care firms also operate in a job-cost setting. Patient treatment may vary significantly across patients. The patient's bill may be thought of as a job order cost sheet in that it reflects the actual services provided during the course of the patient's treatment. Of course, not all of the services provided are shown in the patient's bill. For example, meals provided are rarely charged for as a separate item.

In a typical job order cost setting, standards may not always be applied. When you drop your car off for servicing, the dealer does not prepare a standard job order cost sheet. Dealers have no incentive to do this because they expect that customers will pay the actual costs of the service when they drop by to pick up their cars. If they do not, the dealer may take possession of the car as collateral.

In the past, a similar situation existed among health care firms; the client or patient would pay for the actual cost of services provided. Today this is no longer true for the majority of health care products. Today, most health care firms are paid a fixed fee or price regardless of the range of services provided. Medicare's DRG payment system is the most recent application of this type of payment philosophy.

Because the majority of health care revenue is derived from fixed price payers, we need to define specific STPs wherever possible. Table 9–2 shows a hypothetical STP for DRG #208 (Disorder of Biliary Tract). (This STP is for illustrative purposes only; it should not be regarded as a realistic STP for DRG #208.)

In the Table 9–2 STP, costs are split into fixed and variable components. Thus, the STP requires 25 patient meals at a variable cost of $1.30 per meal and a fixed cost of $1.20 per meal. The basis for these data is the SCP (see

Table 9–2 Standard Treatment Protocol for DRG No. 208/Disorder of Biliary Tract

Service Unit No.	Service Unit Name	Quantity	Variable Cost/Unit	Fixed Cost/Unit	Total Cost/Unit	Total Variable Cost	Total Fixed Cost	Total Cost
1	Admission process	1	$48.00	$52.00	$100.00	$ 48.00	$ 52.00	$ 100.00
7	Nursing care Level 1	1	80.00	40.00	120.00	80.00	40.00	120.00
8	Nursing care Level 2	7	85.00	45.00	130.00	595.00	315.00	910.00
9	Nursing care Level 3	1	110.00	45.00	155.00	110.00	45.00	155.00
29	Pharmacy prescriptions		38.00	19.00	57.00	38.00	19.00	57.00
38	Chest x-ray	1	12.00	8.00	20.00	12.00	8.00	20.00
46	Lab CBC	1	4.00	3.50	7.50	4.00	3.50	7.50
49	Other lab tests		85.00	55.00	140.00	85.00	55.00	140.00
57	Patient meals	25	1.30	1.20	2.50	32.50	30.00	62.50
65	Clean linen changes	5	.60	.50	1.10	3.00	2.50	5.50
93	Room preparation	1	7.00	3.00	10.00	7.00	3.00	10.00
	Totals					$1,014.50	$573.00	$1,587.50

Table 9–1). As noted earlier, this breakout into fixed and variable costs is extremely valuable for management in making its planning and control decisions. For example, if Medicare paid the hospital $1,400 for every DRG # 208 treated, we would conclude that, at least in the short run, the hospital would be financially better off if it continued to treat DRG # 208 cases, since the payment of $1,400 exceeds the variable cost of $1,014.50 and is therefore making a contribution to fixed costs.

Table 9–2 depicts two areas in which no actual quantity is specified: pharmacy prescriptions and other lab tests. In these instances, the total cost of the services is instead divided between fixed and variable costs. Because of the large number of products provided in each of these two areas, it would be impossible to develop a SCP for each product item. However, some of the heavier volume lab tests or pharmacy prescriptions may be separately identified and costed; for example, lab CBC is listed as a separate SU.

Some of the items shown in Table 9–2 may not be reflected in a patient's bill. For example, patient meals, clean linen changes, room preparation, and admission processing would not usually be listed in the bill. Also, separation of nursing care by acuity level may not be identified in the bill; many hospitals do not distinguish between levels of nursing in their pricing structures.

A final point to emphasize is that not all SUs will show up in a STP. Only those SUs that are classified as direct are listed. A direct SU is one that can be directly traced or associated with patient care. The costs associated with the provision of indirect SUs are allocated to the direct SUs. At the same time, the objective should be to create as many direct SUs as possible.

VARIANCE ANALYSIS

In general, given the systems of standards discussed above, four types of variances may be identified in the variance analysis phase of control:

1. Price (rate)
2. Efficiency
3. Volume
4. Intensity

The first three types of variances are a direct result of the development of the SCPs; they are the product of departmental activity. A rate or price variance is the difference between the price actually paid and the standard price multiplied by the actual quantity used:

Price variance = (Actual price – Standard price) × Actual quantity

For example, assume that our dietary department of Table 9–1 produced 1,500 patient meals for the period in question. To produce these meals, it used 180 hours of labor and paid $6.25 per hour. In this case, the price or rate variance would be

($6.25 – $6.00) × 180 hours = $45.00

This variance would be unfavorable because the department paid $6.25 per hour when the expected rate was $6.00.

An efficiency variance reflects productivity in the production process. It is derived by multiplying the difference between actual quantity used and standard quantity by the standard price:

Efficiency variance = (Actual quantity – Standard quantity) × Standard price

In our dietary example, the efficiency variance would be

(180 hours – 155 hours) × $6 = $150

Standard labor is derived by multiplying the variable labor requirement of .05 times the number of meals produced, or 1,500. To this sum is added the budgeted fixed labor requirement of 80 hours (.05 × 1,600 meals). In our example, the department used 25 more hours of labor than had been expected. As a result, it incurred an unfavorable efficiency variance of $150.

The volume variance reflects differences between expected output and actual output. It is a factor to be considered in situations with fixed costs. If no fixed costs existed, the resources required per unit would be constant. This would mean that the cost per unit of production should be constant. For most situations, this is not a reasonable expectation; normally fixed costs are present.

The volume variance is derived by multiplying the expected average fixed cost per unit times the difference between budgeted volume and actual volume:

Volume variance = (Budgeted volume – Actual volume) × Average fixed cost per unit

In the case of direct labor in our dietary example, the volume variance would be an unfavorable $30 ([1,600 Meals – 1,500 Meals] × $ .30).

Notice that in our example, the total of these variances equals the difference between actual costs incurred for direct labor and the standard cost of direct labor assigned to the SU, a patient meal:

Actual direct labor ($6.25 × 180 hours)	$ 1,125
Standard cost ($ .60 × 1,500 meals)	900
Total variance	$ 225
Price variance	$ 45.00
Efficiency variance	150.00
Volume variance	30.00
Total variance	$225.00

The intensity variance is the difference between the quantity of SUs actually required in treating a patient and the quantity called for in the STP. For example, if 20 meals were provided a patient categorized as DRG No. 208, there would be a favorable variance of five meals, given the STP data of Table 9–2.

Intensity variances are generically defined as follows:

Intensity variance = (Actual SUs – Standard SUs) × Price per SU

Thus, in our example, the intensity variance for a patient with respect to meals would be a favorable $12.50 ([20 meals – 25 meals] × $2.50).

It may be useful to split intensity variances into fixed and variable elements. In our example, it is probably not fair to say that $12.50 was realized in savings because five fewer meals were delivered. Five times $1.30, the variable cost, may be a better reflection of short-term realized savings.

One final word on variance analysis: It is important to specify the party responsible for variances. This is, after all, part of the rationale for standard costing—to be able to take corrective action through individuals to correct unfavorable variances. In our example, three variances—price, efficiency, and volume—are distinguished in the department accounts. However, the departmental manager may not be responsible for all of this variation, especially in the volume area. Usually, departmental managers have little control over volume; they merely react to the volume of services requested from their departments.

The intensity variance can be largely associated with a given physician. Most of the SUs are of a medical nature, resulting from physician decisions regarding testing or length of stay. It may be very helpful, therefore, to accumulate intensity variances by physicians. Periodic discussions regarding these variations can be most useful to both the health care executive and the physician. Ideally, physicians should participate actively in the development of STPs.

SUMMARY

Product costing has become much more critical to health care executives today than it was prior to 1983. The emphasis on prospective prices and competitive discounting creates a real need to define costs. For health care purposes, the product is a treated patient. Various aggregations of patients may also be useful. For example, we may want to develop cost data by DRG, by clinical specialty, or by payer category.

To develop a standard cost system in a health care firm, two sets of standards must be defined. First, a series of strategic cost profiles (SCPs) must be developed for all service units or SUs (intermediate departmental products) produced by the firm. This part of standard costing is analogous to that of most manufacturing systems. Second, a set of standard treatment protocols (STPs) must be defined for major patient treatment categories. These STPs must identify all the service units to be provided in the patient treatment. Physician involvement is critical in this area.

The purpose of standard costing is to make planning decisions, such as those involved in pricing and product mix, more precise and meaningful. Standard costing is also useful in making control decisions. Variance analysis is based on the existence of standard cost and the periodic accumulation of actual cost data. Timely analysis of variances can help management achieve desired results.

ASSIGNMENTS

1. An HMO has asked your hospital to provide all of its obstetrical services. The have offered to pay your hospital $2,000 for a normal vaginal delivery without complications (DRG No. 373). You have looked at the STP for this DRG and discovered that your hospital's cost is $2,400. What should you do?

2. Dr. Jones is scheduled to meet with you this afternoon. He has been an active admitter, but you would like to see his practice increase. After reviewing Dr. Jones's financial report shown in Table 9–3 what recommendations would you make?

3. Using the data presented below in Table 9–4, explain why some DRGs have negative values for deductions.

4. In Table 9–4, DRG No. 14 has the largest revenue of all the case types listed, yet it lost money. Why?

5. The data in Table 9–5 represent a cost accountant's effort to define the variable cost for DRG No. 104 (Peptic Ulcer). Evaluate this method.

Table 9–3 Dr. Jones's Financial Report

Case Number	Type Description	Number of Discharges	ALOS	Comp LOS	LOS Var	Total Charges	Deductions	Net Revenue	Variable Cost	Gross Margin	Fixed Cost	Net Income
0316	Renal Failure w/	7	11.7	6.7	5.0	$ 19,371	$ 4,484	$ 14,887	$ 7,372	$ 7,515	$ 6,926	$ 589
0315	Other Kidney Uri	5	42.4	12.7	29.7	28,945	6,270	22,675	12,375	10,300	8,866	1,434
0468	Unrelated OR Pro	5	32.2	11.3	20.9	84,309	12,739	71,570	33,421	38,149	30,955	7,194
0130	Periph Vascular	3	6.0	8.8	-2.8	8,166	1,834	6,332	3,055	3,277	3,297	-20
0138	Cardiac Arrhythm	3	4.3	7.4	-3.1	3,524	1,027	2,497	1,351	1,146	985	161
0182	Esophagitis GI+D	3	7.3	6.7	.6	14,171	3,427	10,744	5,308	5,436	5,503	-67
0331	Other Kid + Urina	3	8.7	7.6	1.1	10,983	2,539	8,444	3,900	4,544	4,390	154
0024	Seizure + Headache	2	16.0	6.8	9.2	4,625	1,156	3,469	1,651	1,818	1,459	359
0127	Heart Failure +	2	4.0	10.4	-6.4	1,827	592	1,235	606	629	348	281
0140	Angina Pectoris	2	7.0	6.6	.4	5,290	1,179	4,111	2,079	2,032	1,765	267
0188	Other Digest/sys	2	9.5	6.5	3.0	4,733	1,148	3,585	1,551	2,034	1,926	108
0296	Nutri + Misc Met	2	8.0	8.9	-.9	2,840	625	2,215	1,103	1,112	995	117
0321	Kid + Urinary Tra	2	23.0	4.6	18.4	12,377	248	12,129	4,103	8,026	4,505	3,521
0442	Other OR Proc In	2	6.5	11.6	-5.1	11,415	2,629	8,786	4,533	4,253	4,082	171
0443	Other OR Proc In	2	8.5	5.6	2.9	8,974	2,227	6,747	3,392	3,355	3,225	130
0452	Complications Tr	2	44.5	6.0	38.5	1,827	482	1,345	562	783	693	90
0467	Other Factors In	2	1.5	3.1	-1.6	1,461	396	1,065	452	613	518	95
0010	Nervous Syst Neo	1	35.0	13.5	21.5	267	99	168	62	106	35	71
0016	Nonspec Cerebrov	1	8.0	11.0	-3.0	4,984	1,093	3,891	2,064	1,827	2,034	-207
0066	Epistaxis	1	7.0	4.6	2.4	302	112	190	86	104	68	36
0085	Pleural Effusion	1	19.0	12.1	6.9	675	251	424	393	31	220	-189
0088	Chronic Obstruct	1	3.0	9.1	-6.1	2,634	694	1,940	1,087	853	946	-93
0112	Vasc Proc No Maj	1	9.0	26.2	-17.2	6,357	1,380	4,977	2,445	2,532	2,482	50
0120	Other OR Procedu	1	71.0	16.4	54.6	10,448	3,461	6,987	2,862	4,125	2,070	1,947
0143	Chest Pain	1	6.0	4.2	1.8	5,659	1,179	4,480	2,333	2,147	2,178	77
0144	Other Circ Diagn	1	2.0	9.3	-7.3	2,085	439	1,646	858	788	713	75
0152	Minor Small + Lar	1	93.0	13.7	79.3	1,084	403	681	241	440	149	291
0171	Other Diges/syst	1	35.0	6.9	28.1	2,136	793	1,343	555	788	358	430
0175	G.I. Hemmorhage A	1	6.0	5.8	.2	3,734	883	2,851	1,676	1,175	1,027	148
0224	Up Extr Proc No	1	23.0	4.3	18.7	10,977	5,544	5,433	3,672	1,761	4,165	-2,404
OP 30	Case types	62	17.9	8.6	9.3	$276,180	$59,333	$216,847	$105,148	$111,699	$96,883	$14,816

Table 9–4 Financial Statement by DRG Category

Number	Description	Total Charges	Total Deductions	Net Revenue	Variable Cost	Gross Margin	Total Margin (%)	Fixed Cost	Net Income	Income Percent (%)
0001	Craniotomy Age 17 No Trau	$14,115	$3,317	$10,798	$4,709	$6,089	43.1	$4,192	$1,897	13.4
0002	Craniotomy Age 17 W/ Trau	1,170	435	735	302	433	37.0	220	213	18.2
0004	Spinal Procedures	5,553	–251	5,804	2,278	3,526	63.4	1,596	1,930	34.7
0005	Extracranial Vasc Procedu	14,814	2,310	12,504	5,641	6,863	46.3	4,898	1,965	13.2
0006	Carpal Tunnel Release	12,488	1,991	10,497	4,441	6,056	48.4	4,649	1,407	11.2
0007	Periph+Cranial Nerv/Syst	2,586	–1,900	4,486	586	3,900	150.8	424	3,476	134.4
0008	Periph+Cranial Nerv/Syst	6,742	605	6,137	2,577	3,560	52.8	2,806	754	11.1
0010	Nervous Syst Neoplasms Ag	36,194	5,602	30,592	13,594	16,998	46.9	13,625	3,373	9.3
0011	Nervous Syst Neoplasms Ag	9,075	2,869	6,206	3,058	3,148	34.6	2,885	263	2.8
0012	Degenerative Nerv/Syst Di	49,084	11,628	37,456	18,392	19,064	38.8	18,500	564	1.1
0013	Multiple Sclerosis & Cere	4,249	532	3,717	1,448	2,269	53.4	1,417	852	20.0
0014	Spec Cerebrovascular Dis	129,884	37,434	92,450	48,146	44,304	34.1	45,014	–710	–.5
0015	Transient Ischemic Attack	39,989	10,813	29,176	13,768	15,408	38.5	14,098	1,310	3.2
0016	Nonspec Cerebrovascular D	7,272	1,713	5,559	2,855	2,704	37.1	2,496	208	2.8
0017	Nonspec Cerebrovascular D	544	11	533	147	386	70.9	223	163	29.9
0018	Cranial+Periph Nerve Diso	12,807	895	11,912	4,305	7,607	59.3	4,680	2,927	22.8
0019	Cranial+Periph Nerve Diso	4,083	–160	4,243	1,311	2,932	71.8	1,535	1,397	34.2
0020	Nerv/Sys Infect No Viral	8,246	619	7,627	2,405	5,222	63.3	2,519	2,703	32.7
0021	Viral Meningitis	3,443	1,334	2,109	1,180	929	26.9	971	–42	–1.2
0022	Hyperten Encephalopathi	589	147	442	194	248	42.1	135	113	19.1
0024	Seizure+Headache Age>69	19,427	2,201	17,226	6,071	11,155	57.4	5,299	5,856	30.1
0025	Seizure+Headache Age =18–6	24,151	2,948	21,203	7,728	13,475	55.7	9,092	4,383	18.1
0026	Seizure+Headache Age =0–17	5,511	424	5,087	2,310	2,777	50.3	2,139	638	11.5
0027	Traumatic Stupor + Coma>	2,572	318	2,254	1,051	1,203	46.7	798	405	15.7
0028	Traumatic Stupor + Coma<	7,220	1,760	5,460	2,227	3,233	44.7	3,357	–124	–1.7
0029	Traumatic Stupor + < 1H	438	9	429	168	261	59.5	70	191	43.6
0032	Concussion Age = 18–69	6,826	277	6,549	2,345	4,204	61.5	2,279	1,925	28.2

Table 9-4 continued

Number	Description	Total Charges	Total Deductions	Net Revenue	Variable Cost	Gross Margin	Total Margin (%)	Fixed Cost	Net Income	Income Percent (%)
0033	Concussion Age = 0-17	1,513	269	1,244	615	629	41.5	613	16	1.0
0034	Other Disorders Nerv/Sys	34,702	9,918	24,784	15,312	9,472	27.2	10,380	-908	-2.6
0035	Other Disorders Nerv/Sys	18,634	764	17,870	8,342	9,528	51.1	7,935	1,593	8.5
0036	Retinal Procedures	13,240	1,999	11,241	4,428	6,813	51.4	5,463	1,350	10.1
0037	Orbital Procedures	3,284	684	2,600	1,437	1,163	35.4	1,089	74	2.2
0038	Primary Iris Procedures	1,092	226	866	574	292	26.7	466	-174	-15.9
0039	Lens Procedures	118,725	27,289	91,436	43,601	47,835	40.2	48,010	-175	-.1
0040	Extraocular Proc No Orbit	4,455	547	3,908	1,819	2,089	46.8	2,131	-42	-.9
0041	Extraocular Proc No Orbit	4,798	228	4,570	1,683	2,887	60.1	1,574	1,313	27.3
0044	Acute Major Eye Infection	6,953	1,841	5,112	2,178	2,934	42.1	2,900	34	.4
0045	Neurological Eye Disorder	8,995	1,432	7,563	3,153	4,410	49.0	3,425	985	10.9

Table 9–5 Format for Defining Variable Cost for DRG No. 104
(Peptic Ulcer)

Department	Average Charges	Ratio of Direct Costs to Charges[a]	Estimated Costs	Estimated Variable Costs (as Percentage of Total Estimated Costs)[b]	Estimated Variable Costs
General nursing	$1,240	.71	$ 880	70	$ 616
Special care unit	1,810	.68	1,231	70	862
Central supply	180	.28	50	75	38
Laboratory	270	.47	127	10	13
EKG	50	.37	19	20	4
EEG	60	.38	23	20	5
Nuclear medicine	190	.37	70	30	21
Diagnostic radiology	95	.38	36	25	9
Operating room	650	.47	306	65	199
Emergency department	105	.49	51	40	21
Transfusion	405	.63	255	70	179
Pharmacy	320	.28	90	75	67
Anesthesiology	180	.44	79	30	24
Respiratory therapy	295	.35	103	25	26
Physical therapy	85	.61	52	25	13
Clinic	110	.53	58	30	17
Totals	$6,045		$3,430		$2,114

Variable cost of other departments (e.g., dietary, housekeeping, admitting, billing, medical records), estimated at $50 per admission plus $30 per day × 9 days.[c]   320

Total estimated variable cost $2,434

[a] Ratio of direct costs (not fully allocated costs) to charges, per the general ledger.
[b] Source: estimates prepared by departmental managers.
[c] Source: estimates prepared by departmental managers.

SOLUTIONS AND ANSWERS

1. Hopefully, the STP for DRG No. 373 separates the costs into variable and fixed elements. If the variable cost is below $2,000, some marginal profit may be earned by your hospital on the additional business. However, a close examination of the STP should be made by the HMO physicians. There may be some patient-management differences, especially with regard to length of stay, that could result in more or less cost. An agreement on the STP with the HMO physicians should be negotiated.

2. Most of the income generated by Dr. Jones is in areas where the LOS is significantly above the normal level. For example, DRG Nos. 468, 321, and 120 accounted for 85 percent of the total income that he generated for the hospital. In each of these three DRG categories his LOS was way above normal. Since these cases were profitable, they must not have been Medicare. If there is a likelihood that some of your major payers may shift to a prospective case payment basis, you may not want to encourage Dr. Jones to increase his practice. The data in his financial report indicate a relatively high LOS in almost all areas.

3. DRG No. 7 has a minus $1,900 deduction. This means that payment received for treating this DRG category exceeded charges by $1,900. This probably reflects payment by Medicare in excess of charges. This situation may change if other hospitals have a similar experience. At the present time, however, DRG No. 7 is a very profitable product for the hospital (134.4 percent).

4. One reason DRG No. 14 lost money can be found in the deductible provision. Approximately 29 percent of the DRG charges were written off. You may want to pay special attention to the firm's STP for this case type. Perhaps the firm's LOS or ancillary services are excessive.

5. The first potential weakness in the cost accountant's method is the use of a cost-to-charge ratio. There is no guarantee that charges for departmental services will always be related to costs. The method also may miss a large block of indirect departmental costs that may be variable. Finally, the method simply does not relate well to the two-stage definition of standard costs involving SCPs and STPs, as discussed in this chapter. In fairness, it must be noted that the cost accountant's method would cost significantly less than other methods. And it is not clear whether the improved accuracy that might result from some other, more sophisticated system would be worth the extra cost.

Chapter 10

The Management
Control Process

Twenty years ago, the word *budgeting* could not have been found in the vocabulary of many hospital managers and other health care facility administrators. Today, this is no longer true. Most hospitals and other health care facilities now develop and use budgets as an integral part of their overall management control process.

To a large extent, the attention being paid to budgeting by health care providers is attributable to changes in the environment. The recent adoption of prospective payment and the increasing price competition among health care providers have forced many health care firms to monitor and control costs with increasing care. Budgeting is of course a logical way for any business organization to control its costs. Indeed, other parties external to health care providers now require health care firms to prepare and submit budgets and other financial forecasts. For example, rate-setting agencies frequently require hospitals and other health care facilities to submit fairly detailed institutional budgets. The certificate of need (CON) also requires a projection of financial information for projects under review.

External forces thus have certainly stimulated the development of budgets in the health care industry, but most likely such budgets would have been developed in any case. Hospitals and health care facilities have grown larger and more complex, in both organization and finances. And budgeting is imperative in organizations in which management authority is delegated to many individuals.

ESSENTIAL ELEMENTS

For our purposes, a budget is defined as a quantitative expression of a plan of action. It is an integral part of the overall management control process of an organization.

Anthony and Herzlinger (*Management Control in Nonprofit Organizations* [Homewood, Ill.: Richard D. Irwin, 1976], p. 16-33) discuss management control in great detail. They define it as "a process by which managers assure that resources are obtained and used effectively and efficiently in the accomplishment of an organization's objectives" (p. 16).

Efficiency and Effectiveness

In the above definition, special emphasis is placed on attaining efficiency and effectiveness. In short, they determine the success or failure of management control.

These two terms have very precise meanings. Often individuals talk about the relative efficiency and effectiveness of their operations as if efficiency and effectiveness were identical, or at least highly correlated. They are not identical, nor are they necessarily correlated. An operation may be effective without being efficient, and vice versa. A well-managed operation should ideally be both effective and efficient. Efficiency is easier to measure and its meaning is fairly well understood; efficiency is simply a relationship between outputs and inputs. For example, a cost per patient day of $110 is a measure of efficiency; it tells how many resources, or inputs, were used to provide one day of care, the measure of output.

Managers and other persons wishing to assess management in the health care industry are increasing their use of efficiency measures. In most situations, efficiency is measured by comparison with some standard. Several basic considerations should be understood if efficiency measures are to be used intelligently. First, output measures may not always be comparable. For example, comparing the costs per patient day of care in a 50-bed rural hospital with those in a 1,000-bed teaching hospital is not likely to be meaningful. A day of care in a teaching hospital typically entails more service. Second, cost measures may not be comparable or useful for the specific decision under consideration. For example, two operations may be identical, but one may be in a newer facility and thus would have a higher depreciation charge, or the two operations may account for costs differently: One hospital may use an accelerated depreciation method, such as the sum of the year's digits, while the other may use straight-line depreciation. Third, the cost concepts used may not be relevant to the decision under consideration. For example, a certificate of need (CON) review to decide which of two hospitals should be permitted to build a 50-bed expansion will obviously consider cost. However, comparing the full costs of a day of care in each institution and selecting the lower one could produce bad results: for this specific decision, the full cost concept is wrong. Incremental or variable cost is the relevant cost concept in this case. The focus of interest is on what the future additional cost would be, not what the historical average cost was.

Effectiveness is concerned with the relationship between an organization's outputs and its objectives or goals. A health care facility's typical goals might include solvency, high quality of care, low cost of patient care, institutional harmony, and growth. Measuring effectiveness is more difficult than measuring efficiency for at least two reasons. First, defining the relationship between outputs and some goals may be difficult because many facilities' goals or objectives are not likely to be quantified. For example, exactly how does an alcoholism program contribute to quality of care? Still, objectives and goals can usually be stated more precisely in quantitative terms. In fact, they should be quantified to the greatest extent possible. In the alcoholism program example, quality scales, such as frequency of repeat visits or new patients treated, might be developed. Second, the output must usually be related to more than one organization goal or objective. For example, solvency and reasonable cost are both legitimate objectives for a hospital. Yet continuing an emergency room operation might affect solvency negatively and at the same time positively affect patient treatment costs. How should decision makers weight these two criteria to determine an overall measure of effectiveness?

Control Unit

Most health care facilities have various responsibility centers over which management control is exercised. These centers are generally referred to as departments. Figure 10–1 presents an organizational chart of a hospital and its departments.

Usually the departments perform special functions that contribute to overall organization goals, directly or indirectly. They receive resources or inputs and produce services or outputs:

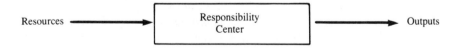

Responsibility centers are the focus of management control efforts. Emphasis is placed on the effectiveness and efficiency of their operations. Measurement problems occur when the responsibility structure is not identical to the program structure. Decision makers are frequently interested

Figure 10–1 Hospital Organization Chart

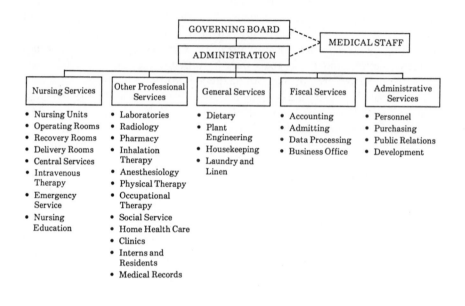

in a program's total cost. Yet in the case of a burn care program, for example, it is unlikely that all the resources used in the program will be assigned to it directly; the costs of medical support services—such as physical therapy, laboratory and radiology, as well as other general and administrative services—will not likely be contained in the burn care unit. Program lines typically run across responsibility center or departmental lines. This necessitates cost allocations for decisions that require program cost information. It should be remembered that where cost allocations are involved, the accuracy of the information as well as its comparability may be suspect. For example, one may be interested in the specific costs of a burn care program, but then find that those costs must be allocated from various departments or responsibility centers, such as laboratory, radiology, and housekeeping.

Responsibility centers vary greatly, depending upon the controlling organization. For a regulatory agency, the responsibility center might be an entire health care facility; for a health care facility manager, it may be an individual department; for a departmental manager, it may be a unit within the department. The only requirement is that a designated person be in charge of the identified responsibility center.

Phases of Management Control

Figure 10–2 illustrates the relationship of various phases of the management control process to each other and to the planning process. Management control relies on the existence of goals and objectives; without them, the structure and evaluation of the management control process is incomplete. Poor or no planning usually limits the value of management control. Effectiveness becomes impossible to assess without stated goals and objectives; in such cases, one can focus only on measuring and attaining efficiency. The organization can assess only whether it has produced outputs efficiently; it cannot evaluate the desirability of those outputs.

For the purposes of this discussion, we shall be concerned with the four phases of management control that Anthony and Herzlinger have identified in their work on management control (see above citation):

1. programming
2. budgeting
3. accounting
4. analysis and reporting

Programming

Programming is the phase of management control that determines the nature and size of programs an organization will use to accomplish its stated goals and objectives. It is the first phase of the management control process and interrelates with planning. In some cases, the line dividing the two activities may in fact be hard to draw. Programming is usually of intermediate length, three to five years. It lasts longer than budgeting, but is shorter than planning.

Programming decisions deal with new and existing programs. The methodology for programming is different in these two areas. Programming decisions for new programs involve capital investment or capital budget decision making (this process is examined more extensively in Chapter 13). The method for making programming decisions for existing programs is often referred to as zero-base review, or zero-base budgeting (this method is discussed later in this chapter).

To illustrate the programming process, assume that a stated objective of a hospital organization is to develop and implement a program of ambulatory

Figure 10–2 The Management Control Process

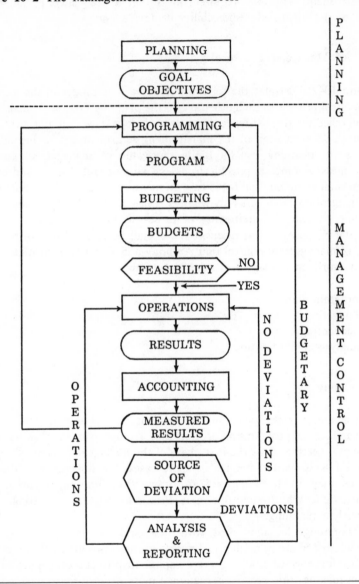

care in the community. The decision makers in the programming phase of management control would take this stated objective and evaluate alternative programs to accomplish it, such as a surgi-center, an outpatient clinic, or a mobile health screening unit. After this analysis, a decision might be made to construct a ten-room surgi-center on a lot adjacent to the hospital. This would be a program decision.

Budgeting

Budgeting is the management control phase of primary interest. It was defined earlier as a quantitative expression of a plan of action. Budgets are usually stated in monetary terms and cover a period of one year.

The budgetary phase of management control follows the determination of programs in the programming phase. In many cases, no real review of existing programs is undertaken; the budgeting phase then may be based on a prior year's budget or on the actual results of existing programs. Proponents of zero-base budgeting have identified this practice as a major shortcoming.

The budgeting phase primarily translates program decisions into terms that are meaningful for responsibility centers. The decision to construct a ten-room surgi-center will affect the revenues and costs of other responsibility centers, such as laboratory, radiology, anesthesiology, and business office. The effects of program decisions thus must be carefully and accurately reflected in the budgets of each of the relevant responsibility centers.

Budgeting may also change programs. A more careful and accurate estimation of revenues and costs may prompt one to reevaluate prior programming decisions as financially unfeasible. For example, the proposed ten-room surgi-center may be shown, through budget analysis, to produce a significant operating loss. If the hospital cannot or will not subsidize this loss from other sources, the programming must be changed. The size of the surgi-center may be reduced from ten rooms to five to make the operation break even.

Accounting

Accounting is the third phase of the management control process. Once programs have been decided on and budgets developed for them along responsibility center lines, the operations begin. The accounting department accumulates and records information on both outputs and inputs during the operating phase.

It is important to note that cost information is provided along both program and responsibility center lines. Responsibility center cost information is used in the reporting and analysis phase to determine the degree of compliance with budget projections. Programmatic cost information is used to assess the desirability of continuing a given program at its present size and scope in the programming phase of management control.

Analysis and Reporting

The last phase of management control is analysis and reporting. In this phase, differences between actual costs and budgeted costs are analyzed to determine the probable cause of the deviations and are then reported to the individuals who can take corrective action. The method used in this phase is often referred to as variance analysis, which is discussed in greater detail in Chapter 11. Those doing the analysis and reporting rely heavily on the information provided from the accounting phase to break down the reported deviations into categories that suggest possible causes.

In general, there are three primary causes for differences between budgeted and actual costs:

1. Prices paid for inputs were different from budgeted prices.
2. Output level was higher or lower than budgeted.
3. Actual quantities of inputs used were different from budgeted levels.

Within each of these causal areas, the problem may arise from either budgeting or operations. A budgetary problem is usually not controllable; no operating action can be taken to correct the situation. For example, the surgi-center may have budgeted for ten RNs at $1,400 each per month. However, if there were no way to employ ten RNs at an average wage less than $1,500 per month, the budget would have to be adjusted to reflect the change in expectations. Alternatively, the problem may arise from operations and be controllable. Perhaps the nurses of the surgi-center are more experienced and better trained than expected. If this is true, and the mix of RNs originally budgeted is still regarded as appropriate, some action should be taken to change the actual mix over time.

THE BUDGETING PROCESS

Elements and Participants

Budgeting is regarded by many as the primary tool that health care facility managers can use to control costs in their organizations. The objectives of budgetary programs, as defined by the American Hospital Association, are four-fold:

1. to provide a written expression, in quantitative terms, of the policies and plans of the hospital

2. to provide a basis for the evaluation of financial performance in accordance with the plans
3. to provide a useful tool for the control of costs
4. to create cost awareness throughout the organization

The budgetary process encompasses a number of interrelated but separate budgets. Figure 10–3 provides a schematic representation of the budgetary process and the relationships between specific types of budgets.

The individuals and roles involved in the budgetary process may vary. In general, the following individuals or parties may be involved:

- governing board
- chief executive officer
- controller
- responsibility center managers
- budgetary committee

The governing board's involvement in the budgetary process is usually indirect. The board provides the goals, objectives, and approved programs that are used as the basis for budgetary development. In many cases, it formally approves the finalized budget, especially the cash budget and budget financial statements; these are critical in assessing financial condition, which is a primary responsibility of the board.

The chief executive officer (CEO) or administrator of the health care facility has overall responsibility for budgetary development. The budget is

Figure 10–3 Integration of the Budgetary Process

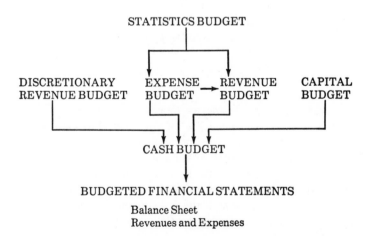

STATISTICS BUDGET

DISCRETIONARY REVENUE BUDGET EXPENSE BUDGET → REVENUE BUDGET CAPITAL BUDGET

CASH BUDGET

BUDGETED FINANCIAL STATEMENTS
Balance Sheet
Revenues and Expenses

the administrator's tool in the overall program of management by exception, which enables the CEO to focus only on those areas where problems exist.

Controllers often serve as budget directors. Their primary function is facilitation: they are responsible for providing relevant data on costs and outputs and for providing budgetary forms that may be used in budget development. They are not responsible for either making or enforcing the budget.

Responsibility centers are the focal points of control. Managers of departments should be actively involved in developing budgets for their assigned areas of responsibility and are responsible for meeting the budgets developed for their areas.

Many large health care facilities use a special budgetary committee to aid in budget development and approval. Typically, this committee is comprised of several departmental managers, headed by the controller or administrator. A committee structure like this can help legitimize budgetary decisions that might appear arbitrary and capricious if made unilaterally by management.

Statistics Budget

Development of the statistics budget is the first step in budgeting. It provides the basis for subsequent development of the revenue and expense budgets. Together, these three budgets are sometimes referred to as the operating budget.

The objective of the statistics budget is to provide measures of work load or activity in each department or responsibility center for the coming budget period. There are three parts to this task:

1. controllable nature of output
2. responsibility for estimation
3. problems in estimation methodology

Controllable Nature of Output

Sales forecasts in many businesses reflect management's output expectations—how much of the business's product can be sold, given certain promotional efforts. There is some question about the extent to which health care facilities can determine their volume of service, at least within the usual budgetary period. Though, in the long run, through the development or discontinuation of certain programs, volume may be changed, most health care facilities implicitly assume in the development of their statistics budget that they cannot affect their overall volume during the coming budgetary period. Instead they assume that they will provide services to meet their actual demand. This leads to a reliance on past-period service levels to forecast demand. Assuming that demand patterns in the budget period will be similar to prior periods can, however, be a costly mistake. First, forseeable but uncontrollable forces may dramatically alter service patterns. For example, retirement of key medical staff with no replacement could drastically reduce admissions. Second, the health care facility may in fact control service levels in the short run and do so in a way that reduces costs. For example, a hospital may decide to use a preadmission testing program that reduces average length of stay in the hospital, thus reducing total volume and total cost.

Responsibility for Estimation

The second issue in the statistics budget is the assignment of responsibility for developing projected output or work-load indicators. Should departmental managers provide this information themselves, or should top management provide it to them? In some situations, departmental managers may tend to overstate demand. Overstatement of demand implies a greater need for resources within their own area and creates potential budgetary slack if anticipated volumes are not realized. The result of the information coming from top management may be the converse: understatement of demand may result in a lower total cost budget and eventually lower total actual costs. Negotiation thus often becomes necessary in determining demand for budgetary purposes.

Problems in Estimation Methodology

The last area of statistics budget development concerns problems of estimation. In most health care facilities, activity in departments depends on a limited number of key variables, such as patient days and outpatient visits.

Such indicators, measured for prior periods and applied through statistical analysis, can be used to project future departmental activity. The major problem becomes one of accurately forecasting values for the indicators.

The use of seasonal, weekly, and daily variations in volume poses an important estimation problem. Too often, yearly volume is assumed to be divided equally between the monthly periods throughout the year, even when that is clearly not the case. Recognition of seasonal, weekly, and daily patterns of variation in volume can in fact create significant opportunities for cost reduction, especially in labor staffing.

Finally, output at the departmental level is often multiple in nature. In fact, a department normally produces more than one type of output; for example, a laboratory may provide literally thousands of different tests. In such situations, a weighted unit of service is needed, such as the relative value units (RVUs) used in areas like laboratory and radiology. The need to use weighted unit measures in the statistics budget is especially important when the mix of services is expected to change. Assume that a hospital is rapidly increasing its volume in outpatient clinics. This expansion in volume will increase activity in many other departments, including pharmacy. If, in such a situation, the filling of an outpatient prescription requires significantly less effort than the filling of an inpatient prescription, the use of an unweighted activity measure for prescriptions could provide misleading information for budgetary control purposes. Far more labor than is actually needed might be budgeted.

Expense Budget

With estimates of activity for individual departments developed in the statistics budget, department managers can proceed to develop expense budgets for their areas of responsibility. Expense budgeting is the area of budgeting "where the rubber meets the road." Management cost control efforts are finally reflected in hard numbers that the departments must live with, in most cases for the budget period. Major categories of expense budgets at the departmental level include payroll, supplies, and other. In some situations, a budget for allocated costs from indirect departments may also be included, although this is usually not done by departmental managers.

In our discussion of expense budgeting, we shall focus on the following four issues of budgeting that are of general interest:

1. length of the budget period
2. flexible or forecast budgets
3. standards for price and quantity
4. allocation of indirect cost

Length of the Budget Period

Generally speaking, there are two alternative budget periods that may be used—*fixed* and *rolling*. Of the two, a fixed budget period is far more frequently used in the health care industry. A fixed budget covers some defined time from a given budget date, usually one year. This contrasts with a rolling budget, in which the budget is periodically extended on a frequent basis, usually a month or a quarter. For example, in a rolling budget period with a monthly update, the entity would always have a budget of at least 11 months in front of them. The same is not true in a fixed budget, in which, at fiscal year end, there may only be one week or one month left.

A rolling budget has a number of advantages, but it requires more time and effort and therefore more cost. Among its major advantages are

- more realistic forecasts, which should improve management planning and control
- equalization of the work load of budget development over the entire year
- improved familiarity and understanding of budgets by departmental managers

Flexible or Forecast Budgets

The use of a flexible budget versus a forecast budget has received much discussion among health care financial people. At the present time, very few hospitals and other health care facilities use a formal system of flexible budgeting. However, flexible budgeting is a more sophisticated method of budgeting than typical forecast budgeting and is being adopted by more and more health care facilities as they become experienced in the budgetary process.

A flexible budget is a budget that adjusts targeted levels of costs for changes in volume. For example, the budget for a nursing unit operating at 95 percent occupancy would be different than the budget for that same unit operating at an 80 percent occupancy. A forecast budget, in contrast, would make no formal differentiation in the allowed budget between these two levels.

The difference between a forecast and a flexible budget is illustrated by the historical data and projected use levels for the laboratory presented in Table 10–1. The forecast levels of volume in relative value units for 1987 are identical to the actual volumes of 1986, except that a 10 percent growth factor is assumed. The departmental manager using this statistics budget must develop a budget for hours worked in 1987. A common approach to this task is to assume that past work experience indicates future requirements. In this case, the average hours work required per relative value unit in 1986 was .5061. A common method for developing a forecast budget is to multiply this value of .5061 by the estimated total work load for the budget period, which is expected to be 72,160, and spread the total product equally over each of the 12 months. This is the forecast budget depicted in Table 10–2.

A major difference between a flexible and a forecast budget is that a flexible budget must recognize and incorporate underlying cost behavioral

Table 10–1 Laboratory Productivity Data

| | 1986 Actual | | 1987 |
	Hours Worked	RVUs	Expected RVUs
January	2,825	5,700	6,270
February	2,700	5,200	5,720
March	2,900	6,000	6,600
April	2,875	5,900	6,490
May	2,825	5,700	6,270
June	2,700	5,200	5,720
July	2,750	5,400	5,940
August	2,625	4,900	5,390
September	2,725	5,300	5,830
October	2,750	5,400	5,940
November	2,750	5,400	5,940
December	2,775	5,500	6,050
Total	33,200	65,600	72,160

Note: 1986 average hours/RVU $= \dfrac{33,200}{65,600} = .5061$

patterns. In this laboratory example, hours worked might be written as a function of relative value units:

Hours worked = (1,400 hours per month) + (.25 × relative value units)

Applying this formula to the budgeted RVUs expected in 1987 yields the flexible budget presented in Table 10–2.

Two points should be made before concluding our discussion of flexible versus forecast budgeting. First, a flexible budget may be represented as a forecast budget for planning purposes. For example, in the laboratory problem of Table 10–2, the flexible budget would provide an estimated hours-worked requirement of 34,837 hours for 1987. However, in an actual control period evaluation, the flexible budget formula would be used. To illustrate, assume that the actual RVUs provided in January 1987 were 6,500 instead of the forecasted 6,270. Budgeted hours in the flexible budget would then not be 2,967, but 3,025:

1,400 + (.25 × 6,500) = 3,025

This value would be compared with the actual hours worked, not the initially forecasted 2,967.

Second, dramatic differences in approved costs can result from the two methods. Recognizing the underlying cost behavioral patterns can change the

Table 10–2 Alternative Hours-Worked Budget for Laboratory

	Forecast Budget[a]	Flexible Budget[b]
January	3,043	2,967
February	3,043	2,830
March	3,043	3,050
April	3,043	3,022
May	3,043	2,967
June	3,043	2,830
July	3,043	2,885
August	3,043	2,747
September	3,043	2,857
October	3,043	2,885
November	3,043	2,885
December	3,043	2,912
Total	36,516	34,837

[a] $(.5061 \times 72{,}160)/12 = 3{,}043.35$
[b] January value = $(1{,}400) + (.25 \times 6{,}270)$

estimated resource requirements approved in the budgetary process. In our laboratory example in Table 10–2, the forecast budget calls for 36,516 hours versus the flexible budget hours requirement of 34,837. The difference results from the method used to estimate hours worked. In a forecast budget method, the prior average hours per RVU relationship is used. In most situations, average hours or average cost should be greater than variable hours or variable cost. In departments with expanding volume, the estimated requirements for resources could be overstated. The converse may be true in departments with declining volume. In many cases, use of forecast budgeting methods is based on the incorporation of prior average cost relationships. Flexible budgeting methods do not make this error, since their use depends on explicit incorporation of cost behavioral patterns that distinctly recognize variable and fixed costs.

Standards for Price and Quantity

Earlier, three factors were identified that can create differences between budgeted and actual costs: volume, prices, and usage or efficiency. The use of flexible budgeting is an attempt to improve the recognition of deviations caused by changes in volume. The use of standards for prices and wage rates, coupled with standards for physical quantities of usage, is an attempt to improve the recognition of deviations from budget that result from prices and usage.

For example, assume that the flexible budget-hours requirement for the laboratory example is still: hours worked = 1,400 + (.25 × RVUs). Assume further that the budget wage rate is $9 per hour and the actual RVUs for January 1987 were 6,500. Total payroll cost for hours worked (excluding vacations and sick pay) are assumed to be $31,000. If the actual hours worked were 3,100, the variance analysis report presented in Table 10–3 would be applicable to the laboratory department.

The total unfavorable variance of $3,775 results from a $3,100 unfavorable price variance and a $675 unfavorable efficiency variance. Splitting the variance in this manner helps management quickly identify possible causes. For example, the $3,100 price variance may be due to a negotiated wage increase of $1 per hour. If this is the case, the departmental manager is clearly not responsible for the variance. If, however, the difference is due to an excessive use of overtime personnel or a more costly mix of labor, then the manager may be held responsible for the difference and should attempt to prevent the problem from occurring again. The unfavorable efficiency variance of $675 reflects excessive use of the labor input during the month in the amount of 75 hours. An explanation for this difference should be sought and steps taken to prevent its recurrence.

Standard costing techniques have been used in industry for many years as an integral part of management control. Although it is true that input and output relationships may not be as objective in the health care industry as they are in general industry, this does not imply that standard costing cannot

---

Table 10–3 Standard Cost Variance Analysis for Labor Costs, Laboratory, January 1987

1. Price variance = (Actual hours worked) × (Actual wage rate)
    − (Actual hours worked) × (Budgeted wage rate)
    = (3,100 × $10.00) − (3,100 × $9.00)
    = $3,100 [Unfavorable]

2. Efficiency variance = (Actual hours worked) × (Budgeted wage rate)
    − (Budgeted hours worked) × (Budgeted wage rate)
    = (3,100 × $9.00) − (3,025 × $9.00)
    = $675 [Unfavorable]

3. Total variance = $3,100 + $675 = $3,775 [Unfavorable]
    Note: Actual wage rate = $31,000/3,100 = $10.00
    Budgeted wage rate = $9.00
    Actual hours worked = 3,100
    Budgeted hours worked = (1,400) + (.25 × 6,500) = 3,025

be used. In fact, there are many areas of activity within a health care facility that have fairly precise input-output relationships—housekeeping, laundry and linen, laboratory, radiology, and many others. Standard costing can prove to be a very valuable tool for cost control in the health care industry, if properly applied (this topic is explored in greater detail in Chapter 11).

Allocation of Indirect Costs

There has probably been more internal strife in organizations over the allocation of indirect costs than over any other single budgetary issue. A comment often heard is, "Why was I charged $3,000 for housekeeping services last month when my department didn't use anywhere near that level of service?"

A strong case can in fact be made for not allocating indirect costs in budget variance reports. In most normal situations, the receiving department has little or no control over the costs of the servicing department. Allocation may thus raise questions that should not be raised. While it is true that indirect costs need to be allocated for some decision-making purposes, such as pricing, they are generally not needed for evaluating individual responsibility center management.

However, an equally strong argument can be made for including indirect costs in the budgets of benefiting departments. They are legitimate costs of the total operation, and departmental managers should be aware of them. If departmental managers can influence costs in indirect areas by their decisions, they should be held accountable for them. For example, maintenance, housekeeping, and other indirect costs can be influenced by the decisions of benefiting departments. Ideally, a charge for these indirect services should be established and levied against using departments, based on their use. Labeling the cost of indirect areas as totally uncontrollable can stimulate excessive and unnecessary use of indirect services and thus have a negative impact on the total cost control program in an organization.

Revenue Budget

The revenue budget can be set effectively only after the expense budget and the statistics budget have been developed. The not-for-profit nature of the health care industry demands that revenue be related to budgeted expenses. Moreover, some of the total revenue actually realized by a health care facility is directly determined by expenses because of the presence of cost reimbursement formulas.

Rate Setting

In this discussion of the revenue budget, we shall focus on only one aspect of revenue budget development—pricing or rate setting. Specifically, we shall illustrate through an additional example the rate-setting model discussed in Chapter 8.

Figure 10–4 illustrates the rate-setting model. Sources of information to define the variables of the model are identified. However, three parameters have no identified source:

1. desired profit
2. proportion of charge payer patients
3. proportion of charge payer patient revenue not collected

In many situations, departmental indicators for these three values are not available. Instead, institution-wide values or averages are substituted. In many cases, this may not be a bad approximation, but some serious inequities can result in departments where the relative proportions of inpatient and outpatient use differ greatly. Typically, departments with high outpatient use experience higher levels of charge reimbursement and higher levels of write-offs on that charge reimbursement, due to the reduced presence of insurance coverage for outpatient types of services. Furthermore, the charge payer patient reimbursement in inpatient areas may be commercial insurance, subject to smaller write-offs. The following data illustrate this:

	Department 1	Department 2	Total
Desired profit	$ 500	$ 500	$ 1,000
Budgeted expense	$10,000	$10,000	$20,000
Estimated volume	100	100	—
Percentage bad debt	4%	20%	12%
Percentage charge payer patients	20%	60%	40%
Percentage bad debt on charge patients	20%	33%	30%

In most situations, separate figures for the percentage of write-offs on charge payer patients and the percentage of charge payers are not available on a departmental basis. Sometimes the best information available may be the percentage of bad debt write-offs on total revenue for the institution as a whole. In the above example, a 4 percent write-off on 20 percent of the patients who pay charges in Department #1 implies that 20 percent of the charge patient revenue in that department is written off. The corresponding figure for Department #2 is 33 percent. Using these data, and substituting the total or aggregate values for the percentage write-offs on charge patients

Figure 10–4 Rate Setting in the Revenue Budget

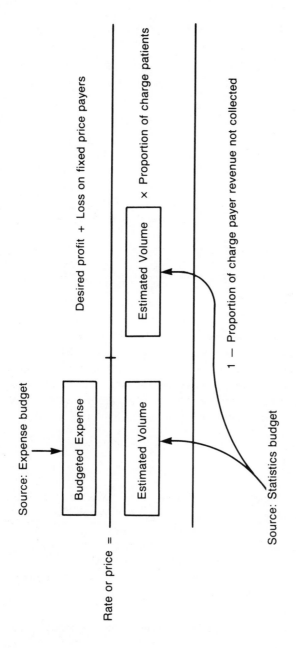

Source: Expense budget

$$\text{Rate or price} = \frac{\boxed{\text{Budgeted Expense}} + \text{Desired profit} + \text{Loss on fixed price payers}}{\boxed{\text{Estimated Volume}} \quad \boxed{\text{Estimated Volume} \times \text{Proportion of charge patients}}}$$

1 – Proportion of charge payer revenue not collected

Source: Statistics budget

Note: The two source items indicate where values for budgeted expense and estimated volume may be found.

and the percentage of charge patients, the following rates would be established:

$$\text{Department } \#1 \text{ price} = \frac{\dfrac{\$10,000}{100} + \dfrac{\$500}{100 \times .4}}{1 - .30} = \$160.71$$

$$\text{Department } \#2 \text{ price} = \frac{\dfrac{\$10,000}{100} + \dfrac{\$500}{100 \times .4}}{1 - .30} = \$160.71$$

However, proper reflection of the departmental values would show the following rates:

$$\text{Department } \#1 \text{ price} = \frac{\dfrac{\$10,000}{100} + \dfrac{\$500}{100 \times .2}}{1 - .2} = \$156.25$$

$$\text{Department } \#2 \text{ price} = \frac{\dfrac{\$10,000}{100} + \dfrac{\$500}{100 \times .6}}{1 - .33} = \$161.69$$

In the former case, the use of aggregate or average values produces an inequitable pricing structure. The price for Department #1 was initially overstated, while the price for Department #2 was initially understated. If equity in rate setting is an objective, reliance on average values can prevent the development of an equitable rate structure along departmental lines. In many cases, the errors may be significant.

Desired Profit Levels

Determining a desired level of profit is not easy. In many cases, it is a subjective process, made to appear objective through the application of a quantitative profit requirement. For example, desired profit may be arbitrarily set at some percentage of budgeted expenses, such as two percent above expenses, or as a certain percentage of total investment. However, desired levels of profit can, in general, be stated as the difference between financial requirements and expenses:

Desired profit = Budgeted financial requirements − Budgeted expenses

Budgeted financial requirements are cash requirements that an entity must meet during the budget period. There are four elements that usually constitute total budgeted financial requirements:

1. budgeted expenses, excluding depreciation
2. requirements for debt principal payment
3. requirements for increases in working capital
4. requirements for capital expenditures

Budgeted expenses at the departmental level should include both direct and indirect (or allocated) expenses. Depreciation charges are excluded because depreciation is a noncash requirement expense.

Debt principal payments include only the principal portion of debt service due. In some cases, additional reserve requirements may be established, which may require additional funding. Interest expense is already included in budgeted expenses and should not be included in debt principal payments.

Working capital requirements were discussed earlier. The maintenance of necessary levels of inventory, accounts receivable, and precautionary cash balances requires an investment. Changes in the total level of this investment must be funded from cash, additional indebtedness, or a combination of the two. Planned financing of increases in working capital is a legitimate financial requirement.

Capital expenditure requirements may be of two types. First, actual capital expenditures may be made for approved projects. Those projects not financed with indebtedness require a cash investment. Second, prudent fiscal management requires that funds be set aside and invested to meet reasonable requirements for future capital expenditures. This amount should be related to the replacement cost depreciation of existing fixed assets.

Any loss incurred on fixed price payers, such as Medicare, must be added to the desired profit target. The amount of the loss would represent the projected difference between allocated costs or expenses and net revenue received from fixed price payers. If revenues exceed costs, the difference would be subtracted from the profit target. For example, if a firm received $5,000,000 in revenue from Medicare and incurred $4,800,000 in costs to provide care to Medicare patients, the difference of $200,000 would be subtracted from the desired profit target. The result would obviously be lower required rates or prices. (Chapter 8 provides more detail on price setting.)

A logical question is, How is the desired profit requirement allocated to individual departments? Usually it is just assigned on the basis of some percentage of budgeted expenses. If a hospital budgets $5 million in expenses and determines that $500,000 profit is required, each department might set its rates to recover 10 percent above its expenses. However, the importance of cost reimbursement and bad debts at the departmental level should also be considered.

Discretionary Revenue Budget and Capital Budget

Discretionary revenue may be important, especially for institutions with large endowments. A good management control system will have a budget for expected return on endowments. Variations from the expected level would then be investigated. In some cases, changes in investment management may be necessary.

Capital budgeting can give many health care managers a major control tool. It can significantly affect the level of cost. This is especially true when not only the initial capital costs associated with given capital expenditures but also the associated operating costs for salaries and supplies are considered. (The capital budgeting process is examined in detail in the next chapter.)

The Cash Budget and Budgeted Financial Statements

The cash budget is management's best indicator of the organization's expected short-run solvency. It translates all of the above budgets into a statement of cash inflows and outflows. The cash budget is usually broken down by periods, such as months or quarters, within the total budget period. An example of a cash budget is shown in Table 10–4.

Departmental expense budgets, departmental revenue budgets, a discretionary revenue budget and a capital budget that do not provide a sufficient cash flow can necessitate major revisions. If the organization cannot or will not finance the deficits, changes must be made in the budgets to maintain the solvency of the organization. A poor cash budget could cause an increase in rates, a reduction in expenses, a reduction in capital expenditures, or many other changes. These changes and revisions must be made until the cash budget reflects a position of short-run solvency.

The two major financial statements that are developed on a budgetary basis are the balance sheet and the statement of revenue and expense. These two statements are indicators of both short- and long-run solvency; however they are more important in assessing long-run solvency. Unfavorable projections in either statement might cause changes in any of the other budgets.

In short, the budgeted financial statements and the cash budget test the adequacy of the entire budgetary process. Budgets that result in an unfavorable financial position, as reflected by the budgeted financial statements and the cash budget, must be adjusted. Solvency is a goal that most organizations cannot sacrifice.

Table 10–4 Cash Budget, Budget Year 1987

	1st Quarter			2nd Quarter	3rd Quarter	4th Quarter
	January	February	March			
Receipts from operations	$300,000	$310,000	$ 320,000	$1,000,000	$1,100,000	$1,100,000
Disbursements from operations	280,000	280,000	300,000	940,000	1,000,000	1,000,000
Cash available from operations	$ 20,000	$ 30,000	$ 20,000	$ 60,000	$ 100,000	$ 100,000
Other receipts						
Increase in mortgage payable				500,000		
Sale of fixed assets		20,000				
Unrestricted income—endowment	-0-		40,000	40,000	40,000	40,000
Total other receipts		$ 20,000	$ 40,000	$ 540,000	$ 40,000	$ 40,000
Other disbursements						
Mortgage payments			150,000		150,000	
Fixed asset purchase				480,000		
Funded depreciation			30,000	130,000	30,000	30,000
Total other disbursements		-0-	180,000	610,000	180,000	30,000
Net cash gain (loss)	$ 20,000	$ 50,000	$(120,000)	(10,000)	(40,000)	110,000
Beginning cash balance	100,000	120,000	170,000	50,000	40,000	-0-
Cumulative cash	$120,000	$170,000	$ 50,000	$40,000	$ -0-	$ 110,000
Desired level of cash	100,000	100,000	100,000	100,000	100,000	100,000
Cash above minimum needs (financing needs)	$ 20,000	$ 70,000	$ (50,000)	$ (60,000)	$(100,000)	$ 10,000

ZERO-BASE BUDGETING

Zero-base budgeting is a term that has recently gained publicity. It has been touted as management's most effective cost-containment tool. It has also been described as the biggest hoax of the century. The truth lies somewhere in the middle.

Zero-base budgeting or zero-base review, as some like to call it, is a way of looking at existing programs. It is part of programming, but it focuses on existing programs instead of new programs. Zero-base budgeting assumes that no existing program is entitled to automatic approval. Many individuals have identified automatic approval with existing budgetary systems that are based on prior year expenditure levels.

Zero-base budgeting looks at the entire budget and determines the efficacy of the entire expenditure. It thus requires a tremendous effort and investment of time. It cannot be done well on an annual basis. This is why many refer to it as zero-base review instead of zero-base budgeting. Some individuals have suggested that a zero-base review of a given activity would be appropriate every five years.

Zero-base budgeting is a process of periodically reevaluating all programs and their associated levels of expenditures. Management decides the frequency of this reevaluation and may vary it from every year to every five years.

Although most decision makers agree with the concept of zero-base budgeting, in practice it poses two significant questions:

1. What arithmetic should be used in zero-base budgeting?
2. Who should be involved in the actual decision-making process?

In each case, the answers are important to the success or failure of the zero-base budget program. Yet there is still not complete agreement among experts regarding the answers.

In this section, we present what we believe to be the basis of the zero-base budgeting concept in terms of the above two questions. We shall illustrate our discussion with a case example of an actual application of the concept in the data-processing department of a hospital. In this example, significant savings were realized through the application of zero-base budgeting.

Arithmetic of the Zero-Base Budgeting Process

Nearly everyone would agree that cost benefit analysis should be the arithmetic of zero-base budgeting. There are two important issues involved in the application of cost benefit analysis to zero base budgeting programs: (1) Are the services that are presently provided being delivered in an efficient manner? (2) Are these services being delivered in an effective manner in terms of the organization's goals and objectives? A procedure for quantitatively answering these two questions involves seven sequential steps:

1. Define the outputs or services provided by the program/departmental area.
2. Determine the costs of these services or outputs.
3. Identify options for reducing the cost through changes in outputs or services.
4. Identify options for producing the services and outputs more efficiently.
5. Determine the cost savings associated with options identified in Steps 3 and 4.
6. Assess the risks, both qualitative and quantitative, associated with the identified options of Steps 3 and 4.
7. Select and implement those options with an acceptable cost/risk relationship.

Definition of Outputs

Table 10–5 lists outputs provided by the data processing department in our case example. Six basic functions or service areas are identified:

1. outpatient systems
2. inpatient systems
3. step-down
4. month-end
5. accounts payable
6. payroll

Determining the specific outputs of each of these areas, as shown in Table 10–5, is, in general, a useful procedure. And determining the basic factors involved in the establishment and maintenance of each department and program is a good first step in defining specific outputs.

Table 10-5 Data Processing Outputs and Costs

	Pages	Runs Per Year	Copies	Total Pages	Weighted Pages	$.0113/pg. Direct Supply Cost	$.2894/wtd. pg.cost Labor&Mach.	Total Cost	Cost Reductions
I. OUTPATIENT SYSTEM									
A. Outpatient Maintenance Report	2	365	4	2,920	1,460	$33.00	$422.49	$455.49	($8.25)
B. Outpatient Error Listing for Admissions	2	365	4	2,920	1,460	33.00	422.49	455.49	(8.25)
C. Outpatient Initial Edit Summary	1	365	4	1,460	730	16.50	211.24	227.74	(4.13)
1. Admissions Summary Total	1	365	4	1,460	730	16.50	211.24	227.74	(4.13)
2. Initial Cash Edit	1								
3. Additional Patients Added to Outpatient History		365	4	1,460	730	16.50	211.24	227.74	(4.13)
D. Daily Transaction Audit Report—Charges	11	365	4	16,060	8,030	181.48	2,323,69	2505.17	(45.37)
E. Outpatient Posting Control	40	365	4	58,400	29,200	659.92	8,449.78	9,189.70	(164.95)
F. Daily Revenue Report	42	365	4	61,320	30,660	692.92	8,872.27	9,565.19	(9,565.19)

Table 10–5 continued

	Pages	Runs Per Year	Copies	Total Pages	Weighted Pages	$.0113/pg. Direct Supply Cost	$.2894/wtd. pg. cost Labor&Mach.	Total Cost	Cost Reductions
G. Outpatient Billing Balance	4	365	4	5,840	2,920	65.99	844.98	910.27	(16.50)
H. Patients Transferred to AR/History File	5	365	4	7,300	3,650	82.49	1,056.22	1,138.71	(20.62)
I. Cash Receipts and Adjustments Report	3	365	4	4,380	2,190	49.49	633.73	683.22	(12.37)
J. AR Transaction Audit	5	365	4	7,300	3,650	82.49	1,056.22	1,138.71	(20.62)
K. AR Error Listing	4	365	4	1,460	730	16.50	211.24	227.74	(4.13)
L. Self-Pay Patient Statement*	100	365	1	36,500	36,500	3,650.00	10,562.22	14,212.22	
M. Revenue and Usage Statistics	42	365	2	30,660	30,660	346.46	8,872.27	9,218.73	
N. General Journal	3	12	2	72	72	81	20.84	21.65	
O. Outpatient Edit Report	5	12	2	120	120	1.36	34.73	36.09	
P. Outpatient Activity Trial Balance	2,500	12	2	60,000	60,000	678.00	17,362.56	18,040.56	
Q. Outpatient Alpha Listing (Telephone)	800	52	4	166,400	83,200	1,880.32	24,076.08	25,906.00	(25,956.40)
R. Outpatient Alpha Listing (Balance)	800	52	4	166,400	83,200	1,880.32	24,076.08	25,956.40	(25,956.40)

Table 10-5 continued

	Pages	Runs Per Year	Copies	Total Pages	Weighted Pages	$.0113/pg. Direct Supply Cost	$.2894/wtd. pg. cost Labor&Mach.	Total Cost	Cost Reductions
II. INPATIENT SYSTEM									
A. Final Census Report	27	365	4	39,420	19,710	$ 445.45	$5,703.60	$6,149.05	($222.75)
B. Volunteer Alpha Listing	6	365	3	6,570	4,380	74.24	1,267.47	1,341.71	
C. Alphabetic Census	6	365	6	13,140	4,380	148.48	1,267.47	1,415.95	
D. Financial Class Census Report	10	365	2	7,300	7,300	82.49	2,112.44	2,194.93	(2,194.93)
E. Utilization Census	6	365	4	8,760	4,380	98.99	1,267.47	1,366.46	(50.00)
F. Social Services Census	10	365	1	3,650	7,300	41.25	2,112.44	2,153.69	
G. Statistical Census Reports	2	365	3	2,190	1,460	24.75	422.49	447.24	(447.24)
H. Clergy Listing	15	365	1	5,475	10,950	61.87	3,168.69	3,230.54	
I. Admission, Discharge and Transfer Report	4	365	8	11,680	2,920	131.98	844.98	976.96	
J. Pap Smear Admissions Control Report	1	365	2	730	730	8.25	211.24	219.49	
K. Census by H-ICDA Code	7	365	2	5,110	5,110	57.74	1,478.71	1,536.45	
L. Daily Charge Transaction Error Listing	5	365	1	1,825	3,650	20.62	1,056.22	1,076.84	

Table 10–5 continued

	Pages	Runs Per Year	Copies	Total Pages	Weighted Pages	$.0113/pg. Direct Supply Cost	$.2894/wtd. pg. cost Labor&Mach.	Total Cost	Cost Reductions
M. Daily Transaction	44	365	1	16,060	32,120	181.48	9,294.76	9,476.24	
N. Daily Dialysis Report	1	365	2	730	730	8.25	211.24	219.49	
O. Inpatient Billing Balance	8	365	2	5,840	5,840	65.99	1,689.96	1,755.95	
P. Outpatient Billing Balance—Dialysis	2	365	2	1,460	1,460	16.50	422.49	438.99	
Q. Summary Patient Statement*	50	365	2	36,500	36,500	1,825.00	10,562.22	12,387.22	
R. Detail Patient Statement*	50	365	2	36,500	36,500	1,825.00	10,562.22	12,387.22	
S. Noncovered Charges	10	365	1	3,650	7,300	41.25	2,112.44	2,153.69	
T. New Accounts Receivable Report	3	365	2	2,190	2,190	24.75	633.73	658.48	
U. Cash Receipts and Adjustments	10	365	3	10,950	7,300	123.74	2,112.44	2,236.18	
V. AR Transaction Audit	10	365	2	7,300	7,300	82.49	2,112.44	2,194.93	
W. Daily Error Listing	3	365	2	2,190	2,190	24.75	633.73	658.48	
X. Schedule of PreAdmission	3	365	2	2,190	2,190	24.75	633.73	658.48	
Y. Medicaid Review Census	2	365	2	1,460	1,460	16.50	422.49	438.99	

Table 10-5 continued

	Pages	Runs Per Year	Copies	Total Pages	Weighted Pages	$.0113/pg. Direct Supply Cost	$.2894/wtd. pg. cost Labor&Mach.	Total Cost	Cost Reductions
III. STEP DOWN									
A. Step Down Cost Center Description Table	2	12	2	48	48				
B. Step Down Allocations Master File	2	12	2	48	48	$ .54	$ 13.89	$ 14.93	
C. Step Down Direct Expense Edit	2	12	2	48	48	.54	13.89	14.43	
D. Step Down Cost Allocation Statistics File	2	12	2	48	48	.54	13.89	14.93	
E. Step Down Cost Allocation—Periodic	2	12	2	48	48	.54	13.89	14.93	
IV. MONTH END									
A. Cummulative Monthly Statistical Census	1	12	2	24	24	.27	6.95	7.22	
B. Monthly Statistical Census by Day	1	12	2	24	24	.27	6.95	7.22	
C. Infection Control Report	1	12	2	24	24	.27	6.95	7.22	

Table 10-5 continued

	Pages	Runs Per Year	Copies	Total Pages	Weighted Pages	$.0113/pg. Direct Supply Cost	$.2894/wtd. pg. cost Labor&Mach.	Total Cost	Cost Reductions
D. Reimbursement Summary	1	12	2	24	24	.27	6.95	7.22	
E. Revenue and Usage Statistics	65	12	2	1,560	1,560	17.63	451.43	469.06	
F. Aged Accounts Receivable Summary	1	12	2	24	24	.27	6.95	7.22	
G. Detail Trial Balance	105	12	2	2,520	2,520	28.48	729.22	757.70	
H. In-House 21 Days Billing	25	12	2	600	600	6.78	173.63	180.41	
I. Dialysis Billing	89	12	2	2,136	2,136	24.14	618.11	642.25	
J. Zero Balance Roster	742	12	4	35,616	17,808	402.46	5,153.21	5,555.67	($5555.67)
K. Bad Debt Report	35	12	2	840	840	9.49	243.08	252.57	
L. General Journal	5	12	2	120	120	1.36	34.73	36.09	
V. ACCOUNTS PAYABLE SYSTEM									
A. Vendor Master Maintenance Report	2	156	2	624	624	7.05	180.57	187.62	
B. AP Initial Edit Listing	1	156	2	312	312	3.53	90.29	93.82	

Table 10–5 continued

	Pages	Runs Per Year	Copies	Total Pages	Weighted Pages	$.0113/pg. Direct Supply Cost	$.2894/wtd. pg. cost Labor&Mach.	Total Cost	Cost Reductions
C. AP Batch Proof	1	156	2	312	312	3.53	90.29	93.82	
D. Cash Requirements Report	50	12	2	1,200	1,200	13.56	347.25	360.81	
E. AP Monthly Reconciliation	30	12	2	720	720	8.14	208.35	216.49	
F. AP Distribution	23	12	2	552	552	6.24	159.74	165.98	
G. AP Trial Balance	50	12	2	1,200	1,200	13.56	347.25	360.81	
H. Vendor Master Listing	2	12	2	48	48	.54	13.89	14.43	
VI. PAYROLL									
A. Payroll Edit Summary									
1. Payroll Update Controls	1	104	2	208	208	$ 2.35	$ 60.19	$ 62.54	
2. Payroll Master File Maintenance	10	104	2	2,080	2,080	23.50	601.90	625.40	
B. Time Card Edit Report	60	52	4	12,480	6,240	141.02	1,805.71	1,946.73	
C. Check Register	58	52	2	6,032	6,032	68.16	1,745.52	1,813.68	
D. Department Benefits Statement	60	52	4	12,480	6,240	141.02	1,805.71	1,946.73	
E. Labor Analysis Report	42	52	2	4,368	4,368	49.36	1,263.99	1,313.35	

Table 10-5 continued

	Pages	Runs Per Year	Copies	Total Pages	Weighted Pages	$.0113/pg. Direct Supply Cost	$.2894/wtd. pg. cost Labor&Mach.	Total Cost	Cost Reductions
F. Payroll Journal Report	10	12	1	120	240	1.36	69.45	70.81	
G. Quarterly 941 Report	27	4	2	216	216	2.44	62.51	64.95	
H. W-2 Forms	1,091	1	1	1,091	2,182	12.33	631.42	643.75	
I. Time Cards*	1,091	52	1	56,732	56,732	4,252.50	16,416.88	20,669.38	($10,334.69)
J. Standard Payroll Checks*	1,091	52	1	56,732	56,732	3,373.65	16,416.88	19,710.53	(9,855.26)
K. Miscellaneous Reports									
1. Employee Longevity Report	10	12	2	240	240	2.70	69.45	72.15	
2. YTD Earnings Report	1,091	4	2	8,728	8,728	98.68	2,525.67	2,524.29	
3. Union Dues Paid	8	12	2	192	192	2.17	55.56	57.73	
4. Estimated Yearly Budget Report by Status and by Grade									
5. Sick Hour Control Report (not done)	60	1	1	60	120	68	34.73	35.41	

Table 10–5 continued

	Pages	Runs Per Year	Copies	Total Pages	Weighted Pages	$.0113/pg. Direct Supply Cost	$.2894/wtd. pg. cost Labor&Mach.	Total Cost	Cost Reductions
6. Prepaid Checks	20	104	1	2,080	2,080	138.76	601.90	740.66	
7. LPN Listing	2	2	2	8	8	.09	2.31	2.40	
8. Employee Address Labels (30/page)	30	2	1	60	60	.68	17.17	17.85	
9. Century Club Membership Labels*(not done)									
				1,077,885	778,900	$24,702.00	$225,367.00	$250,069.00	($90,138.00)

*Items for which supplies were directly costed.
Total pages for these items were 225,044 and total direct supply cost was $15,065.

Determination of Costs

The concept of cost that is most relevant in zero-base budgeting is avoidable cost. An attempt is made to discover what the costs of a department's services are now and what cost would be incurred if those services were discontinued. In this context, the direct cost of the department is most useful. Indirect cost in most situations should be ignored because it is unavoidable. In our data processing case example, the three direct cost components are supply cost, labor and machine cost, and other. Of these three, only labor and machine cost and supply cost can be avoided, given a reduction in services.

The average supply cost per page was derived by dividing total supply cost, less supply cost that could be traced to a specific report, by the total number of pages, less pages associated with reports for which supply cost could be directly traced:

$$\text{Supply cost/Page} = \frac{\$24,702 - \$15,065}{1,077,885 - 225,044} = \$.0113$$

The six reports for which supply cost was directly traceable are:

		System
1.	self-pay patient statement	I-L
2.	summary patient statement	II-Q
3.	detail patient statement	II-R
4.	time cards	VI-I
5.	standard payroll checks	VI-J
6.	prepaid checks	VI-K(1)

Labor and machine cost is divided by weighted pages to determine cost per weighted page. Weighted pages is an index that reflects the fact that little or no additional labor and machine cost is incurred for multiple copies of reports. The index uses a base report of two copies to provide the conversion. Thus, a four-copy report consisting of 3 pages would require 12 total pages, but it would be stated as a 6-page report when expressed in weighted pages. In certain situations, the index is modified to reflect a more realistic assessment of cost variation. In our data-processing department, the labor and machine cost per weighted page was

$$\text{Labor and machine cost/Weighted page} = \frac{\$225,367}{778,900} = \$.2894$$

Options for Modifying Output

Table 10–6 identifies 11 options for modifying the output of the data processing department. Typical output changes could occur through elimination of the service, reduction in the frequency of the service, reduction in the quality of service, or reduction in the amount of service. All of these types of changes, except reduction in quality, occurred in the data processing case example.

Options for Producing Services More Efficiently

Only after some determination of the need for services is made can efficiency be seriously examined. In our case example, there are no efficiency options identified. Yet the identification of improved ways to provide services

Table 10–6 Options for Reducing Output in a Data Processing Department

Option	Risk	Savings
1. Reduce outpatient report copies I-A-K from four copies to three copies per day.	small	$ 314.48
2. Change usage demand on outpatient report I-F from daily to monthly.	small	9,251.02
3. Eliminate two copies of inpatient report II-A—Final census.	small	222.75
4. Discontinue inpatient report II-D— Financial class census.	small	2,194.93
5. Eliminate two copies of inpatient report I-E—Utilization census.	small	50.00
6. Eliminate outpatient report I-Q—Alpha listing with telephone number.	small	25,956.40
7. Eliminate outpatient report I-R—Alpha listing with balance.	small	25,956.40
8. Eliminate inpatient report II-G— Statistical census.	small	447.24
9. Eliminate zero balance roster report— Month end, Report II-J	small	5,555.67
10. Pay biweekly rather than weekly; cut preparation and usage of time cards by 50%	medium	10,334.69
11. Pay biweekly rather than weekly; reduce paychecks preparation and usage by 50%.	medium	9,855.26
Total estimated savings		$90,138.84

is an important activity in efforts to minimize costs. In a complete zero-base review, efficiency should be considered.

Determination of Cost Savings

Table 10–6 also identifies the cost savings associated with the options for modifying the output of the data processing department. Avoidable cost is the cost concept that is used. The savings are limited to just supply costs when a report is not discontinued but only the number of copies is changed. When a report is discontinued or its frequency is reduced, then labor and machine costs are also reflected in the savings to be realized. Some may question whether significant labor and machine savings could be realized in changes this small. Since many costs of this type are step or semifixed, the actual incremental cost associated with a very slight reduction in volume may indeed be negligible. Still, in reviews of this type, where significant changes in work effort are envisioned, the average cost estimate may be a reasonable expectation of savings. In this example, total cost savings from the identified 11 options is projected to be approximately $90,000.

Risk Assessment

Risk is a function of two factors: the probability of an adverse consequence and the potential severity of that consequence. In most situations, both these factors are highly subjective. Nevertheless, some idea of risk, even subjectively determined, is necessary in the overall assessment of the option's desirability.

Management Decision Making

After concluding the above analysis, someone needs to make decisions concerning the specific options to be selected. This responsibility falls to those in the management structure who are involved in the zero-base review.

In general, with regard to management's participation in the decision-making process of a zero-base budgeting program, three major aspects must be considered:

1. In the case of general service or indirect departments, panels of managers from the using departments should be involved in identifying options for changes in outputs. These individuals have an obvious

interest in and a need to know the changes that are likely to be made. In addition, their assessment of risk is important.

2. Individuals from the specific program area under evaluation should also be involved in the zero-base review. Their involvement is essential for two reasons: (1) In many cases, the best ideas for changes in output or methods of production will come from those who are intimately involved in the delivery of the product. (2) Participation of these individuals in the review process will help ensure cooperation in any decisions that are made.

3. Final decisions on options should be made by top management because it has a total perspective of the organization. Placing responsibility in lower level management may create problems of suboptimization.

SUMMARY

This chapter has focused specifically on budgeting and management control as practiced at the institutional or organizational level. The basic unit in management control is usually a department. However, the application of the principles of management control can be much broader. The control unit may be an entire hospital or region, and the controller may be a health system agency or a rate-setting organization. Even on this broad scale, the general principles of management control and budgeting discussed in this chapter are applicable.

ASSIGNMENTS

1. Under what conditions is a flexible budget likely to be more effective than a forecast budget?

2. Can an organization be efficient but not effective? Discuss the circumstances in which this could be true.

3. The first step in the budgeting process is to develop the statistics budget. Why is this true?

4. Ann Walker, CPA, is the controller for your hospital. For a long time, Ms. Walker has been concerned about management control in the hospital, and she has finally developed a new departmental labor control system. It is based on the following data for the obstetrics nursing unit:

Period	Patient Days	Hours Worked	Rate	Total Cost
1	350	1,550	$4.50	$ 6,975
2	400	1,700	4.60	7,820
3	300	1,400	4.40	6,160
4	375	1,625	4.60	7,475
5	450	1,850	4.60	8,510
Total	1,875	8,125		$36,940

Average rate = $4.55 = $36,940/8,125

Average hours/Patient day = 4.33 = 8,125/1,875

Using these data, Ms. Walker developed a two-factor variance model for labor costs in the obstetrics department. In Period 1, the variances in this model would be as follows:

Labor rate variance = ($4.50 - $4.55) $\times$ 1,550 = $77.50 (Favorable)

Labor usage variance = (1,550 - 1,515.5) $\times$ $4.55 = $156.98 (Unfavorable)

A similar model for labor control has been adopted in all other departments. As the chief executive officer of the hospital, are you satisfied with this labor control system? What suggestions for revisions would you make?

5. Floyd Farley is the maintenance department head. His department is participating in a wage incentive program in which he and his staff receive 20 percent of the department's income as supplemental income. Net income is defined as $12 times maintenance man hours charged, less direct departmental expense. Do you see any problems with this system? If so, how might they be solved?

6. You have been asked to prepare a flexible budget for a 40-bed nursing unit. A schedule of staffing requirements by occupancy is presented below:

Schedule of Personnel Requirements

	Below 60% Occupancy	60–80% Occupancy	80–100% Occupancy
First shift			
Head nurse	1	1	1
Registered nurse	1	1	2
Licensed practical nurse	1	1	1
Aides	1	2	2
Second shift			
Registered nurse	2	2	2
Licensed practical nurse	1	1	1
Aides	2	3	3

	Below 60% Occupancy	60–80% Occupancy	80–100% Occupancy
Third shift			
Registered nurse	1	1	1
Licensed practical nurse	1	1	1
Aides	0	1	2

Daily personnel costs by job title and shift:

Head nurse	$70
Registered nurse—First shift	54
Second and third shift	62
Licensed practical nurse—First shift	34
Second and third shift	40
Aides—First shift	28
Second and third shift	30

Prepare a budget for management that shows expected personnel costs for this nursing unit by occupancy level.

7. You must establish a pricing schedule for laboratory procedures. From a total hospital perspective, management has decided that the hospital must earn five percent above costs. The hospital has established that they lose ten percent on each fixed-price payer (Medicare or Medicaid). That is, for every $100 of cost incurred to treat a fixed-price payer, the hospital receives only $90 in payment. You must build both the required profit and the expected loss on fixed-price payers into your rate structure. Payer mix for the laboratory is expected to be as follows:

	Budgeted Relative Value Units (RVUs)		
	Inpatient	Outpatient	Total
Medicare	200,000	50,000	250,000
Medicaid	40,000	10,000	50,000
Blue Cross	80,000	20,000	100,000
Commercial insurance and HMOs	60,000	10,000	70,000
Bad debt and charity	15,000	15,000	30,000
Total RVUs	395,000	105,000	500,000

Medicare pays on a fixed price per DRG for all inpatients. There is thus no separate payment for laboratory tests. Medicaid pays average cost for both inpatient and outpatient tests. Medicare also pays average costs for outpatient tests. Blue Cross pays 95 percent of charges for both inpatient and outpatient procedures. All other commercial insurance and HMO patients pay 100 percent of charges. If budgeted expenses are $1,000,000 ($2.00 per RVU), what price must be set to meet management's profit expectations?

8. How would you calculate the amount of revenue to be realized as cash from patient sources in a fiscal period?

9. What is the major conceptual difference between zero-base budgeting and conventional budgeting?

10. In a hospital operation, what key variables are important in projecting volume at departmental levels?

SOLUTIONS AND ANSWERS

1. Two conditions are necessary for a flexible budget to be more useful than a forecast budget: First, there must be some indication that costs are variable, at least in part. Second, there must be some variability in activity levels, that is, volume is not expected to be constant in each period.

2. Efficiency relates to the costs per unit of output produced. Effectiveness relates to the attainment of organizational objectives given its outputs. It is quite possible for a firm to be efficient but not effective. For example, a hospital might provide inpatient care at an extremely low cost. However, this might not be effective if the provision of the inpatient care is at rates that threaten the hospital's goal of financial solvency.

3. Figure 10–3 indicates that the statistics budget provides input for the development of the expense budget and the revenue budget. Projection of both expenses and revenues is a function of expected volume and variability of volume over the budget period. In cases where volume is expected to vary significantly, management may try to make more of their costs variable to maximize their ability to control costs, given volume changes. For example, more variable staffing may be used through the use of part-time employees, nursing pools, or overtime.

4. The primary weakness of Ms. Walker's model is its failure to incorporate fixed labor requirements. A flexible budgeting system should be put into effect instead. Using a high-low method, the following budget parameters for hours required can be estimated:

$$\text{Variable hours} = \frac{1,850 - 1,400}{450 - 300} = 3.0 \text{ hours per patient day}$$

Fixed hours per period = $1,850 - 3.0 \times 450 = 500$ hours per period

The deviation in hours worked per period is removed when the fixed labor requirement is recognized:

Period	Actual Hours	Budgeted Hours (500 + 3.0 × PD)	Difference
1	1,550	1,550	0
2	1,700	1,700	0
3	1,400	1,400	0
4	1,625	1,625	0
5	1,850	1,850	0

5. Mr. Farley has an incentive to engage his staff in what might be needless maintenance. This could be controlled by setting limits on the absolute level of incentive payment that could be earned, for example, by basing the incentive payments on the difference between actual and budgeted costs or by establishing control systems for authorizing maintenance work.

6. The following budget could be developed to show daily standard personnel costs by occupancy level for the nursing unit:

	Occupancy		
	Below 60%	60–80%	80–100%
First shift			
Head nurse	$70	$70	$ 70
Registered nurse	54	54	108
Licensed practical nurse	34	34	34
Aides	28	56	56
Second shift			
Registered nurse	124	124	124
Licensed practical nurse	40	40	40
Aides	60	90	90
Third shift			
Registered nurse	62	62	62
Licensed practical nurse	40	40	40
Aides	0	30	60
Total Standard Personnel Costs	$512	$600	$684

7. Using the formula in Figure 10–4, the following rate structure can be established to meet management's profit expectations:

$$\text{Price} = \frac{\frac{\$1,000,000}{500,000} + \frac{(\$50,000 + \$40,000)}{500,000 \times .40}}{1 - .175} = \$2.9697$$

Desired profit = .05 × $1,000,000 = $50,000

Loss on fixed price payers = .4 × $1,000,000 × .10 = $40,000

Proportion of charge payers = (100,000 + 70,000 + 30,000)/500,000 = .40

Proportion of charge payers

$$\text{Revenue not collected} = \frac{30,000 + .05 \times 100,000}{100,000 + 70,000 + 30,000} = .175$$

Medicare inpatient (.4 × $1,000,000 × .9)	$ 360,000
Medicare outpatient (.1 × $1,000,000)	100,000
Medicaid (.1 × $1,000,000)	100,000
Blue Cross (100,000 × $2.9697 × .95)	282,121
Commercial insurance and HMO (70,000 × $2.9697)	207,879
Bad debt and charity	0
Total revenue	$1,050,000
Less expenses	1,000,000
Budget profit	$ 50,000

8. Cash realized from patient sources could be expressed as follows:

Cash flow = Net patient revenue + Beginning patient accounts receivable
— Ending patient account receivables

9. Zero-base budgeting starts from a zero base. That is, all expenditures must be justified in the budgeting review. Conventional budgeting looks primarily at expenditures that are above prior levels.

10. The volume of actual cases treated (discharges or admissions) and outpatient activity are the key variables that affect departmental volumes. For example, laboratory tests are usually related to discharges and outpatient visits. Patient days are derived from discharges by assuming an average length of stay. Refinements in forecasting can be achieved by projecting case mix. Finally, more or fewer ancillary services per discharge may be required, depending on the type of case.

Chapter 11

Cost Variance Analysis

Cost variance analysis is of great potential importance to the health care industry. Successful utilization of cost variance analysis requires the existence of a sound system of standard setting, or budgeting, and a related system of cost accounting. Perhaps the major factor impeding the widespread adoption of more effective cost variance analysis in the health care industry has been the lack of interaction between it and our systems of cost accounting.

Cost accounting systems usually serve two basic informational needs. First, they supply data essential for product/service costing. Second, they provide information for managerial cost control activity. This second role is the major topic of this chapter.

COST CONTROL

The following conceptual model will be used to discuss the major alternatives to cost control in organizations:

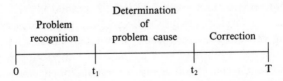

In general, there are three distinct time phases in an out-of-control situation:

1. recognition of problem (0 to t_1)
2. determination of problem cause (t_1 to t_2)
3. correction of problem (t_2 to T)

The unit of time used in the above representation may be minutes, hours, days, weeks, or even months. The important point is that, the longer the problem remains uncorrected (0 to T), the greater the cost to the organization.

The term *efficiency cost* is sometimes used to describe the total cost incurred by an organization from an out-of-control situation. Efficiency cost may be represented as follows:

$$\text{Efficiency cost} = T \times R \times P$$

where:

T = total time units that the problem remains uncorrected
R = loss or cost per time unit
P = probability that the problem occurrence is correctible

The objective of management should be to minimize the efficiency cost in any given situation. In the accomplishment of this objective, two major alternatives are available to management: (1) the preventive approach and (2) the detection-correction (DC) approach.

In the preventive approach, management attempts to minimize the efficiency cost by minimizing the probability of a problem occurring (P). One of the major methods for reducing the value of P centers on staffing. Management attempts not only to hire the most competent individuals available but also to provide them with relevant training programs and materials to ensure consistently high levels of performance. The nature of the reward structure, both monetary and nonmonetary, also enters into this management strategy. The preventive approach is obviously employed by most organizations, but the emphasis on it is usually greater in small organizations. In these organizations, the control span is usually smaller and the evaluation of individual performance is more direct.

The DC approach seeks to minimize efficiency cost by minimizing the time that a problem remains uncorrected (T). This method is directly related to the effectiveness of variance analysis. Effective variance analysis should result in a reduction of both the recognition of problem phase (0 to t_1) and the determination of cause phase (t_1 to t_2). The actual correction phase (t_2 to T) rests primarily upon the effective motivation of management.

The development of cost variance analysis systems to reduce the recognition and determination phases usually involves the expenditure of funds. Prudent management dictates that the marginal expenditures of funds for system improvements be evaluated by their expected reductions in efficiency cost. For example, the frequency of reporting could be altered to reduce the problem recognition phase, or the number of cost areas reported could be increased to improve both recognition and determination times. However, these improvements are likely to result in increased cost and may not be justified. Areas of relatively small dollar expenditure or largely uncontrolled costs are thus not prime candidates for major system improvements.

INVESTIGATION OF VARIANCES

In the DC approach to cost control, cost variances are the clues that both signal a potential problem exists and suggest a possible cause. These variances are usually an integral part of any management-by-exception plan of operations. A decision to investigate a given variance is not an automatic occurrence. It involves some financial commitment by the organization and thus should be weighed carefully against the expected benefits. Unfortunately, management rarely knows whether any given variance is due to a random or noncontrollable cause, or to an underlying problem that is correctible or controllable.

Many organizations have developed rules to determine which variances will be investigated. Common examples of such rules are to investigate:

- all variances that exceed an absolute dollar size (for example, $500)
- all variances that exceed budgeted or standard values by some fixed percent (for example, ten percent)
- all variances that have been unfavorable for a defined number of periods (for example, three periods)
- some combination of the above

Actual specification of criteria values in the above rules is highly dependent upon management judgment and experience. A variance of $1,000 may be considered normal in some circumstances and abnormal in others.

At some point, management may wish to determine whether the historical criteria values should be changed. In that case, some method of testing whether the historic values are acceptable or not acceptable must be developed. In general, there are two possible theories that may be used to develop this information, (1) classical statistical theory and (2) decision theory.

Classical Statistical Theory

One of the most commonly employed means to determine which cost variances to investigate is the control chart. The control chart is often used to monitor a physical process by comparing output observations with predetermined tolerance limits. If actual observations fall between predetermined upper and lower control limits on the chart, the process is assumed to be in control.

Control charts can be established for determining when a cost variance should be investigated. The major assumption underlying the traditional development of control charts is that observed cost variances are distributed in accordance with a normal probability distribution. In a normal distribution, it can be anticipated that approximately 68.3 percent of the observations will fall within one standard deviation (σ) of the mean ($\bar{x}$), 95.5 percent will fall within two standard deviations ($\bar{x} \pm 2\sigma$), and 99.7 percent will fall within three standard deviations ($\bar{x} \pm 3\sigma$).

The control limits for any given variance will then be set at:

$$\bar{x} \pm K\sigma$$

If the costs of investigation are high relative to the benefits in a given situation, then K may be set to a high value (for example, 3.0). This will ensure that few investigations will be made and that some out-of-control situations may be continued. Conversely, if benefits are high relative to the costs of investigation, then lower values of K may be selected that will ensure that more investigations will be performed and that some individuals in control situations will be investigated.

To develop the control chart, the underlying distribution must be specified. An assumption that the distribution is normal means that the analyst must define both the mean ($\bar{x}$) and the standard deviation (σ). In most situations, this specification will result from an analysis of prior observations. To illustrate this process, assume that the following pattern of labor variances occurred during the 13 biweekly pay periods:

Pay Period	Variance (x_i)
1	800
2	400
3	– 500
4	– 100
5	200
6	– 700
7	500
8	– 300
9	– 200
10	300
11	200
12	– 200
13	– 400
	0

The mean ($\bar{x}$) of these observations is calculated as follows:

$$\bar{x} = \frac{\Sigma x_i}{n} = \frac{0}{13} = 0$$

An estimate of the standard deviation (s) is calculated as follows:

$$s = \sqrt{\frac{\Sigma(x_i - \bar{x})^2}{n-1}} = \$437.80$$

If the labor cost variances in this example are expected to follow a normal distribution in the future with $\bar{x} = 0$ and $\sigma = \$437.80$, control limits for investigation at the 95 percent level could be defined by multiplying the estimated standard deviation by two. The following control chart would result:

$$\bar{x} + 2\sigma = 875.60$$
$$\bar{x} = 0$$
$$\bar{x} - 2\sigma = -875.60$$

Any observation falling within the control limits would not be investigated, while variances falling outside the established limits would be investigated.

The major deficiency in the classical statistical approach is that it does not relate the expected costs of investigation and benefits with the probability that the variance signals are out of control. The control chart can signal when a situation is likely to be out of control, but it cannot directly evaluate whether an investigation is warranted.

Decision Theory

Decision theory provides a framework for directly integrating the probability of the system being out of control and the costs and benefits of investigation into a definite decision rule. Central to this approach is the payoff table, which specifically considers costs and benefits. An example of a payoff table is presented below:

	States	
Actions	In Control	Out of Control
Investigate	I	I + C
Do not investigate	O	L

where:

I = cost of investigation
C = cost of correcting an out-of-control situation
L = cost of letting an out-of-control situation continue
   (expected loss)

The payoff table is a conceptualization of the actual decision evaluation process. It may be applied in any cost variance situation. The objective is to minimize the actual cost for a given situation. To accomplish this, estimates of the probabilities for the two states, in control and out-of-control, are required.

Assume that P denotes the probability that the system is in control and that (1–P) represents the probability that the system is out of control. The expected cost of the two courses of action can be defined as follows:

Expected cost of investigating	$= (P \times I) + (1-P)(I+C)$ $= I + (1-P)C$
Expected cost of not investigating	$= (P \times O) + (1-P)L = (1-P)L$

By setting the two expected costs equal to each other, we can determine the value of P to which the decision maker is indifferent. Calculation of this break-even probability would be:

$$P^* = 1 - \frac{I}{L-C}$$

Evaluation of this formula provides a nice summarization of earlier comments concerning the costs and benefits of investigating variances. In situations of high investigation costs (I) and low net benefits (L–C), the critical value of P (P*) becomes quite low. This, of course, means that, in order to justify an investigation, the probability that the system is actually in control (P) must be very low, or, alternatively, the probability that the system is actually out of control (1–P) must be quite large.

To employ the decision theory model just described, the analyst must have estimates of I, C, L, and P. In most situations, there is a reasonable expectation that I and C will be relatively constant. These costs are usually directly related to the labor involved in the analysis. L, however, usually varies, depending upon the size of the cost variance. In short, the loss depends upon the proportion of the variance to be saved in future periods and the number of periods over which the loss is expected to occur if the situation is not corrected.

The value of P is in many respects the most difficult of the parameter values to specify. Either objective or subjective approaches may be used. An objective method may be used to develop an estimated probability distribution for the system. If the underlying distribution is assumed to be normal, estimating the mean and standard deviation from prior observations will enable the analyst to specify the distribution from this estimated distribution. The probability of any given observation being in control (P) can then be defined.

Subjective estimates of P are possible on both an a priori and an ex post facto basis. A subjective normalized distribution of variances can be built in advance as a basis for the estimate. The analyst might ask departmental managers between which two values they would expect 50 percent of actual observations to fall. If the budget cost for labor in a department is $4,000 per pay period, the department manager might specify that 50 percent of the time the manager would expect actual observations to fall between $3,700 and $4,300. Using this information, a normalized distribution could be defined as follows:

3700	4000	4300
−2/3	0	+2/3

Subjective estimates of P may also be made after the fact and then related directly to the actual size of the cost variance. This assessment can then be related to a table of critical values of P necessary for an investigation decision of a given variance. This permits analysts to employ directly sensitivity analysis in their decisions. For example, assume that I is $100 and that C is $200. Assume further that L is equal to two times the absolute size of the variance. The following table of critical values of P could then be defined:

Critical Value of P(P*)	Size of Variance
0.50	$200
0.75	300
0.83	400
0.88	500
0.90	600

This table is relatively straightforward. As the dollar size of the variance increases, the probability that the system is under control must increase to justify a "do not investigate" decision. For example, if a $600 variance occurred, the analyst must believe that there is at least a 90 percent probability that the system is under control.

VARIANCE ANALYSIS CALCULATIONS

Variance analysis is simply an examination of the deviation of an actual observation from a standard. For the purposes of this chapter, two types of standards for comparative purposes are used, (1) prior period values and (2) budgeted values. In each case, the objective of cost variance analysis is to explain why actual costs are different, either from budgeted values or from prior period actual values. This objective is a very important element in the cost control process in the organization.

Prior Period Comparisons

Relevant Factors

An evaluation of the difference between current levels of cost and prior costs should suggest to management which factors have contributed to the change. In general, three major factors influence costs: (1) input prices, (2) productivity of inputs, and (3) output levels.

Input prices usually may be expected to increase over time. It is important, however, from management's perspective to evaluate what portion, if any, of that increase was controllable or avoidable. Rapidly increasing prices for some commodities may signal opportunities for resource substitutions, for example, by switching to a less expensive mix of labor or substituting one supply item for another. Measuring productivity has in fact become increasingly important in the health care industry as a result of the new emphasis on cost containment. One of the major difficulties in evaluating productivity, however, has been the changing nature of health care services. Comparison of productivity within a hospital for two time periods requires that the services in each period be identical. For example, a comparison of full-time equivalents (FTEs) per patient day in 1986 with FTEs per patient day of care in 1983 is meaningless unless a patient day of care in 1986 is identical to a patient day of care in 1983. Finally, changes in output levels also influence the level of costs. This influence may occur in two ways. First, the absolute level of output provided may affect the quantity of resources necessary to produce the output level. Second, service intensity may affect resource requirements. Any increase in the number of services required per unit of output will directly affect costs. For example, a change in the number of laboratory procedures performed per patient day of care will probably affect the total cost per patient day of care.

This discussion can be summarized in the following cost function:

$$\text{Total cost} = P \times \frac{I}{X} \times \frac{X}{Q} \times Q$$

where:

P = input prices
I = physical quantities of inputs
X = services required per unit of output
Q = output level

In the above cost equation, P represents the effect of input prices, I/X represents the effect of productivity, X/Q represents the effect of service intensity, and Q represents the influence of output. Changes in cost can result from changes in any one of these four terms.

American Hospital Association Cost Indexes

A simple application of the preceding cost model was developed by the American Hospital Association (AHA) in its attempts to explain better the factors causing the escalation in hospital costs. To accomplish this objective, the measure of output chosen was cost per adjusted patient day (APD). Cost per APD in any period (t) was defined as follows:

$$APD^t = \sum_{i=1}^{n} C_i^t X_i^t = C^t X^t$$

where:

C_i^t = direct cost per unit of service (i) in period (t)
X_i^t = units of service (i) utilized in one patient day in period (t)
C^t = a 1 by n vector of C_i^t
X^t = an n by 1 vector of X_i^t

From this equation, two indexes that partition the causes of cost changes into two areas were derived as follows:

$$\frac{APD^t}{APD^o} = \frac{C^t X^t}{C^o X^o} = HCI \times HII$$

The hospital cost index (HCI) is defined as:

$$HCI = \frac{C^t X^o}{C^o X^o}$$

The HCI measures the change in cost attributed to both price increases and productivity changes. The other index, the hospital intensity index (HII) is defined as:

$$HII = \frac{C^o X^t}{C^o X^o}$$

The HII measures the change in cost due to changes in service intensity.

To illustrate, these two indexes may be applied in the following cost comparison for a hospital:

	Lab Tests PD	Nursing Hours PD	Cost Per Lab Test	Cost Per Nursing Hour	Cost Per Patient Day (APD)
1983	3.2	3.1	$2.00	$4.50	$20.35
1986	4.5	3.5	2.50	5.20	29.45

During the three-year period, costs increased 44.7 percent ($29.45/$20.35-1), which is a rather sizable increase. However, a calculation of the two AHA indexes gives a somewhat different picture:

$$\text{HCI} = \frac{(\$2.50 \times 3.2) + (5.20 \times 3.1)}{(\$2.00 \times 3.2) + (4.50 \times 3.1)} = \frac{\$24.12}{\$20.35} = 1.185$$

$$\text{HII} = \frac{(\$2.00 \times 4.5) + (4.50 \times 3.5)}{(\$2.00 \times 3.2) + (4.50 \times 3.1)} = \frac{\$24.75}{\$20.35} = 1.216$$

Breaking down the increase in costs for the hospital would now yield the following:

Percentage increase due to cost increases	18.5%
Percentage increase due to intensity	21.6
Joint cost and intensity	4.6
Total increase	44.7%

Departmental Analysis of Variance

The preceding AHA indexes are very useful for analyzing cost changes at the total facility level. In such situations, a measure of output for the facility as a whole—such as patient days, admissions, discharges, visits, or enrollees—would be used. However, though this type of analysis may be very useful, it is also often desirable to analyze the reasons for cost changes at the departmental level. In general, the primary reason for a cost change at the departmental level between two time periods can be stated as a function of three factors:

1. changes in input prices
2. changes in input productivity (efficiency)
3. changes in departmental volume

The following variances can be calculated to compute the effects of these three factors:

Price variance = (Present price − Old price) × Present quantity

Efficiency variance = (Present quantity − Expected quantity at old productivity) × Old price

Volume variance = (Present volume − Old volume) × Old cost per unit

These formulas may be applied to the following laundry example. It is assumed that the laundry has only two inputs: soap and labor.

	1983	1986
Pounds of laundry	140,000	180,000
Units of soap	1,400	1,800
Soap units per pound of laundry	.01	.01
Price per soap unit	$ 40.00	$ 50.00
Productive hours worked	19,600	27,000
Productive hours per pound of laundry	.14	.15
Wage rate per productive hour	5.25	6.00
Total cost	$158,900	$252,000
Cost per pound	$ 1.135	$ 1.40

Price variances:
   Soap = ($50.00 – $40.00) × 1,800 = $18,000 (Unfavorable)
   Labor = ($6.00 – $5.25) × 27,000 = $20,250 (Unfavorable)

Efficiency variances:
   Soap = (1,800 – [.01 × 180,000] × $40.00 = 0
   Labor = (27,000 – [.14 × 180,000] × $5.25 = $9,450 (Unfavorable)

Volume variances:
   Volume variance = (180,000 – 140,000) × $1.135 = 45,400 (Unfavorable)

With these calculations, the following table can be generated to summarize the factors that created cost changes in the laundry department:

Causes of Laundry Department
Cost Change—1983 to 1986

	Dollars	Percentage Change
Increase in wages	$20,250	21.8
Increase in soap price	18,000	19.3
Decline in labor efficiency	9,450	10.1
Increase in volume	45,400	48.8
Total change in cost	$93,100	

The table indicates that increased volume was the largest source of the total change in cost. It is often useful to factor this volume variance into two areas:

Intensity = (Change in volume due to intensity difference) × Old cost per unit
Pure volume = (Change in volume due to change in overall service) × Old cost per unit

Here, the intensity variance represents the change in volume due to increased intensity of service. For example, assume that, in 1986, 2.25 pounds of laundry were provided per patient day. The corresponding value for 1983 was 2.00 pounds per patient day. Also assume that total patient days were 70,000 in 1983 and 80,000 in 1986. The two volume variances would be:

$$\text{Intensity variance} = ([2.25 - 2.00] \times 80,000) \times \$1.135 = \$22,700$$
$$\text{Pure volume} = 2.00 \times (80,000 - 70,000) \times \$1.135 = \$22,700$$

The system of cost variance analysis described above should be a useful framework in which to discuss factors causing changes in departmental costs. Aggregation of some resource categories will probably be both necessary and desirable. There would be little point in calculating price and efficiency variances for each of a hundred or more supply items. Only major supply categories should be examined. The supply items that are aggregated together could not be broken out in terms of individual price and efficiency variances because there would be no common input quantity measure. For example, the addition of numbers of pencils, sheets of paper, and boxes of paper clips would not produce a comparable unit of measure. For these smaller areas of supply or material costs, a simple change in cost per unit of departmental output may be just as informative as detailed price and efficiency variances.

VARIANCE ANALYSIS IN BUDGETARY SETTINGS

A final area in which variance analysis can be applied is in the operation of a formalized budgeting system. The presentation that follows assumes a budgeting system that is based upon a flexible model. This means that management must have identified in the budgetary process those elements of cost that are presumed to be fixed and those that are presumed to be variable. Although relatively few health care organizations employ flexible budgeting models at the present time, a trend toward their adoption is clearly visible. In this context, the variance analysis models examined here may be applied in any budgetary situation, fixed or flexible.

The cost equation for any given department may be represented as follows:

$$\text{Cost} = (F + V) \times Q$$

where:

F = fixed costs
V = variable costs per unit of output
Q = output in units

The fixed and variable cost coefficients are the sum of many individual resource quantity and unit price products. These terms can be represented as follows:

$$F = I_f \times P_f$$
$$V = I_v \times P_v$$

where:

I_f = physical units of fixed resources
P_f = price per unit of fixed resources
I_v = physical units of variable resources
P_v = price per unit of variable resources

In most budgeting situations, there are three levels of output or volume that are critical in cost variance analysis. The first is the actual level of volume produced in the budget reporting period. This level of activity is critical because, if management has established a set of expectations concerning how costs should behave, given changes in volume from budgeted levels, an adjustment to budgeted cost can be made.

The second critical level is that of budgeted or expected volume. It is upon this expected volume level that management establishes its commitments for resources, and therefore incurs cost. An unjustified faith in volume forecasts can lock management into a very sizable fixed cost position, especially with respect to labor costs.

The third critical level is that of standard volume. Standard volume is equal to actual volume, unless there is some indication that not all of the output was necessary. For example, a utilization review committee may determine that a certain number of patient days were medically unnecessary or that some surgical procedures were not warranted. Alternatively, in some indirect departments, such as maintenance, it may be important to identify the difference between actual and standard, or necessary output. The cost effect of these output decisions needs to be isolated and control directed at the individual(s) responsible.

The expected level of costs to be incurred at each of the three levels of volume (actual, budgeted, and standard) may be expressed as follows:

$$FB^a = (F + V) \times Q^a$$
$$FB^b = (F + V) \times Q^b$$
$$FB^s = (F + V) \times Q^s$$

where:

FB^a = flexible budget at actual output level
FB^b = flexible budget at budgeted output level
FB^s = flexible budget at standard output level
Q^a = actual output
Q^b = budgeted output
Q^s = standard output

The major categories of variances can now be defined to explain the difference between actual cost (AC) and applied cost ($Q^s \times FB^b/Q^b$):

Variance Name	Definition	Cause
Spending	$(AC - FB^a)$	Price and efficiency
Utilization	$(Q^a - Q^s) \times (FB^b/Q^b)$	Excessive services
Volume	$(Q^b - Q^a) \times (F/Q^b)$	Difference from budgeted volume

For control purposes, it is important to break down the spending variance further into individual resource categories, and also to isolate the change due to price and efficiency factors. This will not only better isolate control for budget deviations but also improve the problem definition and determination phase times discussed earlier in the detection-correction approach to cost control. The spending variances are broken down as follows:

$$\text{Efficiency} = (I^a - I^b)\, P^b$$

$$\text{Price} = (P^a - P^b)\, I^a$$

where:

I^a = actual physical units of resource

I^b = budgeted physical units of resource

P^a = actual price per unit of resource

P^b = budgeted price per unit of resource

With this background, we must now relate the structure we developed for standard costing in Chapter 9 to our analyses of budgetary variances. Two sets of standards are involved: (1) standard cost profiles (SCPs) and (2) standard treatment protocols (STPs). SCPs are developed at the departmental level. They reflect the quantity of resources that should be used and the prices that should be paid for those resources to produce a specific departmental output unit, defined as a service unit (SU). Below is a SCP for a nursing unit, with the SU defined as a patient day:

Standard Cost Profile
Nursing Unit No. 6
Patient Day = Service Unit
Expected Patient Days = 630

Resource	Quantity Variable	Quantity Fixed	Unit Cost	Variable Cost	Average Fixed Cost	Average Total Cost
Head nurse	0.00	.30	$15.00	$ 0.00	$ 4.50	$ 4.50
RN	2.00	1.00	12.00	24.00	12.00	36.00
LPN	2.00	0.00	8.00	16.00	0.00	16.00
Aides	3.00	1.00	5.00	15.00	5.00	20.00
Supplies	2.00	0.00	2.20	4.40	0.00	4.40
Totals				$59.40	$21.50	$80.90

Using this table, a standard variance analysis could be performed for any time period. For example the following data reflect actual experience in the most recent month:

Actual Months Cost
Nursing Unit No. 6
Actual Patient Days = 600

Resource	Quantity Used	Unit Cost	Total Cost
Head nurse	180	$15.50	$ 2,790.00
RN	1,800	12.50	22,500.00
LPN	1,200	8.10	9,720.00
Aides	2,400	4.80	11,520.00
Supplies	1,300	2.40	3,120.00
Total			$49,650.00

In this example, the nursing unit would have incurred actual expenditures of $49,650 during the month. It would have charged to the treated patient its standard cost times the number of patient days:

Costs charged to patients = $48,540 = $80.90 × 600

The total variance to be accounted for would be the difference, or $1,110.00, which is an unfavorable variance. The individual variances that constitute this total are shown in the following calculations:

1. Spending variances
   - Efficiency variances ($[I^a - I^b]P^b$)
     a. Head nurse = (180 − 189) × $15.00 = $135.00 (Favorable)
     b. RN = (1,800 − 1,830) × $12.00 = $360.00 (Favorable)
     c. LPN = (1,200 − 1,200) × $8.00 = 0

    d. Aides = (2,400 − 2,430) × $5.00 = $150.00 (Favorable)

    e. Supplies = (1,300 − 1,200) × $2.20 = $220.00 (Unfavorable)

• Price variances ([P^a − P^b] I^a)

    a. Head nurse = ($15.50 − $15.00) × 180 = $90.00 (Unfavorable)

    b. RN = ($12.50 − $12.00) × 1,800 = $900.00 (Unfavorable)

    c. LPN = ($8.10 − $8.00) × 1,200 = $120.00 (Unfavorable)

    d. Aides = ($4.80 − $5.00) × 2,400 = $480.00 (Favorable)

    e. Supplies = ($2.40 − $2.20) × 1,300 = $260.00 (Unfavorable)

2. Volume Variance ([Q^b − Q^a] [F/Q^b])

• Volume variance = (630 − 600) × $21.50 = $645.00 (Unfavorable)

Totaling up the above individual variances validates the accuracy of our calculations:

Price—Head nurse	$ 90.00 (Unfavorable)
Price—RN	900.00 (Unfavorable)
Price—LPN	120.00 (Unfavorable)
Price—Aides	480.00 (Favorable)
Price—Supplies	260.00 (Unfavorable)
Efficiency—Head nurse	135.00 (Favorable)
Efficiency—RN	360.00 (Favorable)
Efficiency—LPN	0.00
Efficiency—Aides	150.00 (Favorable)
Efficiency—Supplies	220.00 (Unfavorable)
Volume	645.00 (Unfavorable)
Total	$1,110.00 (Unfavorable)

A few further words about the calculation of the efficiency variances may be in order. The formula states that the difference between actual quantity (I^a) and budgeted quantity (I^b) is multiplied by budgeted price (P^b). The most difficult calculation is that for budgeted quantity. It represents the quantity of resource that should have been used at the actual level of output, or the sum of the budgeted fixed requirement plus the variable requirement at actual output (600 patient days). The following table shows the calculation of fixed and variable requirements for the individual resource categories:

1	2	3	4	5	6
		Budgeted		Budgeted	
	Average	Fixed		Variable	
	Fixed	Requirement	Average Vari-	Requirement	
Resource	Require-	(Col. 2 ×	able Require-	(Col. 4 ×	Total Requirements
Category	ment/Unit	630)	ment/Unit	600)	(Col. 3 + Col. 5)
Head					
nurse	.30	189	0.00	0	189
RN	1.00	630	2.00	1,200	1,830
LPN	0.00	0	2.00	1,200	1,200
Aides	1.00	630	3.00	1,800	2,430
Supplies	0.00	0	2.00	1,200	1,200

The calculation for volume variance may also require some further explanation. This variance is simply the product of the difference between budgeted and actual volume ($Q^a - Q^b$) and the average fixed cost budgeted (F/Q^b). The average fixed cost, as calculated in the standard cost profile, amounted to $21.50. You will notice that, in our example, volume variance is unfavorable because actual volume of patient days (600) was less than budgeted patient days (630). Because actual volume was less than budgeted, average fixed cost per unit will rise. The reverse situation would have existed if actual volume had exceeded budgeted volume. In that situation, the volume variance would have been favorable.

The third type of variance, utilization variance, results from a difference between actual volume and standard volume, or the quantity of volume actually needed. The measure of standard volume is generated from the standard treatment protocols (STPs), which define how much output or how many service units are required per treated patient type.

Let us generate a hypothetical set of data to apply to our nursing unit example. Assume that the patients treated in Nursing Unit No. 6 are all DRG No. 209 (Major Joint Procedures) and are all associated with one physician, Dr. Mallard. Our STP for DRG No. 209 calls for a 14-day length of stay. A review of Dr. Mallard's patient records reveals that only 560 patient days of care should have been used (40 cases at 14 days per case). Dr. Mallard had 20 patients with lengths of stay greater than 14 days. These 20 patients accounted for an excess of 80 patient days. Dr. Mallard also had 10 patients with shorter lengths of stay. These patients offset 40 days of the 80-day surplus. Thus, while 600 patient days of care were provided, only 560 should have been used. This creates an unfavorable utilization variance, calculated as the product of budgeted cost per unit and the difference between actual and standard volume. In our example of Nursing Unit No. 6, the utilization variance would be:

Utilization variance = (600 − 560) × $80.90 = $3,236.00 (Unfavorable)

This variance is not charged to the nursing department. It is charged to the manager of patient treatment, in this case Dr. Mallard.

The following schematic depicts the flow of costs and the variances associated with each account:

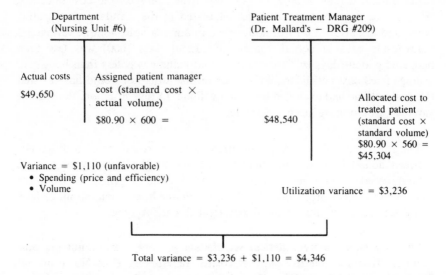

Department
(Nursing Unit #6)

Patient Treatment Manager
(Dr. Mallard's — DRG #209)

Actual costs

$49,650

Assigned patient manager
cost (standard cost ×
actual volume)

$80.90 × 600 =

$48,540

Allocated cost to
treated patient
(standard cost ×
standard volume)
$80.90 × 560 =
$45,304

Variance = $1,110 (unfavorable)
• Spending (price and efficiency)
• Volume

Utilization variance = $3,236

Total variance = $3,236 + $1,110 = $4,346

This delineation of variances represents a very powerful analytical tool for analyzing cost variances from budgeted cost levels. The existence of a flexible budget model is not a prerequisite to its employment. The only real prerequisite is that major resource cost categories be separated into price and utilization components. Since effective cost control appears to be predicated on a separate analysis of price and utilization decisions, this does not seem too difficult a task, in view of the potential payoff. Finally, it should be noted that there is no requirement for a formalization of these variances into the budget reporting models. They can be calculated on an ad hoc basis to investigate and explain large cost variances.

SUMMARY

In general, within the framework for cost control, two approaches are possible: (1) preventive and (2) detection-correction. The detection-correction approach is usually based upon some system of variance analysis. From a decision-theory perspective, the investigation of a variance is based upon the cost of investigation, the probability that a correctible problem exists, the potential loss if the problem is not corrected, and the costs of problem correction. It may not always be possible to develop truly objective measures for these values, but sensitivity analysis may offer a useful aid in such situations.

ASSIGNMENTS

1. Two general approaches to internal control are preventive and detection. Preventive approaches stress the elimination of problems, whereas detection approaches stress the early recognition and correction of problems. What sorts of things could you do if you used a preventive approach to reduce costs?

2. What is a coefficient of variation, and how can that information be used in budgeting?

3. Which would you investigate first—a budget variance that is 1.0 standard deviations away from the expected value or one that is 1.5 standard deviations away from the value? Why?

4. When is the utilization of a flexible budget likely to be most effective?

5. Standard cost accounting systems often separate variance into price and efficiency components. Why?

6. Utilization of a multivariable flexible budget may reduce the time involved in investigating variances. Why might this be true?

7. Ned Zechman is the dietary manager of a large convalescent center. He is disturbed by variances, all highly unfavorable, in his food budget for the past three months. Ned has been reducing both the quantity and quality of delivered meals, but to date there has been no reflection of this in his monthly budget variance report. A recent organizational change brought in Pat Schumaker, who is now responsible for all purchasing activity, including dietary. All purchased food costs are charged to dietary at the time of purchase. What do you think might explain Ned's problem, and how would you determine the cause?

8. Assume the budgeted cost for a department is $10,000 and the amount represented by the standard deviation is $500. The decision to investigate a variance requires a comparison of expected benefits with expected costs. Suppose an unfavorable variance of $1,000 is observed. The normal distribution indicates the probability of observing this variance is .0228 if the system is in control. Further assume that the benefits would be 50 percent of the variance and that investigation costs are $200. Should this variance be investigated? Assume the variance is still $1,000, but it is favorable. Should it still be investigated?

9. Departmental costs may be out of control if either the variance is outside specified limits or the number of successive observations, above or below expected costs, is excessive. The binomial distribution can be used as a basis for determining what is or is not excessive. If we assume that the probability of being either above or below budgeted costs is .50, then the probability of n successive observations of actual costs being greater than budgeted costs is $.50^n$. What is the probability of observing six successive periods in which actual costs are greater than budgeted costs?

10. You are evaluating the performance of the radiology department manager. The service unit (SU) or output for this department is the number of x-rays. A static budget was prepared at the start of the year. You are now examining that budget in relation to actual experience. The relevant data are:

	Actual	Original Budget	Variance	
Volume of x-rays	100,000	120,000	20,000	(Unfavorable)
Variable costs	$1,200,000	$1,320,000	$120,000	(Favorable)
Fixed costs	600,000	600,000	—	
Total costs	$1,800,000	$1,920,000	$120,000	(Favorable)

The departmental manager is pleased because he has a favorable $120,000 cost variance. Evaluate the effectiveness claims of the manager, using the budgetary variance model described in the chapter.

11. The following data were assembled for a laundry department during the period 1984–1985:

	1984	1985
Weighted patient days	24,140	24,539
Pounds of laundry	333,225	328,624
Pounds per day	13.80385	13.39191
Number of FTEs	3.0	3.0
FTEs per pound	.00000900292	.00000912897
Average salary	$7,260.67	$7,873.00
Salary cost per pound	$.065367	$.071872
Supply units	3,332	3,286
Supply units per pound	.01	.01
Cost per supply unit	$2.6946	$3.1848
Total cost	$30,761	$34,085
Cost per pound	$.092313	$.10372

Break out the total change in cost ($3,324) into the variance categories described in the chapter, that is, price, efficiency, intensity volume, and pure volume variances.

SOLUTIONS AND ANSWERS

1. The following are some of the things you could do, using a preventive approach: improve employee training, increase inspection of material, improve equipment maintenance, and increase supervision.

2. The coefficient of variation is the ratio of the standard deviation to the mean. A large value implies great variability in the results. In a budgeting context, operations with large prior coefficients of variation typically require a more sophisticated budget model, such as a flexible budget, to account for deviations from average performance.

3. The budget variance that is 1.5 standard deviations from expected performance is more likely to be controllable and should be investigated first. However, adjustments for the relative differences in investigation costs and variance size should be considered.

4. A flexible budget is likely to be most effective when costs in a department are not fixed and are expected to vary with changes in output or other variables.

5. Standard cost accounting systems separate variances into price and efficiency components because, in many situations, one person does not have decision responsibility for both purchases and usage. Even in situations where one person does have responsibility for both components, the separation is useful because it provides information for focused management correction.

6. To the extent that a multivariable budget model reflects cost behavior more accurately, it may provide a better indication of when actual costs are out of control. This may reduce the number of times needless investigations or justification efforts are conducted.

7. Prices paid for food may have increased significantly either because of recent changes in food prices or because of ineptness or fraud on the part of Mr. Schumaker. An audit of purchasing costs should be initiated, especially if other departments in the center have similar problems.

8. The following calculations should be made as a basis for deciding if an investigation should be conducted:

   Expected benefits = .5 $\times$ \$1,000 $\times$ (1 – .0228)* = \$488.60
   Expected costs = \$200
   *(1 – .0228) = Probability that the variance is not a random occurrence

   Yes, the variance should be investigated, since the expected benefits are greater than the expected costs. Even if the variance is favorable, it should be investigated, because it may indicate that the budget is not accurate. A reduction of the budget may promote a future reduction in costs.

9. The probability of observing six successive periods in which actual costs are greater than budgeted costs is $.50^6 = .0156$.

10. In your evaluation, you can calculate spending and volume variances for the radiology department. The total variance would be calculated as

   Actual cost less assigned cost,

   $$\text{or } \$1,800,000 - \left(100,000 \times \frac{\$1,920,000}{\$120,000}\right) = \$200,000 \text{ (Unfavorable)}$$

   The radiology department has an unfavorable variance of \$200,000, as opposed to a favorable variance of \$120,000. The \$200,000 unfavorable variance can be broken into spending and volume variances:

   Spending variance =
   \$1,800,000 – \$600,000 – (\$11 $\times$ \$100,000) = \$100,000 (Unfavorable)

   $$\text{Volume variance} = (\$120,000 - \$100,000) \times \frac{\$600,000}{\$120,000} = \$100,000 \text{ (Unfavorable)}$$

   The department manager may not be responsible for the volume variance, but the unfavorable spending variance of \$100,000 should be analyzed to see what caused it. More detail would permit further breakouts by price and efficiency variances.

11. The causes of the change in cost and the resulting variances for the laundry department are as follows:

Labor price	1,837	(Unfavorable)	55.26%
Supply price	1,611	(Unfavorable)	48.47
Labor efficiency	301	(Unfavorable)	9.06
Pure volume	508	(Unfavorable)	15.28
Intensity volume	933	(Favorable)	(28.07)
	3,324		100.00%

Labor price = (\$7,873.00 – \$7,260.67) $\times$ 3.0 = \$1,837 (Unfavorable)
Supply price = (\$3.1848 – \$2.6946) $\times$ 3,286 = \$1,611 (Unfavorable)
Labor efficiency = (3.0 – .00000900292 $\times$ 328,624) $\times$ \$7,260.67 = \$301 (Unfavorable)
Pure volume = (13.80385 $\times$ [24,539 – 24,140]) $\times$ \$.092313 = 508 (Unfavorable)
Intensity volume = ([13.39191 – 13.80385] $\times$ 24,539) $\times$ \$.092313 = \$933 (Favorable)

Chapter 12

Financial Mathematics

In this chapter, we examine the concepts and methods of discounting sums of money received at various points in time through the use of compound interest formulas and tables. This material is of special importance in the context of the next two chapters on capital budgeting (Chapter 13) and capital financing (Chapter 14). The present abbreviated discussion of financial mathematics is intended as a review for those who have had prior exposure; if this material is new, some background reading may be necessary.

The two major questions in the financial decision-making process of any business are: (1) Where shall we invest our funds? and (2) How shall we finance our investment needs? Investment decisions involve the expenditure of funds today in the expectation of realizing returns in future periods. Financing decisions involve the receipt of funds today in return for a promise to make payments in the future. The evaluation of the relative attractiveness of alternative investment and financing opportunities is a major task of management. Differences in the timing of either receipts or payments can have a significant impact upon the ultimate decision to invest or finance in a certain way. A payment that is made or received in the first year has a greater value than an identical payment made or received in the tenth year. The concept underlying this point is often referred to as the time value of money. A time value for money simply assigns a cost or interest rate for money.

Money or funds can be thought of as a commodity, like any other commodity that can be bought or sold. The price for the commodity called money is often stated as an interest rate, for example, 10 percent per year. An interest rate of ten percent per year implies exchange rates between money at different time periods. When the interest rate is ten percent, a dollar received one year from today is worth only .9091 of a dollar received today, and a dollar received ten years from today is worth only .3855 of a dollar today. Compound interest rate tables are merely values that provide relative weighting for money received or paid in different time periods at specified prices or interest rates. With these relative weightings, money received or paid can be added or subtracted to produce some logical meaningful result. The major purpose of compound interest tables is to permit addition and subtraction of money paid or received in different time periods. The resulting sums of individual yearly or period values are usually expressed in dollars at one of two time points: (1) present value and (2) future value.

The compound interest tables we shall use in this chapter are categorized as either present value or future value tables. The present value tables provide the relative weights that should be used to restate money of future time periods back to the present. Future value tables provide the relative weighting for restating money of one time period to some designated future time period.

SINGLE-SUM PROBLEMS

Future Value—Single Sum

There are a number of situations in which a business would be interested in the future value of a single sum. For example, a nursing home may want to invest $100,000 today in a fund to be used in two years for replacement. It would like to know what sum of money would be available two years from now.

This type of problem is easily solved, using the values presented in Table 12–1. The first step in solving the problem is to set up a time graph. This involves the four variables that make up any simple compound interest problem:

1. number of time periods in which the compounding takes place (n)
2. present value of future sum (p)
3. future value of present sum (f)
4. interest rate per time period (i)

If you know the values of any three of these variables, you can solve for the fourth. The time graph is a simple device that helps you to conceptualize the problem and identify the known values to permit solution. In the above nursing home investment example, a ten percent interest rate per period would be reflected in the following time graph:

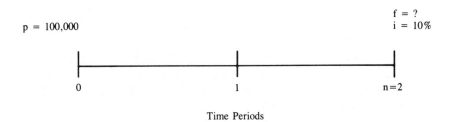

f = ?
i = 10%

p = 100,000

0   1   n=2

Time Periods

The value 0 on this time graph represents the present time, while the values 1 and 2 represent Year 1 and Year 2. In the nursing home example, we know three of the four variables and can therefore solve the problem through substitution in the following formula:

$$f = p \times f(i,n)$$

The factor $f(i,n)$ is the future value of $1.00 invested today for n periods at i rate of interest per period. These values can be found in Table 12–1, using the above generic formula. The following calculation can then be made to solve the problem:

$$f = \$100,000 \times f(10\%,2) \text{ or}$$
$$f = \$100,000 \times 1.210 \text{ or}$$
$$f = \$121,000$$

In some situations it may be the interest rate that we wish to determine. Assume that we can invest $8,576 today in a discounted note that will pay us $10,000 two years from today. The following time graph summarizes the problem:

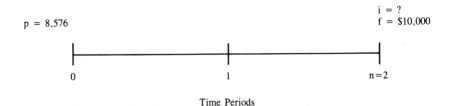

i = ?
f = $10,000

p = 8,576

0   1   n=2

Time Periods

The following calculation can then be made to solve the problem:

$$\$10,000 = \$8,576 \times f(i,2) \text{ or}$$
$$f(i,2) = 1.166$$

A check of the values in Table 12–1 indicates that the interest rate would be eight percent (f[8%,2] equals 1.166). If the above value had not matched exactly a figure in the table, some interpolation would have been required.

A microcomputer or a calculator with a financial mathematics function could also be used to solve the above types of problems. It is still useful, however, to set up a time graph to conceptualize the problem before entering numbers into the calculator or computer.

Present Value—Single Sum

In some situations, it is the present value of a future sum that is of interest. This type of problem is similar to those we examined with regard to the future value of a single sum. In fact, the same table of values could be used, except that now we would use division rather than multiplication. The general equation used to solve present value—single sum problems is:

$$p = f \times p(i,n)$$

The factor $p(i,n)$ represents the present value of $1.00 received in n periods at an interest rate of i. Values for $p(i,n)$ can be found in Table 12–2.

Assume that your HMO has a $100,000 debt service obligation due in two years. You are interested in learning how much money must be set aside today to meet the obligation if the expected yield on the investment is 12 percent. The relevant time graph would be:

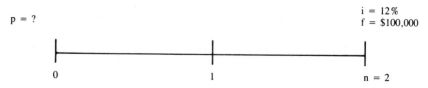

p = ?

i = 12%
f = $100,000

```
0                  1                  n = 2
```

and the calculation to solve the problem would be:

$$p = f \times p(i,n) \text{ or}$$
$$p = \$100,000 \times p(12\%,2) \text{ or}$$
$$p = \$100,000 \times .797 \text{ or}$$
$$p = \$79,700$$

It is important to note that the values of Table 12–1 and Table 12–2 are reciprocals of each other. That is:

$$f(i,n) = 1/p(i,n)$$

Table 12–1 Future Value of $1.00 Received in n Periods

Period	2%	4%	5%	6%	8%	10%
1	1.0200	1.0400	1.0500	1.0600	1.0800	1.1000
2	1.0404	1.0816	1.1025	1.1236	1.1664	1.2100
3	1.0612	1.1249	1.1576	1.1910	1.2597	1.3310
4	1.0824	1.1699	1.2155	1.2625	1.3605	1.4641
5	1.1041	1.2167	1.2763	1.3382	1.4693	1.6105
6	1.1262	1.2653	1.3401	1.4185	1.5869	1.7716
7	1.1487	1.3159	1.4071	1.5036	1.7138	1.9488
8	1.1717	1.3686	1.4775	1.5938	1.8509	2.1436
9	1.1951	1.4233	1.5513	1.6895	1.9990	2.3589
10	1.2190	1.4802	1.6289	1.7908	2.1589	2.5938
11	1.2434	1.5395	1.7103	1.8983	2.3316	2.8532
12	1.2682	1.6010	1.7959	2.0122	2.5182	3.1385
13	1.2936	1.6651	1.8856	2.1329	2.7196	3.4524
14	1.3195	1.7317	1.9799	2.2609	2.9372	3.7976
15	1.3459	1.8009	2.0709	2.3966	3.1722	4.1774
16	1.3728	1.8730	2.1829	2.5404	3.4259	4.5951
17	1.4002	1.9479	2.2920	2.6928	3.7000	5.0545
18	1.4282	2.0258	2.4066	2.8543	3.9960	5.5600
19	1.4568	2.1068	2.5270	3.0256	4.3157	6.1160
20	1.4859	2.1911	2.6533	3.2071	4.6610	6.7276
30	1.8114	3.2434	4.3219	5.7435	10.0627	17.4495
40	2.2080	4.8010	7.0400	10.2857	21.7245	45.2597

Table 12–2 Present Value of $1.00 Due in n Periods

Period	4%	6%	8%	10%	12%	14%	16%	18%	20%	22%	24%	26%	28%	30%	40%
1	0.962	0.943	0.926	0.909	0.893	0.877	0.862	0.847	0.833	0.820	0.806	0.794	0.781	0.769	0.714
2	0.925	0.890	0.857	0.826	0.797	0.769	0.743	0.718	0.694	0.672	0.650	0.630	0.610	0.592	0.510
3	0.889	0.840	0.794	0.751	0.712	0.675	0.641	0.609	0.579	0.551	0.524	0.500	0.477	0.455	0.364
4	0.855	0.792	0.735	0.683	0.636	0.592	0.552	0.516	0.482	0.451	0.423	0.397	0.373	0.350	0.260
5	0.822	0.747	0.681	0.621	0.567	0.519	0.476	0.437	0.402	0.370	0.341	0.315	0.291	0.269	0.186
6	0.790	0.705	0.630	0.564	0.507	0.456	0.410	0.370	0.335	0.303	0.275	0.250	0.227	0.207	0.133
7	0.760	0.665	0.583	0.513	0.452	0.400	0.354	0.314	0.279	0.249	0.222	0.198	0.178	0.159	0.095
8	0.731	0.627	0.540	0.467	0.404	0.351	0.305	0.266	0.233	0.204	0.179	0.157	0.139	0.123	0.068
9	0.703	0.592	0.500	0.424	0.361	0.308	0.263	0.225	0.194	0.167	0.144	0.125	0.108	0.094	0.048
10	0.676	0.558	0.463	0.386	0.322	0.270	0.227	0.191	0.162	0.137	0.116	0.099	0.085	0.073	0.035
11	0.650	0.527	0.429	0.350	0.287	0.237	0.195	0.162	0.135	0.112	0.094	0.079	0.066	0.056	0.025
12	0.625	0.497	0.397	0.319	0.257	0.208	0.168	0.137	0.112	0.092	0.076	0.062	0.052	0.043	0.018
13	0.601	0.469	0.368	0.290	0.229	0.182	0.145	0.116	0.093	0.075	0.061	0.050	0.040	0.033	0.013
14	0.577	0.442	0.340	0.263	0.205	0.160	0.125	0.099	0.078	0.062	0.049	0.039	0.032	0.025	0.009
15	0.555	0.417	0.315	0.239	0.183	0.140	0.108	0.084	0.065	0.051	0.040	0.031	0.025	0.020	0.006
16	0.534	0.394	0.292	0.218	0.163	0.123	0.093	0.071	0.054	0.042	0.032	0.025	0.019	0.015	0.005
17	0.513	0.371	0.270	0.198	0.146	0.108	0.080	0.060	0.045	0.034	0.026	0.020	0.015	0.012	0.003
18	0.494	0.350	0.250	0.180	0.130	0.095	0.069	0.051	0.038	0.028	0.021	0.016	0.012	0.009	0.002
19	0.475	0.331	0.232	0.164	0.116	0.083	0.060	0.043	0.031	0.023	0.017	0.012	0.009	0.007	0.002
20	0.456	0.312	0.215	0.149	0.104	0.073	0.051	0.037	0.026	0.019	0.014	0.010	0.007	0.005	0.001

Table 12-2 continued

Period	4%	6%	8%	10%	12%	14%	16%	18%	20%	22%	24%	26%	28%	30%	40%
21	0.439	0.294	0.199	0.135	0.093	0.064	0.044	0.031	0.022	0.015	0.011	0.008	0.006	0.004	0.001
22	0.422	0.278	0.184	0.123	0.083	0.056	0.038	0.026	0.018	0.013	0.009	0.006	0.004	0.003	0.001
23	0.406	0.262	0.170	0.112	0.074	0.049	0.033	0.022	0.015	0.010	0.007	0.005	0.003	0.002	
24	0.390	0.247	0.158	0.102	0.066	0.043	0.028	0.019	0.013	0.008	0.006	0.004	0.003	0.002	
25	0.375	0.233	0.146	0.092	0.059	0.038	0.024	0.016	0.010	0.007	0.005	0.003	0.002	0.001	
26	0.361	0.220	0.135	0.084	0.053	0.033	0.021	0.014	0.009	0.006	0.004	0.002	0.002	0.001	
27	0.347	0.207	0.125	0.076	0.047	0.029	0.018	0.011	0.007	0.005	0.003	0.002	0.001	0.001	
28	0.333	0.196	0.116	0.069	0.042	0.026	0.016	0.010	0.006	0.004	0.002	0.002	0.001	0.001	
29	0.321	0.185	0.107	0.063	0.037	0.022	0.014	0.008	0.005	0.003	0.002	0.001	0.001	0.001	
30	0.308	0.174	0.099	0.057	0.033	0.020	0.012	0.007	0.004	0.003	0.002	0.001	0.001		
40	0.208	0.097	0.046	0.022	0.011	0.005	0.003	0.001	0.001						

In effect, this means that only one of the two tables is necessary to solve either a present-value or future-value problem involving a single sum.

ANNUITY PROBLEMS

Future Value

In many business situations, there is more than one payment or receipt. In the case of multiple payments or receipts, when each payment or receipt is constant per time period, we have an annuity situation. The time graph for an annuity looks like this:

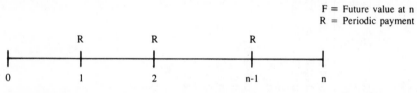

F = Future value at n
R = Periodic payment

In this graph, F represents the future value of the invested annuity deposits at the end of period n. The values for R represent the periodic deposits that are constant each time period. It should be emphasized that the deposits are made at the end of each time period. Such a system of deposits is often described as an ordinary annuity. The values presented in Tables 12–3 and 12–4 assume an ordinary annuity situation in which deposits or receipts occur at the end of the period.

The basic equation for a future value annuity is:

$$F = R \times F(i,n)$$

The factor $F(i,n)$ represents the future value of \$1.00 invested each period for n periods at i rate of interest. Values for $F(i,n)$ can be found in Table 12–3. Again, if three of the four variables (F, R, i, and n) in the above equation are known, the equation can be solved to determine the fourth. Thus, if we know F, i, and n, we can solve for R.

Assume that a hospital wants to know the future value in three years of \$50,000 annual deposits in a trust fund for professional malpractice insurance if the fund earns eight percent per year. The time graph for this problem would be:

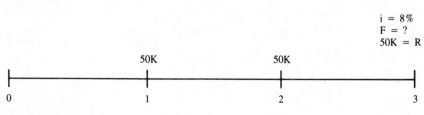

i = 8%
F = ?
50K = R

The calculation to solve the problem would be:

F = R × F(i,n) or
F = $50,000 × F(8%,3) or
F = $50,000 × 3.2464 or
F = $162,320

Table 12–3 Future Value of $1.00 Received Each Period for n Periods

Period	2%	4%	5%	6%	8%	10%
1	1.0000	1.0000	1.0000	1.0000	1.0000	1.0000
2	2.0200	2.0400	2.0500	2.0600	2.0800	2.1000
3	3.0604	3.1216	3.1525	3.1836	3.2464	3.3100
4	4.1216	4.2465	4.3101	4.3746	4.5061	4.6410
5	5.2040	5.4163	5.5256	5.6371	5.8666	6.1051
6	6.3081	6.6330	6.8019	6.9753	7.3359	7.7156
7	7.4343	7.8983	8.1420	8.3938	8.9228	9.4872
8	8.5830	9.2142	9.5491	9.8975	10.6366	11.4360
9	9.7546	10.5828	11.0266	11.4913	12.4876	13.5796
10	10.9497	12.0061	12.5779	13.1808	14.4866	15.9376
11	12.1687	13.4864	14.2068	14.9716	16.6455	18.5314
12	13.4121	15.0258	15.9171	16.8699	18.9771	21.3846
13	14.6803	16.6268	17.7130	18.8821	21.4953	24.5231
14	15.9739	18.2919	19.5986	21.0151	24.2149	27.9755
15	17.2934	20.0236	21.5786	23.2760	27.1521	31.7731
16	18.6393	21.8245	23.6575	25.6725	30.3243	35.9503
17	20.0121	23.6975	25.8404	28.2129	33.7502	40.5456
18	21.4123	25.6454	28.1324	30.9057	37.4502	45.6001
19	22.8406	27.6712	30.5390	33.7600	41.4463	51.1601
20	24.2974	29.7781	33.0660	36.7856	45.7620	57.2761
30	40.5681	56.0849	66.4388	79.0582	113.2832	164.4962
40	60.4020	95.0255	120.7998	154.7620	259.0565	442.5974

The values in Table 12–3 could also be determined through simple addition of the values for a single sum in Table 12–1. This can be easily seen by a further examination of our hospital example. The following table summarizes the relevant data:

Year	Future Value Factor (8%)	Future Value	Year Invested		
			1	2	3
1	1.1664	$58,320	$50,000		
2	1.0800	54,000		$50,000	
3	1.0000	50,000			$50,000
Total	3.2464	$162,320			

Notice that the future value total in the table above is identical to that in the earlier annuity formula. Also note that the summation of the individual future value factors yields the value of the annuity factor (3.2464). In general, a future value annuity factor can be expressed as follows:

$$F(i,n) = f(i,1) + f(i,2) + \ldots\ldots + f(i,n - 1) + 1.0$$

In many situations, a financial mathematics problem may be part annuity and part single sum. In such cases, the use of a time graph will help you spot this duality and solve the problem correctly. Assume that a hospital has a sinking fund payment requirement for the last 10 years of a bond's life. At the end of that period of time, there must be $45 million available to retire the debt. The hospital has created a $5 million fund today, 20 years before debt retirement, to offset part of the future sinking fund requirement. If the investment yield is expected to be ten percent per year, what annual deposit must be made to the sinking fund? The following time graph summarizes the problem:

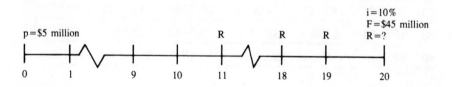

The first step is to determine the future value of the $5 million deposit;

$$f = \$5,000,000 \times f(10\%,20) \text{ or}$$
$$f = \$5,000,000 \times 6.7275 \text{ or}$$
$$f = \$33,637,500$$

Table 12–4 Present Value of $1.00 Received Each Period for n Periods

Period	4%	6%	8%	10%	12%	14%	16%	18%	20%	22%	24%	25%	26%	28%	30%	40%
1	0.962	0.943	0.926	0.909	0.893	0.877	0.862	0.847	0.833	0.820	0.806	0.800	0.794	0.781	0.769	0.714
2	1.886	1.833	1.783	1.736	1.690	1.647	1.605	1.566	1.528	1.492	1.457	1.440	1.424	1.392	1.361	1.224
3	2.775	2.673	2.577	2.487	2.402	2.322	2.246	2.174	2.106	2.042	1.981	1.952	1.923	1.868	1.816	1.589
4	3.630	3.465	3.312	3.170	3.037	2.914	2.798	2.690	2.589	2.494	2.404	2.362	2.320	2.241	2.166	1.879
5	4.452	4.212	3.993	3.791	3.605	3.433	3.274	3.127	2.991	2.864	2.745	2.689	2.635	2.532	2.436	2.035
6	5.242	4.917	4.623	4.355	4.111	3.889	3.685	3.498	3.326	3.167	3.020	2.951	2.885	2.759	2.643	2.168
7	6.002	5.582	5.206	4.868	4.564	4.288	4.039	3.812	3.605	3.416	3.242	3.161	3.083	2.937	2.802	2.263
8	6.733	6.210	5.747	5.335	4.968	4.639	4.344	4.078	3.837	3.619	3.421	3.329	3.241	3.076	2.925	2.331
9	7.435	6.802	6.247	5.759	5.328	4.946	4.607	4.303	4.031	3.786	3.566	3.463	3.366	3.184	3.019	2.379
10	8.111	7.360	6.710	6.145	5.650	5.216	4.833	4.494	4.192	3.923	3.682	3.571	3.465	3.269	3.092	2.414
11	8.760	7.887	7.139	6.495	5.988	5.453	5.029	4.656	4.327	4.035	3.776	3.656	3.544	3.335	3.147	2.438
12	9.385	8.384	7.536	6.814	6.194	5.660	5.197	4.793	4.439	4.127	3.851	3.725	3.606	3.387	3.190	2.456
13	9.986	8.853	7.904	7.103	6.424	5.842	5.342	4.910	4.533	4.203	3.912	3.780	3.656	3.427	3.223	2.468
14	10.563	9.295	8.244	7.367	6.628	6.002	5.468	5.008	4.611	4.265	3.962	3.824	3.695	3.459	3.249	2.477
15	11.118	9.712	8.559	7.606	6.811	6.142	5.575	5.092	4.675	4.315	4.001	3.859	3.726	3.483	3.268	2.484
16	11.652	10.106	8.851	7.824	6.974	6.265	5.669	5.162	4.730	4.357	4.033	3.887	3.751	3.503	3.283	2.489
17	12.166	10.477	9.122	8.022	7.120	6.373	5.749	5.222	4.775	4.391	4.059	3.910	3.771	3.518	3.295	2.492
18	12.659	10.828	9.372	8.201	7.250	6.467	5.818	5.273	4.812	4.419	4.080	3.928	3.786	3.529	3.304	2.494
19	13.134	11.158	9.604	8.365	7.366	6.550	5.877	5.316	4.844	4.442	4.097	3.942	3.799	3.539	3.311	2.496
20	13.590	11.470	9.818	8.514	7.469	6.623	5.929	5.353	4.870	4.460	4.110	3.954	3.808	3.546	3.316	2.497

Table 12–4 continued

Period	4%	6%	8%	10%	12%	14%	16%	18%	20%	22%	24%	25%	26%	28%	30%	40%
21	14.029	11.764	10.017	8.649	7.562	6.687	5.973	5.384	4.891	4.476	4.121	3.963	3.816	3.551	3.320	2.498
22	14.451	12.042	10.201	8.772	7.645	6.743	6.011	5.410	4.909	4.488	4.130	3.970	3.822	3.556	3.323	2.498
23	14.857	12.303	10.371	8.883	7.718	6.792	6.044	5.432	4.925	4.499	4.137	3.976	3.827	3.559	3.325	2.499
24	15.247	12.550	10.529	8.985	7.784	6.835	6.073	5.451	4.937	4.507	4.143	3.981	3.831	3.562	3.327	2.499
25	15.622	12.783	10.675	9.077	7.843	6.873	6.097	5.467	4.948	4.514	4.147	3.985	3.834	3.564	3.329	2.499
26	15.983	13.003	10.810	9.161	7.896	6.906	6.118	5.480	4.956	4.520	4.151	3.988	3.837	3.566	3.330	2.500
27	16.330	13.211	10.935	9.237	7.943	6.935	6.136	5.492	4.964	4.525	4.154	3.990	3.839	3.567	3.331	2.500
28	16.663	13.406	11.051	9.307	7.984	6.961	6.152	5.502	4.970	4.528	4.157	3.992	3.840	3.568	3.331	2.500
29	16.984	13.591	11.158	9.370	8.022	6.983	6.166	5.510	4.975	4.531	4.159	3.994	3.841	3.569	3.332	2.500
30	17.292	13.765	11.258	9.427	8.055	7.003	6.177	5.517	4.979	4.534	4.160	3.995	3.842	3.569	3.332	2.500
40	19.793	15.046	11.925	9.779	8.244	7.105	6.234	5.548	4.997	4.544	4.166	3.999	3.846	3.571	3.333	2.500

This means that the amount of money that must be generated by the ten sinking fund deposits must equal $11,362,500. The following calculation provides the solution:

$$F-f = R \times F(i,n) \text{ or}$$
$$\$11,362,500 = R \times F(10\%,10) \text{ or}$$
$$\$11,362,500 = R \times 15.9376 \text{ or}$$
$$R = \$712,937$$

Present Value

In determining the present value of an annuity, the procedure is analogous to that used to determine the future value of an annuity, except that our attention is now on present value rather than future value. The following time graph represents the typical present-value annuity problem:

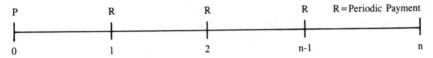

As noted earlier, this is an ordinary annuity situation because the payments are at the end of the period. The basic equation used to solve a present value annuity problem is:

$$P = R \times P(i,n)$$

The factor $P(i,n)$ represents the present value of $1.00 received at the end of each period for n periods when i is the rate of interest. Values for $P(i,n)$ are found in Table 12–4.

Assume that a hospital is considering buying an older hospital and consolidating its operations in another nearby facility. An actuary has estimated that pension payments of $100,000 per year for the next four years will be required to satisfy the obligation to vested employees. The hospital wants to know what the present value of this obligation is so that it can be subtracted from the negotiated purchase price. The obligation's discount rate is assumed to be 12 percent. Here is the time graph for the problem:

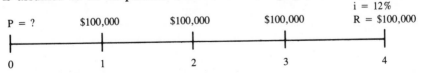

The calculation to solve the problem is:

$$P = \$100,000 \times P(12\%,4) \text{ or}$$
$$P = \$100,000 \times 3.037$$
$$P = \$303,700$$

Present value annuity problems can be thought of as a series of individual single-sum problems. The present value annuity factor $P(i,n)$ is the sum of the individual single-sum values of Table 12–2. The data below summarize this calculation in our hospital example:

Year	Present Value Factor (12%)	Present Value	Year of Payment 1	2	3	4
1	.893	$ 89,300	$100,000			
2	.797	79,700		$100,000		
3	.712	71,200			$100,000	
4	.636	63,600				$100,000
Total	3.038	$303,800				

The small differences between the annuity values and the single-sum values in the above table are due to rounding errors.

The present value annuity factor $(P(i,n))$ can be expressed as follows:

$$P(i,n) = p(i,1) + p(i,2) + \ldots + p(i,n)$$

In most business situations, ordinary annuity problems do not arise. A classic exception to the ordinary annuity situation is a lease with front-end payments. Assume that a clinic wants to lease a computer for the next five years with quarterly payments of $1,000 due at the beginning of each quarter. If the clinic's discount rate is 16 percent per annum, what is the present value of the lease liability? The relevant time graph is presented below:

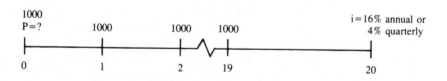

The above graph tells us that the clinic has a 19-period ordinary annuity with each period three months. The effective interest rate for each quarter is 4 percent. The present value of the first payment is $1,000, since it occurs at the start of the first quarter. The following calculation provides the solution to the problem:

$$P = \$1,000 + \$1,000 \times P(4\%,19) \text{ or}$$
$$P = \$1,000 + \$1,000 \times 13.134 \text{ or}$$
$$P = \$14,134$$

SUMMARY

In the area of financial mathematics, compound interest rate tables provide us with values with which we can weight money flows that are received or paid in different time periods. The relative weighting assigned to each period's money flow is a function of the price of money or the interest rate. The relative weightings permit us to add or subtract money flows from different time periods and produce a meaningful measure. The value of money is usually expressed in terms of present value or value at some future specified date.

ASSIGNMENTS

1. Steven Hudson has agreed to settle a debt of $100,000 by paying $14,903 per year for ten years. What effective rate of interest is Steven paying under this agreement?

2. Findling Hospital is planning a major expansion project. The construction cost of the project is to be paid from the proceeds of serial notes. The notes are of equal amount and include a provision for interest at an annual rate of eight percent payable semiannually over the next 10 years. It is expected that receipts from the hospital will provide for the repayment of principal and interest on the notes. Allan Klein, controller of the hospital, has estimated that the cash flow available for repayment of principal and interest will be $450,000 per year. The construction project is expected to cost $3,420,000. Can the hospital meet the peak debt service with existing cash flows?

3. Jerry Scott has just accepted a position with a state agency that has a retirement pension plan calling for joint contributions by the employee and the employer. Jerry is now 10 years from retirement age of 65 and expects to contribute $400 per year to the plan, which would make him eligible for payments of $1,000 per year for the remainder of his life, starting in 10 years.

   Since this retirement plan is optional, Jerry is considering the alternative of investing annually an amount equal to his $400 per year contribution. If Jerry can assume that his investments would earn eight percent annually, and that his life expectancy is 80 years, should he invest in his own plan or should he make contributions to his employer's fund?

4. Meany Hospital wishes to provide for the retirement of an obligation of $10,000,000 that becomes due July 1, 1995. The hospital plans to deposit $500,000 in a special fund each July 1st for eight years, starting July 1, 1987. In addition, the hospital wishes to deposit on July 1, 1987, an amount that, with accumulated interest at ten percent compounded annually, will bring the total value of the fund to the required $10,000,000 at the end of 1995. What dollar amount should the hospital deposit?

5. Jim Hubert, an investment banker with The Ohio Company, is arranging a financing package with Bill Andrews, president of Liebish Hospital. The financing package calls for $20 million in bonds to be repaid in 20 years. A decision must be made regarding the amount that must be deposited on an annual basis in a sinking fund. It is estimated that the sinking fund will earn interest at the rate of eight percent compounded annually. What dollar amount must be set aside annually in the sinking fund to meet the $20 million repayment in the 20th year?

6. General Hospital is evaluating a zero-interest capital financing alternative. General would borrow $100,000,000 and receive $62,100,000 in cash. The $100,000,000 note would carry no interest payment but would be due at the end of the fifth year. The lendor would require an annual sinking fund payment over the next five years to meet the maturity value of

$100,000,000. If the fund is scheduled to earn interest at the rate of six percent annually, what amount must be deposited annually?

7. ABC Hospital is embarking upon a major renovation program. The total cost of construction will be $50,000,000. Payments will be $10,000,000 at the end of Year 1, $30,000,000 at the end of Year 2, and $10,000,000 at the end of Year 3. ABC wants to set aside sufficient funds today to meet the expected construction draws. If the fund can be expected to earn eight percent per annum, what amount should be set aside?

8. If you issue $100,000 of 10 percent bonds with interest payable semiannually over the next five years, what is the market value of the bonds if the required market rate of interest is 12% annually? Assume that no payment of principal is made until maturity.

9. You have agreed to buy an adjacent medical office building with quarterly payments of $100,000 for the next six years. Payments are due at the beginning of each quarter. If the cost of money to you is 16% per annum, would you pay $1,200,000 in cash today to the present owners?

10. You plan to invest $1 million per year for the next three years to meet future professional liability payments. If the fund earns interest at a rate of ten percent per annum, how large will the balance be in five years? Assume that no payments for claims are made until then.

SOLUTIONS AND ANSWERS

1. The following graph and calculations show the effective rate of interest Steven is paying:

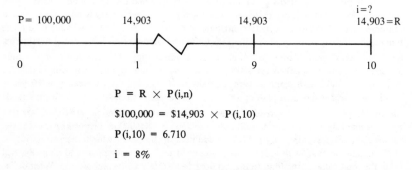

$$P = R \times P(i,n)$$
$$\$100,000 = \$14,903 \times P(i,10)$$
$$P(i,10) = 6.710$$
$$i = 8\%$$

2. In this hospital expansion project, it is necessary to recognize that debt service will be at the maximum or peak in the first year. This is the pattern that results with a serial note. Thus:

Debt principal payment = $3,420,000/20 = $171,000

Interest in first six months = .04 × $3,420,000 = $136,800

Interest in second six months = .04 × ($3,420,000 − $171,000) = $129,960

Total first-year debt service = $171,000 + $136,800 + $171,000 + $129,960 = $608,760

Thus, Findling Hospital's project cannot be financed with the existing cash flow of $450,000.

3. The following graph and calculations are relevant to Jerry's retirement fund decision:

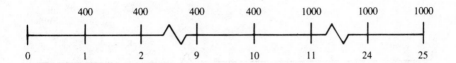

Calculation of the value of the state agency's payments at Year 10:

$$P = \$1,000 \times P(8\%,15)$$
$$P = \$1,000 \times 8.559$$
$$P = \$8,559$$

Calculation of the value of Jerry's deposits at Year 10:

$$F = \$400 \times F(8\%,10)$$
$$F = \$400 \times 14.4866$$
$$F = \$5,795$$

Thus, Jerry is better off with the state agency's retirement plan. His deposits of $400 would not provide a fund large enough to give him $1,000 a year for 15 years.

4. The relevant calculations for Meany Hospital are as follows:

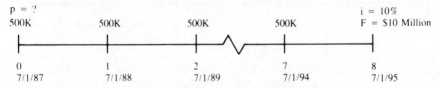

Calculation of the value of annual deposits at July 1, 1995:

$$F = \$500,000 \times f(10\%,8)$$
$$+ \; [\$500,000 \times F(10\%,7)] \; f(10\%,1)$$
$$F = \$500,000 \times 2.1436 + (\$500,000 \times 9.4872) \times 1.10$$
$$F = \$1,071,800 + \$5,217,960 = \$6,289,760$$

Calculation of the required deposit at July 1, 1987:

Required amount at July 1, 1995, must equal $10,000,000 − $6,289,760, or $3,710,240

$$P = \$3,710,240 \times p(10\%,8) = \text{required deposit at July 1, 1987}$$
$$P = \$3,710,240 \times .467$$
$$P = \$1,732,682 = \text{deposit required at July 1, 1987}$$

5. The following graph and calculations show the dollar amount that must be set aside annually in the sinking fund to meet the $20-million repayment in the 20th year:

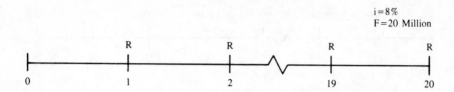

$$F = R \times F(i,n)$$
$$\$20,000,000 = R \times F(8\%,20)$$
$$\$20,000,000 = R \times 45.7620$$
$$R = \$437,044$$

6. The following graph and calculations show the amount General Hospital will have to deposit in the sinking fund each year:

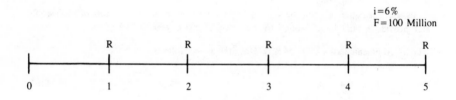

$$F = R \times F(i,n)$$
$$\$100,000,000 = R \times F(6\%,5)$$
$$\$100,000,000 = R \times 5.6371$$
$$R = \$17,739,618$$

7. The following graph and calculations show the amount that ABC Hospital must set aside to meet expected construction draws:

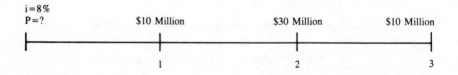

$$P = \$10,000,000 \times P(8\%,1) + \$30,000,000 \times P(8\%,2) + \$10,000,000 \times P(8\%,3)$$
$$P = \$10,000,000 \times .926 + \$30,000,000 \times .857 + \$10,000,000 \times .794$$
$$P = \$42,910,000$$

8. The market value of the bonds may be calculated as follows:

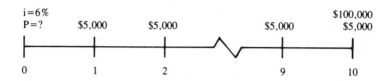

$$P = \$5,000 \times P(6\%,10) + \$100,000 \times p(6\%,10)$$
$$P = \$5,000 \times 7.360 + \$100,000 \times .558$$
$$P = \$92,600$$

9. To determine whether you should pay $1,200,000 in cash today to the present owners, the following graph and calculations are relevant:

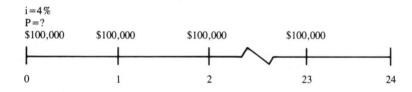

$$P = \$100,000 + \$100,000 \times P(4\%,23)$$
$$P = \$100,000 + \$100,000 \times 14.857$$
$$P = \$1,585,700$$

Yes, you should make the $1,200,000 cash payment to the present owners. The present value of an outright purchase price of $1,200,000 is less than the present value of the installment sale arrangement.

10. The following graph and calculations show the amount of the fund balance in five years:

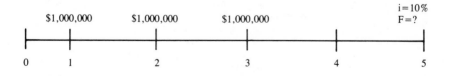

$$F = \$1,000,000 \times F(10\%,3) \times f(10\%,2)$$
$$F = \$1,000,000 \times 3.310 \times 1.210$$
$$F = \$4,005,100$$

Chapter 13

Capital Project Analysis

Capital project analysis falls in the programming phase of the management control process. Whereas zero-base budgeting or zero-base review can be thought of as the programming phase of management control concerned with old or existing programs, capital project analysis is the phase primarily concerned with new programs. Here, it is broadly defined to include the selection of investment projects.

Capital project analysis is an ongoing activity, but it is not usually summarized annually in the budget. The capital budget is the yearly estimate of resources that will be expended for new programs during the coming year. Capital budgeting may be thought of as less comprehensive and shorter-term than capital project analysis.

PARTICIPANTS IN THE ANALYTIC PROCESS

The capital decision-making process in the health care industry is complex for several reasons. First, the stated goals and objectives of a health care facility are likely to be more complex and less quantifiable than those of a for-profit firm in which profit is the major, if not exclusive, goal. Second, the number of individuals involved in the process, either directly or indirectly, is likely to be greater in the health care industry than in most other industries. Figure 13–1 illustrates the relationships of various parties involved in the capital decision-making process of a health care facility.

Figure 13–1 Capital Decision-Making Participants

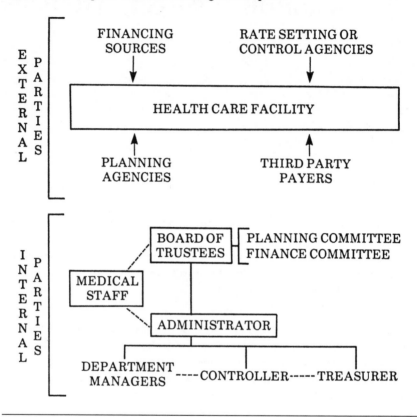

External Participants

Financing Sources

The availability of external funding for many new programs is an important variable in the capital decision-making process. A variety of individual organizations are involved in the credit determination process, including investment bankers, bond rating agencies, bankers, and feasibility consultants. Many of these entities and their roles are discussed in the next chapter. At this juncture, it is important to recognize that, collectively, these entities may influence the amount of money that can be borrowed and the terms of the borrowing and this can affect the nature and size of capital projects undertaken by a given health care facility.

Rate-Setting and Rate-Control Agencies

Many states have agencies that set and control the rates hospitals and other health care facilities can charge for services. The influence exerted by rate-setting or rate-control organizations on capital decision making is indirect but still extremely important. Control of rates can limit both short-term and long-term profitability. This control can reduce a health care facility's ability to repay indebtedness and thus limit its access to the capital markets. More directly, rate-setting organizations can limit the amount of money available for financing capital projects by reducing the amount of profits that may be retained. One of the major effects of rate control is to reduce significantly the level of capital expenditures by hospitals.

Third Party Payers

Like rate-setting and rate-control agencies, third party payers can indirectly influence the capital decision-making process. Through their reimbursement provisions, third party payers can affect both capital expenditure levels and sources of financing. For example, many individuals feel that third party cost reimbursement provides a strong incentive for increased capital spending: in most situations, such cost reimbursement provides for the reimbursement of depreciation and interest expense, which may then be used to repay financial requirements associated with any indebtedness. As a result, the risk associated with hospital indebtedness is reduced. In the past, third party cost reimbursement has favorably affected the availability of credit. Conversely, recent departures from cost reimbursement have had an adverse impact on credit availability.

Planning Agencies

In most states, state approval of capital expenditures is still required. In some areas, planning agencies at the local level initially review certificate of need (CON) applications. Their recommendations are then passed on to the state authority responsible for final approval or disapproval. An unfavorable decision by the state can be appealed in court.

Internal Participants

Board of Trustees

Ultimately, the board of trustees is responsible for the capital expenditure and capital financing program of the health care facility. However, in most situations, the board delegates this authority to management and special board committees. The board's major function should be to establish clearly defined goals and objectives. The statement of goals and objectives is a prerequisite to the programming phase of management control, which includes capital expenditure analysis. Without a clear statement of goals and objectives, capital expenditure programs cannot be adequately defined and analyzed.

Planning Committee

Many health care facility boards of trustees have established planning committees whose primary function is to define, analyze, and propose programs to help the organization attain its goals and objectives. These committees are specialized groups, within the board of trustees, that are directly involved in capital expenditure analysis.

Finance Committee

Some boards of trustees have also established finance committees that have authority in several key financial functional areas, including budgeting and capital financing. In the latter two areas, a finance committee may be involved with translating programs, perhaps identified by the planning committee, into financing requirements. These requirements may be operational or capital. The ensuring of adequate financing to meet program requirements is the financial committee's major responsibility. Many of the finance committee's budgetary functions are delegated to the controller, many of its capital financing functions to the treasurer.

Administration

The administration is responsible on a day-to-day basis for implementing approved capital expenditure programs and developing related financing plans. The administration must develop an organizational system that responds to the requests of departmental managers and medical staff for capital expenditures. Much of the authority vested in the administrator's position is delegated by the board of trustees. The administration may also seek board approval for its own programs.

Departmental Managers

Departmental managers make most of the internal requests for capital expenditure approval. In many health care facilities, formal systems for approving capital expenditures have been developed to receive, process, and answer departmental requests. The allocation of a limited capital budget to competing departmental areas is a difficult task for management. Careful definition of the criteria for capital decision making can help make this problem less political and more objective.

Medical Staff

Medical staff demands for capital expenditures are a problem unique to the health care industry. Medical staff members, in most situations, are not employees of the health care facility but rather use it to treat their private patients. Because of their ability to change a facility's use patterns dramatically and thus affect financial solvency, administrators listen to, and frequently honor, their wishes. Health care facilities are thus faced with strong pressure from individuals who have little financial interest in their organization and whose financial interest may in fact be contrary to that of the health care facility.

Controller

The controller facilitates capital expenditure approval. The controller is usually responsible for developing capital expenditure request forms and for assisting departmental managers in preparing their capital expenditure proposals. The controller usually serves as an analyst, assisting the administrator in allocating the budget to competing departmental areas. In many small health care facilities, the controller's function may be merged with that of the treasurer.

Treasurer

The treasurer is responsible for obtaining funds for both short- and long-term programs. The treasurer may work with the financial committee to negotiate for funds necessary to implement approved programs.

CLASSIFICATION OF CAPITAL EXPENDITURES

A capital expenditure is a commitment of resources that is expected to provide benefits over a reasonably long period of time, at least two or more years. Any system of management control must take into account the various types of capital expenditure. Different types raise different problems; they may require specific individuals to evaluate them or special methods of evaluation.

The more important classifications of capital expenditures are:

- time period over which the investment occurs
- type of resources invested
- dollar amount of capital expenditures
- type of benefits received

Time Period of Investment

Determining the amount of resources committed to a capital project depends heavily upon the definition of the time period. For example, how would you determine the capital expenditures needed by a project that had a very low initial investment cost but a significant investment cost in future years? Should just the initial capital expenditure be considered, or should total expenditures over the life of the project be considered? If the latter is the answer, is it appropriate just to add the total expenditures together, or should expenditures made in later years be weighted to reflect their lower present value? If so, at what discount rate? These are not simple questions to answer, but they are very important in evaluating capital projects.

A classic example of this type of problem in the health care industry is the initiation of programs that have been funded by grants. In many such situations, there appears to be little or no investment of capital expenditure, since the amounts are funded almost totally through the grant. The programs thus appear to be highly desirable. However, if there is a formal or informal commitment to continue the programs for a longer period of time, capital expenditures and additional operating funds for later periods may be required. In such cases, it is imperative that the grant-funded projects be classified separately and their long-run capital cost requirements be identified. The health care facility may very well not have a sufficient capital base to finance a program's continuation. Thus, granting agencies should assess the health care facility's financial capability to continue funded programs after the grant period expires.

Type of Resources Invested

When discussing capital expenditures, many individuals are apt to limit their attention to just the expenditure or resources invested in capital assets, that is tangible fixed assets. This narrow focus has several shortcomings, however, and may result in ineffective capital expenditure decisions.

First, focusing on tangible fixed assets implies ownership, yet many health care facilities lease a significant percentage of their fixed assets, especially in the major movable equipment area. If a lease is not construed to be a capital expenditure, it may escape the normal review and approval system, that is, with regard to both the internal review and approval process and the review and approval process of a health systems agency. Lease payments should be considered as a capital expenditure. Furthermore, the contractual provisions of the lease should be considered in determining the total expenditure amount. Weight should be given to future payments or to the alternative purchase price of the asset.

Second, the capital costs of a capital expenditure are only one part of total cost; indeed, in the labor intensive health care industry, capital costs may be just the tip of the iceberg. All of the operating costs associated with beginning and continuing a capital project should be considered. Programs with very low capital investment costs may not look as good when their operating costs are considered.

Life cycle costing is a method for estimating the cost of a capital project that reflects total costs, both operating and capital, over the project's estimated useful life. The life cycle cost of all contemplated programs should be considered—failure to do this can cause errors in the capital decision-making process, especially in the selection of alternative programs. Consider, for example, two alternative renal dialysis projects; both may have the same capacity, but one may have a significantly greater investment cost because it uses equipment requiring less monitoring and lower operating costs. Failure to consider the operating cost differences between these two projects may bias the decision in favor of the project with lower capital expenditures, and result in higher expenses in the long run.

Amount of the Expenditure

Different systems of control and evaluation are required for different-sized projects. It would not be economical to spend $500 in administrative time evaluating the purchase of a $100 calculator. Nor would it be wise to spend only $500 to evaluate a $25 million building program. Obviously control over capital expenditures should be conditioned by the total amount involved; and, if appropriate, the amount should be based on the total life cycle cost.

Controlling capital expenditures in most organizations, including health care facilities, typically follows one of three patterns:

1. approval required for all dollar-sized capital expenditures
2. approval required for all dollar-sized capital expenditures above a preestablished limit
3. no approval required for individual capital expenditure projects below a total budgeted amount

Retaining final approval of all capital expenditures lets management exert maximum control over the resource spending area. However, the cost of management time to develop and review expenditure proposals is high. In most organizations of any size, management review of all capital expenditure requests is not productive. However, some review is needed, so a limit must be established. For example, a given responsibility center or department need not submit any justification for individual capital expenditure projects requiring less than $200 in investment cost. In such cases, there is usually some formal or informal limitation on the total dollar size of the capital budget that will be available for small dollar capital expenditures. This prevents responsibility center managers from making excessive investments in capital expenditures that have no formalized reviewing system.

Another form of management control over capital expenditures is an absolute dollar limit; that is, any responsibility center manager may spend up to an authorized capital budget on any items in question. The real negotiation involves determining the size of the capital budget that will be available for individual departments. However, this system, while least costly in terms of review time, does not ensure that the capital expenditures actually made are necessarily in the best interests of the organization.

Types of Benefits

Depending upon the types of benefits envisioned for a capital expenditure, different systems of management control and evaluation may be necessary.

For example, investment in a medical office building brings different benefits than investment in an alcoholic rehabilitation unit. Such differences make it inappropriate to rely exclusively on any one method of evaluating projects. This is important: *traditional methods of evaluating capital budgeting may not be appropriate in the health care industry.* Traditional methods evaluate only the financial aspects of a capital expenditure. However, projects in the health care industry may produce benefits that are far more important than a reduction in cost or an increase in profit.

The major categories of investment in which benefits may be differentially evaluated are:

- operational continuance

- financial

- other

The first category of investment produces benefits that permit continuance of operations of the facility along present lines. Here, the governing board or management must usually make two decisions: (1) Are continued operations in the present form desirable? (In most cases the answer is affirmative.) (2) Which alternative investment project can achieve continued operations in the most desirable way (for example, with lowest cost, patient safety, and so on)? A classic example of this type of investment is one based on a licensure requirement for installation of a sprinkler system in a nursing home. Failure to make the investment may imply discontinuance of operations.

The second category of investment provides benefits that are largely financial, in terms of either reduced cost or increased profits to the organization. Many individuals may believe that these two are identical, that is, that reduced costs imply increased profits. However, as we will see, this may not be true if cost reimbursement for either operating or capital costs is present. The important point to remember is that, if the major benefits are financial, traditional capital budgeting methods may be more appropriate.

The third category of investments is a catch-all category. Investments here would range from projects that activate major new medical areas, like outpatient or mental health services, to projects that improve employee working conditions, like employee gymnasiums. In this category, benefits may be harder to quantify and evaluate. Traditional capital budgeting methods may thus be appropriate only in the selection of least costly ways to provide designated services.

THE CAPITAL PROJECT DECISION-MAKING PROCESS

Making decisions on which capital projects will be undertaken is not an easy task. In many respects, this may represent the most difficult and important management decision area. The allocation of limited resources to specific project areas will directly affect the efficiency and effectiveness, and ultimately the continued viability, of the organization.

For our purposes we can divide the capital decision-making process into four interrelated activities or stages:

1. generation of project information
2. evaluation of projects
3. decisions about which projects to fund
4. project implementation and reporting

Generation of Project Information

In this stage of the decision-making process, information is gathered that can later be analyzed and evaluated. This is an extremely important stage because inadequate or inaccurate information can lead to bad decision making. Specifically, there are six major categories of information that should be included in most capital expenditure proposals:

1. information on alternatives available
2. information on resources available
3. cost data
4. benefit data
5. data regarding prior performance
6. risk projection information

Alternatives Available

A major deficiency in many capital expenditure decisions is the failure to consider possible alternatives. Too many times, capital expenditures are presented on a "take it or leave it" basis; yet there usually are alternatives. For example, different manufacturers might be selected, different methods of financing could be used, or different boundaries in the scope of the project could be defined.

Resources Available

Capital expenditure decisions are not made in a vacuum. In most situations, there are constraints on the amount of available funding. This is the whole rationale behind capital expenditure decision making: Scarce resources must be allocated among a virtually unlimited number of investment opportunities. There is little question about the necessity of information concerning the availability of funding at the top level of management. However, there is some question about its importance at the departmental level. On one hand, a budgetary constraint may temper requests for capital expenditures. On the other hand, it may encourage a departmental manager to submit only those projects that are in the department's best interests. These may, in fact, conflict with the broader goals and objectives of the organization as a whole.

Cost Data

It goes without saying that cost information is an important variable in the decision-making process. In all cases, the life cycle costs of a project should be presented. Limiting cost information just to capital costs can be counterproductive.

Benefit Data

We can divide benefit data into two categories: quantitative and nonquantitative. It is believed by some that much of the benefit data in the health care industry is nonquantitative. To a large extent, quantitative data are viewed as synonymous with financial data. And since financial criteria are sometimes viewed as less important in the nonprofit health care industry, the assumption is that quantitative data are also less important. This is not true. Quantitative data can and should be used: Effective management control is predicated upon the use of numbers that relate to the organization's stated goals and objectives. It may not be easy to develop quantitative estimates of benefits, but it is not impossible. For example, assume that a hospital in an urban area opens a clinic in a medically underserved area. One of the stated goals for the clinic is the reduction of unnecessary use of the hospital's emergency room for nonurgent care. A realistic and quantifiable benefit of this project should be a numerical reduction in the use of the hospital's emergency room for nonurgent care by individuals from the clinic area. However, no quantitative assessments are either projected or reported; the only quantitative statistics used are those of a financial nature. The management control process in this situation is less valuable than it should have been.

Prior Performance

Information on prior operating results of projects proposed by responsibility center managers can be useful. A comparison of prior, actual results with forecast results can give a decision maker some idea of the manager's reliability in forecasting. In too many cases, project planners are likely to overstate a project's benefits if the project interests them. Review of prior performance can help a manager evaluate the accuracy of the projections.

Risk Projections

Nothing is certain in this world except death and taxes, especially when evaluating capital expenditure projects. It is important to ask "what if" questions. For example, how would costs and benefits change if volume changed? Volume of service is a key variable in most capital expenditure forecasts, and its effects should be understood. In some situations requiring projections for the highest, the lowest, and the most likely, projections of volume can help answer the questions. The same type of calculations can be made for other key factors, such as prices of key inputs and technological changes. This is an important area to understand because some capital expenditure projects are inherently more risky than others. Specifically, programs with extremely high proportions of fixed or sunk costs are far more sensitive to changes in volume than those with low percentages of fixed or sunk costs.

Evaluation of Projects

Although financial criteria are clearly not the only factors that should be evaluated in capital expenditure decisions, there are few, if any, capital expenditure decisions that can omit financial considerations. Our focus is on two prime financial criteria: solvency and cost.

Solvency

A project that cannot show a positive rate of return in the long run should be questioned. If implemented, such a program will need to be subsidized by some other existing program area. For example, should a hospital subsidize an outpatient clinic? If so, to what extent? This is the kind of policy and *financial* question the governing board of the organization needs to determine. The fairness of some patients subsidizing other patients is one of the basic qualitative issues in capital project analysis. Operation of an insolvent program can eventually threaten the solvency of the entire organization. Thus, organizations that plan to subsidize insolvent programs must be in good financial condition. And assessment of financial condition can only be done after the organization's financial statements are examined.

Cost

Cost is the second important financial concern. An organization needs to select the projects that contribute most to the attainment of its objectives, given resource constraints. This type of analysis is often called cost benefit analysis. Benefits differ from project to project. In evaluating alternative programs, decision makers must weight those benefits according to their own preferences and then compare them to cost.

There is a second dimension to the cost criterion. All projects that are eventually selected should cost the least to provide the service. This type of evaluation is sometimes called cost effectiveness analysis. Least cost should be defined as the present value of both operating and capital costs (methods for determining this are discussed later in the chapter).

Decisions About Which Projects to Fund

At this juncture of the capital expenditure decision-making process, it is time to make the decisions. In front of the decision makers is a list of possible projects that may be funded. Each project should represent the lowest cost of providing the desired service or output. In addition, various benefit data on each project should be described. These data should be consistent with the criteria that the decision makers used in their capital expenditure decision making.

To illustrate this process, assume that the governing board is deciding on how many, if any, of three proposed programs it will fund in the coming year. The three programs are a burn care unit, a hemodialysis unit, and a commercial laboratory. Assume further that the governing board has decided that there are only four criteria of importance to them:

1. solvency
2. incremental management time required
3. public image
4. medical staff approval

Since none of the three projects clearly dominates, it is not clear which, if any, should be funded. Thus, the decision makers must weight the criteria according to their own preferences and determine the overall ranking of the three projects. For example, one manager might weight solvency and management time very high, relative to public image and medical staff, and might thus select the commercial laboratory project. Another manager might weight medical staff and public image more heavily and thus select the hemodialysis or burn care unit projects.

In this example, the three projects can be ranked in terms of their relative standing on each of the four criteria:

	Projects		
	---	---	---
Criteria	Hemodialysis Unit	Burn Care Unit	Commercial Laboratory
Solvency	2	3	1
Management time	2	3	1
Public image	2	1	3
Medical staff	1	2	3

Project Implementation and Reporting

Most capital expenditure control systems are concerned primarily, if not exclusively, with analysis and evaluation prior to selection. However, a very real concern should be focused on whether the projected benefits are actually being realized as forecast. Without this feedback on the actual results of prior investments, the capital expenditure control system's feedback loop is not complete.

Here are some of the specific advantages of establishing a capital expenditure review program:

- Capital expenditure review could highlight differences between planned versus actual performance that may permit corrective action. If actual performance is never evaluated, corrective action may not be taken. This could mean that the projected benefits might never be realized.

- Use of a review process may result in more accurate estimates. If individuals realize that they will be held responsible for their estimates, they may tend to be more careful with their projections. This will ensure greater accuracy in forecast results.

- Forecasts by individuals with a continuous record of biased forecasts can be adjusted to reflect that bias. This should result in a better forecast of actual results.

JUSTIFICATION OF CAPITAL EXPENDITURES

In most health care organizations, there is a very formalized process for approval of a capital expenditure. Usually, this approval process is initiated by a department or responsibility center manager through the completion of a capital expenditure approval form. An example of a completed capital expenditure approval form is shown in Exhibit 13–1. Both the approval form and the approval process may vary across health care organizations, depending upon the nature of the management control process in each case.

The approval form in Exhibit 13–1 is in fact more comprehensive than that employed in most health care organizations. Thus, it provides a detailed summarization of the key aspects involved in capital expenditure approval:

- amount and type of expenditure

- attainment of key decision criteria

- detailed financial analysis

In most firms, small capital expenditures are usually not subjected to detailed analysis and do not require justification. For example, capital expenditures under $2,000 are not reviewed according to the instructions in Exhibit 13–1. This does not mean that a department has an unlimited capital expenditures budget if it spends less than $2,000 per item; the department is most likely subject to some overall level for small capital expenditures. For example, a department such as physical therapy might have an $8,000 limit on small capital expenditure items. No justification for capital expenditure items under $2,000 would be required if the aggregate limit of $8,000 is not violated.

Exhibit 13–1 Completed Capital Expenditure Approval Form

APPRAISAL SHEET FOR
CAPITAL EXPENDITURE PROPOSALS

Department and #   Surgery #818

Date of request for purchase   1/7/87

Summary description of item or package of items (attach original request for purchase)
IABP Model 10 with cardiac output computer and recorder (Intra Aortic Balloon
Pump)

Total capital expenditure, including training, renovation, and purchase of equipment (attach
list) $19,500

Undepreciated value of equipment being replaced   0

  Total cost of implementation $19,500

Appraisal Instructions

  Level I—Complete a Level I assessment for:
   1. a new item having a total capital expenditure exceeding $2,000, or
   2. a replacement item having a total capital expenditure exceeding $20,000, or
   3. a proposed capital expenditure requiring an evaluation before a purchase (or lease)
       decision may be made.

  Level II—Complete both a Level I and a Level II assessment for any proposed capital
           expenditure that:
   1. exceeds $100,000, or
   2. initiates or modifies the scope or type of health services rendered in the community
       and may require a certificate of need, or
   3. requires a more extensive evaluation than offered by a Level I review.

Appraisal Outcome   By (initials)   Date   Priority Status

Request denied   _____   _____   _____
Request accepted & pending   _____   _____   _____
Request approved   _____   _____   _____

I. Level I Review—Complete the following assessment for any proposed capital expenditure
           requiring either a Level I or Level II review.
A. Need
   1. Indicate whether the proposed capital expenditure contributes *directly* to the achieve-
      ment of any of the following management goals (check those that apply)
            _____ Revenue
            _____ Hospital improvement study
            _____ Productivity
            ___X____ Quality assurance
            _____ Employee development
            _____ Management services consultant package
            _____ Other goal (specify) _____

Exhibit 13–1 continued

2. Indicate whether the proposed capital expenditure contributes *directly* to the achievement of any of the following hospital goals (check one or more goals)

    X   Patient care

         Medical and allied health education

    X   Community service

         Cost containment

    X   The leadership role

         Clinical research

3. Provide the following information on historical and projected utilization of items for the provision of patient care services. (See the Finance Department for assistance in completing this section.)

    a. For replacement items only:

        (1) Identify units of service, if any, provided through the utilization of existing equipment; the actual volume of services provided during the most recent year for which statistics are available; the current patient charge, if any, for these services; and the annual revenue realized.

Unit of Service	Historical Annual Volume	Patient Charge	Annual Revenue
1.			
2.			
3.			
4.			
Total	Units		$

        (2) Serial # of item _____

        (3) Fixed asset tag # _____

    b. For both new and replacement items:

        (1) Identify the units of service, if any, to be offered through acquisition of the proposed item and the estimated volume of services to be provided annually. If known, provide the proposed patient charge per unit of service.

Unit of Service	Estimated Annual Volume	Proposed Patient Charge
1. Ped. open heart	161	$459.16(Avg)
2.		
3.		
4.		

        (2) Identify any other services whose volume of utilization will be affected through acquisition of the proposed item.

        (3) Percentage of charge patients for department (from cost report) __93.1__

        (4) Estimated useful life of equipment: _____10_____ years.

Exhibit 13–1 continued

4. Document the reasons justifying the acquisition of the proposed capital expenditure, particularly as they relate to the achievement of hospital, departmental, and management goals and objectives.
   We presently borrow General Hospital's Balloon Pumps 3 or 4 times per month. This is a life-saving device. Without it, some patients cannot survive open-heart surgery.

B. Economic feasibility
   1. Estimate any change in the annual operating costs associated with acquisition of this proposed capital expenditure. (See the Finance Department for assistance in completing this section.)

	Change in Annual Operating Cost
Personnel	
Employee Benefits @23%	
Physician Cost	
Materials and Supplies	
Maintenance Contracts	
Insurance	
Other Depreciation	$1,950
Total Change in Annual Operating Cost	$1,950

Provide documentation in support of the above estimates.

   2. Financial analysis (to be completed by Finance):

Estimated Cost to Purchase
IAPB Model 10 with Cardiac Output Computer

Cash Expenditure	Cost Reimbursement @ 26%	Net Cash (Disbursed) Received	Present Value @ 6%
$(19,500)	$ 507	$(18,993)	$(17,918)
	507	507	451
	507	507	426
	507	507	402
	507	507	379
	507	507	357
	507	507	337
	507	507	318
	507	507	300
	507	507	283
$(19,500)	$5,070	$(14,430)	$(14,665)

Total present value (cost) $(14,665)

   3. Space analysis:
      a. Change in the number of square feet of space required for item: N/A
      b. Is existing departmental space available for the item?
         (Circle one)   Yes   No
         If not, document plan for acquiring additional space.

Exhibit 13–1 continued

C. Acceptability
  1. Physician impact of the capital expenditure decision:
     a. What is the *scope* of any physician attitude change? (check one)
        _____ 1 No change. (skip to Section C–2)
        ____X____ 2 One or two physicians will be affected.
        _____ 3 The majority of the physicians in a hospital service will be affected.

     b. What is the *intensity* of the effect on physician attitude? (check two answers—one for acceptance and one for nonacceptance)
        Not accepted:
        _____ 4 The physicians affected will move their practices to other hospitals.
        ____X____ 3 The physicians affected will tend to reduce their practices at the hospital.
        _____ 2 The physicians affected, at the very least, will be disgruntled and will tend to discuss in the community and with other physicians the lack of the expenditure or project.
        _____ 1 The physicians will be aware of the lack of support for the project and will be less likely to believe that the hospital is maintaining a proper level of patient care.
        _____ 0 No effect.
        Accepted:
        _____ 0 No effect.
        _____ 1 The physicians affected will be aware of the expenditure or project and will be satisfied that the hospital is maintaining a high level of patient care.
        ____X____ 2 The physicians affected will be very impressed and will tend to discuss the expenditure or project favorably in the community and with other physicians.
        _____ 3 The physicians affected will tend to increase their practices moderately in the hospital.
        _____ 4 The physicians affected will move their practices to the hospital.

  2. Employee impact of the capital expenditure decision:
     What is the effect on the attitude of hospital employees?
     (Check two answers—one for acceptance and one for nonacceptance.)
     Not accepted:
        _____ 4 Major and widespread negative impact on employee morale and attitude toward the hospital.
        _____ 3 Widespread disappointment with the hospital and some general negative effect on the hospital's image among employees.
        ____X____ 2 Negative reaction from a limited group of employees (one or two departments).
        _____ 1 Limited reaction from a few employees.
        _____ 0 No effect.

Exhibit 13–1 continued

Accepted:

———————— 0 No effect.

———————— 1 Limited reaction from a few employees.

——— X ——— 2 Positive reaction from a limited group of employees (one or two departments).

———————— 3 Positive impact on nearly all employees.

———————— 4 Major and widespread impact with long-term effect on employee attitude toward the hospital.

3. Community impact of the capital expenditure decision:

What is the expected community impact?

(Check the answers below which best describe the expected community impact; check one for acceptance and one for nonacceptance.)

Not accepted:

———————— 4 Intense and widespread negative reaction in the community will result in a severe blow to the hospital's image.

——— X ——— 3 A widespread negative effect on the hospital's general image and reputation will result.

———————— 1 The attitudes of relatively few people will be negatively affected.

———————— 0 No effect.

Accepted:

———————— 0 No effect.

———————— 1 Relatively few people will be positively affected.

———————— 2 Certain groups in the community will be favorably impressed.

——— X ——— 3 A widespread positive effect on the hospital's image and reputation will result.

———————— 4 Significant and widespread positive community reaction will contribute significantly to the hospital's general image and reputation.

APPRAISAL SCORE SHEET FOR
CAPITAL EXPENDITURE PROPOSALS

	Assigned Value	Raw Score	Priority Instructions	Priority Score
A. Need evaluation				
1. If proposal directly contributes to one or more management goals (I–A–1)	+1	+1		
2. If proposal directly contributes to one or more hospital goals (I–A–2)	+1	+1		

Exhibit 13–1 continued

	Assigned Value	Raw Score	Priority Instructions	Priority Score
(For Level II reviews only)				
3. Performance expectations (II–A–4)				
If negative or questionable	−1			
If positive	+1			
4. If certificate–of–need approval is necessary, but unlikely (II–A–5)	−3	___		___
Subtotal, need raw score		2	Enter positive raw score as priority score.	2
B. Economic Evaluation				
1. If annual operating costs (including depreciation) are reduced (I–B–1–a)	+1			
2. Return on investment (I–B–2–a)				
If greater than 7.5%	+2			
If positive	0			
If negative	−2	−2		
3. If significant additional space is required (I–B–3)	−1			
(For Level II reviews only)				
4. If external financing is required (II–B–1)	−1	___		___
Subtotal, economic raw score		−2	Enter positive raw score as priority score.	
C. Acceptability Evaluation				
1. Physician attitude				
a. Scope (enter score for response to question I–C–1–A)	1 to 3	1	If scope score is greater than 2, enter raw score in priority score column.	

Exhibit 13–1 continued

	Assigned Value	Raw Score	Priority Instructions	Priority Score
b. Intensity (add responses to question I–C–1–b)	0 to 8	5	If raw score exceeds 4, the excess is priority score.	1
2. Employee attitude (add responses to question I–C–2)	0 to 8	4	If raw score exceeds 4, the excess is priority score.	
3. Community attitude (add responses to question I–C–3)	0 to 8	6	If raw score exceeds 4, the excess is priority score.	2
Subtotal, acceptability raw score		16		3
Total Raw Score		16	Total priority score	5

Note: A capital expenditure proposal may be approved, disapproved, or deferred on the basis of an appraisal of the raw scores for need, economy, and acceptability, considered either independently or together. An approved capital expenditure proposal is ranked according to its priority score for future appropriation of capital expenditure funds.

Special recognition is also often given to replacement items. In the Exhibit 13–1 example, a replacement expenditure below $20,000 is not subject to review. The rationale for this higher limit relates to the operational continuance of capital expenditures. Replacement expenditures are often viewed as essential to the continuation of existing operations. They are therefore not as closely evaluated as expenditures for new pieces of equipment.

In any decision-making process, it is important to define carefully the criteria that will be used in the selection process. The example in Exhibit 13–1 has three categories of criteria:

1. need (management goals, hospital goals)
2. economic feasibility
3. acceptability (physicians, employees, community)

Most capital expenditure forms would probably ask for data in the area of economic or financial feasibility. The Exhibit 13–1 form provides data in other areas as well, and also includes a means for scoring the project. For the specific project being appraised, a raw score of 16 and a priority score of 5 resulted. Different values could be obtained by changing the form's measures and their relative weightings.

The important point to recognize is that project selection usually involves the consideration of criteria other than financial. Failure to collect data on the attainment of those additional criteria for specific projects will often lead to more subjectivity in the process. Without such relevant data, individuals may make inferences that are not legitimate.

A key aspect of the capital expenditure approval process is the financial or economic feasibility of the project. In most capital expenditure forms, there is some summary statistic that measures the project's overall financial performance. In general, such measures are usually categorized as either (1) discounted cash flow methods or (2) nondiscounted cash flow methods. In the present discussion, we shall not be concerned with nondiscounted cash flow methods because they are usually regarded as less sophisticated than discounted cash flow methods.

DISCOUNTED CASH FLOW METHODS

In this section, we shall examine three discounted cash flow (DCF) methods that are relatively easy to understand and use:

1. net present value
2. profitability index
3. equivalent annual cost

Before examining these three methods, a word of caution is in order: In our view, the calculation of specific DCF measures is an important, but not a critical, phase of capital expenditure review. We strongly believe that the most important phase in the capital expenditure review process is the generation of quality project information. Specifically, the set of alternatives being considered must include the best ones; it does a firm little good to select the best five projects from a list of ten inferior ones. Beyond that, the validity of the forecasted data is critical; small changes in projected volumes, rates, or costs can have profound effects on cash flow. Determination of possible changes in both these parameters is far more important than discussions over the appropriate discount rate or cost of capital.

Each of the above three DCF methods is based on a time value concept of money. Each is useful in evaluating a specific type of capital expenditure or capital financing alternative. Specifically, their areas of application are:

Method of Evaluation	Area of Application
Net present value	Capital financing alternatives
Profitability index	Capital expenditures with financial benefits
Equivalent annual cost	Capital expenditures with nonfinancial benefits

Net Present Value

A net present value analysis is a very useful way to analyze alternative methods of capital financing. In most situations, the objective in such a situation is clear: the commodity being dealt with is money, and it is management's goal to minimize the cost of financing operations. (We shall consider shortly how this goal may conflict with solvency when the effects of cost reimbursement are considered.)

Net present value equals discounted cash inflows less discounted cash outflows. In a comparison of two alternative financing packages, the one with the highest net present value should be selected.

For example, assume that an asset can be financed with a four-year annual $1,000 lease payment, or can be purchased outright for $2,800. Assume further that the discount rate is ten percent, which may reflect either the borrowing cost or the investment rate, depending on which alternative is relevant. (We shall discuss the issue of an appropriate discount rate shortly.) The present value cost of the lease is $3,169. This amount is greater than the present value cost of the purchase, $2,800. With no consideration given to cost reimbursement, the purchase alternative is the lowest cost alternative method of financing.

However, for accuracy, the effects of cost reimbursement should be considered. Reimbursement of costs would mean that the facility would be entitled to reimbursement for depreciation if the asset were purchased, or entitled to the rent payment if the asset were leased. (Some third party cost payers limit reimbursement on leases to depreciation and interest if the lease is treated as an installment purchase.) Assuming that straight-line depreciation is used and that 80 percent of capital expenses are reimbursed by third party cost payers, the present value of the reimbursed cash inflow (using the discount factors from Table 12–4) would be as follows:

		Annual Reimbursement	Discount Factor	% of Cost Reimbursement	
Present value of reimbursed depreciation	=	$\dfrac{\$2,800}{4}$	× 3.170 ×	.80	= $1,775
Present values of reimbursed lease payments	=	$1,000	× 3.170 ×	.80	= $2,536

If the asset were purchased, the organization would pay out $2,800 immediately. For each of the next four years, it would be reimbursed for the noncash expense item of depreciation in the amount of $700 per year ($2,800/ 4). However, since only 80 percent of the patients are capital cost payers, only $560 per year would be received (.80 × $700). If the asset were leased, the organization would be permitted reimbursement of the lease payment in the amount of $1,000 per year. However, since only 80 percent of the patients are capital cost payers, only $800 (.80 × $1000) would be paid.

The net present value of the above two financing methods for considering cost reimbursement would be as follows:

		Present Value of Reimbursement (Cash Inflows)	Present Value of Payments (Cash Outflows)		Net Present Value
Net present value of purchase	=	$1,775	–$2,800	=	–$1,025
Net present value of lease	=	$2,536	–$3,169	=	–$633

In this case, cost reimbursement has changed the relative desirability of the two financing alternatives. If the organization's objective is cost minimization, the purchase alternative should be selected, since the present value of costs are lower under this alternative. If, however, the organization is primarily interested in solvency, the effect of cost reimbursement should be considered, and the lease alternative becomes the best financing package.

Profitability Index

The profitability index method of capital project evaluation is of primary importance in cases where the benefits of the projects are mostly financial, for example, a capital project that saves costs or expands revenue with a primary purpose of increased profits. In these situations, there is usually a constraint on the availability of funding. Thus, those projects with the highest rate of return per dollar of capital investment are the best candidates for selection. The profitability index attempts to compare rates of return. The numerator is the net present value of the project, and the denominator is the investment cost:

$$\text{Profitability index} = \frac{\text{Net present value}}{\text{Investment cost}}$$

To illustrate the use of this measure, let us assume that a hospital is considering an investment in a laundry shared with a group of neighboring hospitals. The initial investment cost is $10,000 for the purchase of new equipment and delivery trucks. Savings in operating costs are estimated to be $2,000 per year for the entire ten-year life of the project. If the discount rate is assumed to be ten percent, the following calculations could be made, ignoring the effect of cost reimbursement and using the discount factors of Table 12–4.

$$\text{Present value of operating savings} = \$2,000 \times 6.145 = \$12,290$$

$$\text{Net present value} = \$12,290 - \$10,000 = \$2,290$$

$$\text{Profitability index} = \frac{\$2,290}{\$10,000} = .229$$

Values for profitability indexes that are greater than zero imply that the project is earning at a rate greater than the discount rate. Given no funding constraints, all projects with profitability indexes greater than zero should be funded. However, in most situations funding constraints do exist, and only a portion of those projects with profitability indexes greater than zero are actually accepted.

The above calculations give no consideration to the effects of cost reimbursement. If we assume that 80 percent of the facility's capital expenses are reimbursed and 20 percent of its operating expenses are reimbursed, then the following additional calculations must be made:

$$\text{Present value of reimbursed depreciation} = \frac{\$10,000}{10} \times 6.145 \times .80 = \$4,916$$

$$\text{Present value of lost reimbursement from operating savings} = \$2,000 \times 6.145 \times .20$$
$$= \$2,458$$

$$\text{Net present value} = \$2,290 + \$4,916 - \$2,458 = \$4,748$$

$$\text{Profitability index} = \frac{\$4,748}{\$10,000} = .4748$$

The above calculations require some clarification. We are adjusting the initially calculated net present value of $2,290 to reflect the effects of cost reimbursement. Depreciation is the first item to be considered. Since 80 percent of the facility's patients are on capital cost reimbursement formulas, it can expect to receive 80 percent of the annual depreciation charge of $1,000 ($10,000/10) or $800 per year as a reimbursement cash flow. The present value of this stream, $4,916, is added to the initial net present value of $2,290.

The second item to be considered is the operating savings. If the investment is undertaken, the facility can anticipate a yearly savings of $2,000 for the next ten years. However, that savings will reduce its reimbursable costs by $2,000 annually, which means that 20 percent of that amount, or $400, will be lost annually in reimbursement. The present value of that loss for the ten years is $2,458, which is subtracted from the initial net present value. The effect of cost reimbursement thus reduces increased costs associated with new programs, but it also reduces the cost savings associated with new programs.

The preceding example illustrates an important financial concept discussed earlier in Chapter 2. Because some third party payers still reimburse actual capital costs, a strong financial incentive exists for investment in projects that reduce operating costs. In the above example, the laundry facility's profitability index increased from .229 to .4748 when the effects of capital and operating cost reimbursement were considered.

Equivalent Annual Cost

Equivalent annual cost is of primary value in the selection of capital projects where alternatives exist. Usually these are capital expenditure projects that are classified as operational continuance or other. (The profitability index measure just discussed is used for projects in which the benefits are primarily financial in nature.)

Equivalent annual cost is the expected average cost, considering both capital and operating cost, over the life of the project. It is calculated by dividing the sum of the present value of operating costs over the life of the project and the present value of the investment cost by the discount factor for an annualized stream of equal payments (as derived from Table 12–4):

Equivalent annual cost =

$$\frac{\text{Present value of operating cost} + \text{Present value of investment cost}}{\text{Present value of annuity}}$$

To illustrate use of this measure, assume that an extended care facility must invest in a sprinkler system to maintain its license. After investigation, two alternatives are identified. One sprinkler system would require a $5,000 investment and an annual maintenance cost of $500 in each year of its estimated 10-year life. An alternative sprinkler system can be purchased for $10,000 and would require only $200 in maintenance cost each year of its estimated 20-year life. Ignoring cost reimbursement and assuming a discount factor of ten percent, the following calculations can be made.

Equivalent annual cost of $5,000 sprinkler system:

$$\text{Present value of operating costs} = \$500 \times 6.145 = \$3,073$$
$$\text{Present value of investment} = \$5,000$$

$$\text{Equivalent annual cost} = \frac{\$3,073 + \$5,000}{6.145} = \$1,314$$

Equivalent annual cost of $10,000 sprinkler system:

$$\text{Present value of operating costs} = \$200 \times 8.514 = \$1,703$$
$$\text{Present value of investment} = \$10,000$$

$$\text{Equivalent annual cost} = \frac{\$1,703 + \$10,000}{8.541} = \$1,375$$

From this analysis, it can be seen that the $5,000 sprinkler system would produce the lowest equivalent annual cost, $1,314 per year, compared to the $1,375 equivalent annual cost of the $10,000 system.

Two points should be made with respect to this analysis. First, the equivalent annual cost method permits comparison of two alternative projects with different lives. In this case, a 10-year life project was compared with a project with a 20-year life. There is an assumption here that the technology will not change and that in ten years the relevant alternatives will still be the two systems being analyzed. However, in situations of estimated rapid technology changes, some subjective weight should be given to projects of shorter duration. In the above example, this is no problem, since the project with the shorter life also has the lowest equivalent annual cost.

Second, equivalent annual cost is not identical to the reported or accounting cost. The annual reported accounting cost for the two alternatives would be the annual depreciation expenses plus the maintenance cost. Thus:

$$\text{Accounting expense per year (\$5,000 sprinkler system)} = \frac{\$5,000}{10} + \$500 = \$1,000$$

$$\text{Accounting expense per year (\$10,000 sprinkler system)} = \frac{\$10,000}{20} + \$200 = \$700$$

Reliance on information like the above that does not incorporate the time value concept of money can produce misleading results, as it does in the above example. The second alternative is not the lowest cost alternative when the cost of capital is included. In this case, the savings of $5,000 in investment cost between the two systems can be used either to generate additional investment income or to reduce outstanding indebtedness. It is assumed that the appropriate discount rate for each of these two alternatives would be 10 percent.

Once again, the effects of cost reimbursement should be considered. In our example, we assume that 50 percent of the extended care facility's capital costs will be reimbursed and 10 percent of its operating costs will be reimbursed. The following adjustments result:

Equivalent annual cost of $5,000 sprinkler system:

Present value of reimbursed operating costs = $500 $\times$ 6.145 $\times$ .10 = $307.25

Present value of reimbursed depreciation = $\dfrac{\$5,000}{10}$ $\times$ 6.145 $\times$ .50 = $1,536.25

Equivalent annual cost = $1,314 $-$ $\dfrac{(\$307.25 + \$1,536.25)}{6.145}$ = $1,014

Equivalent annual cost of $10,000 sprinkler system:

Present value of reimbursed operating costs = $200 $\times$ 8.514 $\times$ .10 = $170.25

Present value of reimbursed depreciation = $\dfrac{\$10,000}{20}$ $\times$ 8.514 $\times$ .5 = $2,128.50

Equivalent annual cost = $1,375 $-$ $\dfrac{(\$170.25 + \$2,128.50)}{8.514}$ = $1,105

Again, some clarification of the calculations may be useful. To reflect the effect of cost reimbursement, consideration must be given to the reimbursement of reported expenses for the two alternative sprinkler systems. The reported expense items for both sprinkler systems are depreciation and maintenance cost, which is referred to as an operating cost. Depreciation for the $5,000 sprinkler system will be $500 per year ($500/10) and 50 percent of this amount, $250, will be reimbursed each year. The present value of the reimbursed depreciation ($250 $\times$ 6.145) is $1,536.25. Using the same procedure, the present value of reimbursed depreciation for the $10,000 sprinkler system is $2,128.50 ($250 $\times$ 8.514). In a similar fashion, the maintenance costs for the two sprinkler systems will also be reimbursed. For the $5,000 system, the annual $500 maintenance cost will yield $50 in new reimbursement (.10 $\times$ $500) per year. The present value of this reimbursement inflow is $307.25. Using the same calculations for the $10,000 sprinkler system yields a present value of $170.25. The present values of both reimbursed depreciation and maintenance costs are then annualized and subtracted from the initially calculated equivalent annual cost to derive new equivalent annual costs that reflect cost-reimbursement effects.

In this case, cost reimbursement did not change the decision. The lower-cost sprinkler system, after consideration of the effects of reimbursement, is still the best alternative. In fact, the relative difference has increased.

SELECTION OF THE DISCOUNT RATE

In the three DCF methods just discussed, to specify the discount rate, we simply selected a number arbitrarily for each of our examples. In an actual case, however, the question of how to select the appropriate discount rate requires careful attention.

Before discussing methods of determining the appropriate discount rate, it may be useful to evaluate the role of the discount rate in project selection. A natural question at this point is, Would an alternative discount rate affect the list of capital projects selected? For example, if we used a discount rate of 10 percent and later learned that 12 percent should have been used, would our list of approved projects change? The answer is maybe. In some cases, alternative values for the discount rate would alter the relative ranking and therefore the desirability of particular projects.

Again, we believe that the definition of the discount rate is an important issue, but not a critical one—especially for health care organizations. This is true for several reasons. First, in the case of health care organizations, the financial criterion is not likely to be the only criterion. Other areas—such as need, quality of care, and teaching—may also be important. Second, a change in the relative ranking of projects is much more likely to result from an accurate forecast of cash flows than it is from an alternative discount rate. Efforts to improve forecasting would appear to be far more important than esoteric discussions over the relevancy of cost-of-capital alternatives.

In this context, we can examine three primary methods for defining a discount rate or the cost of capital for use in a DCF analysis:

1. cost of specific financing source
2. yield achievable on other investments
3. weighted cost of capital

The cost of a specific financing source is sometimes used as the discount rate. Usually, the identified financing source is debt. For example, if a hospital can borrow money at 11 percent in the revenue bond market, that rate would become its cost of capital or discount rate.

Another alternative is to use the yield rate possible on other investments. In many cases, this rate might be equal to the investment yield possible in the firm's security portfolio. For example, if the firm currently earned 13 percent on its security investments, then 13 percent would be its discount rate. This method, based on an opportunity cost concept, is relatively easy to understand.

The last alternative is to use the weighted cost of capital. This is the most widely discussed and used method of defining the discount rate. In its simplest form, it is calculated as:

Cost of capital = (% Debt × Cost of debt) + (% Equity × Cost of equity)

The advantage of this method is that it clearly represents the cost of capital to the firm. A major problem with its use, however, is the definition of the cost of equity capital. This is an especially difficult problem for nonprofit firms. How do you define the cost of equity capital? Detailed exploration of this issue and other aspects of discount rate selection are beyond the scope of the present discussion.

Readers who are interested in examining these topics in greater depth are referred to any good introductory finance textbook.

SUMMARY

The capital decision-making process in the health care industry is very complex, involving a great many independent decision makers. In this chapter, we examined the process and focused on methods for evaluating capital projects. Although capital expenditure decisions in the health care industry are not usually decided exclusively on the basis of financial criteria, most health care decision makers regard financial factors as important elements in the process. In that context, the three discounted cash flow methods we have examined can serve as useful tools in capital project analysis for health care facilities.

ASSIGNMENTS

1. A health care firm's investment of $1,000 in a piece of equipment will reduce labor costs by $400 per year for the next five years. Eighty percent of all patients seen by the firm have a third party payer arrangement that pays for capital costs on a retrospective basis. Ten percent of all patients reimburse for actual operating costs. What is the annual cash flow of the investment? Assume a five-year life and straight-line depreciation.

2. A hospital has just experienced a breakdown in one of its boilers. The boiler must be replaced very quickly if the hospital is to continue operations. Should this investment be subjected to any analysis?

3. Few firms ever track the actual results achieved from a specific capital investment against projected results. What are the likely effects of such a management policy?

4. Santa Cruz Community Hospital is considering investing $90,000 in new laundry equipment to replace its present equipment, which is completely depreciated and outmoded. An alternative to this investment is a long-term contract with a local firm to perform the hospital's laundry service. It is expected that the hospital would save $20,000 per year in operating costs if the laundry service were performed internally. The expected life and

depreciable life of the projected equipment are both six years. Salvage value of the present equipment is expected to be zero.

Assuming that Santa Cruz Community Hospital can borrow or invest money at eight percent, calculate the payback, the net present value, and the profitability index. Ignore any reimbursement effects.

5. Frances Gebauer, president of Lucas Valley Hospital System, is investigating the purchase of 36 TV sets for rental purposes. The sets have an expected life of two years and cost $500 apiece. The possible rental income flows are:

Year 1		Year 2	
Rental Income	Conditional Probability	Rental Income	Conditional Probability
$12,000	.40	$4,000	.40
		7,000	.60
$15,000	.60	6,000	.30
		8,000	.70

If funds cost Lucas Valley ten percent, calculate the expected net present value of this project.

6. Mr. Dobbs, administrator at Innovative Hospital, is considering opening a new Health Screening Department in the hospital. However, he is terribly concerned about the financial consequences of this action, since his Board has indicated that, because the current financial position of the hospital is not good, the project must pay for itself.

Mr. Dobbs is thus especially interested in the establishment of a rate for the service and has called upon you for your expert financial advice. He has prepared the following cost and utilization data for your review:

Year	Variable Cost	Fixed Costs[a]	Patients Screened
1	$ 96,000	$120,000	2,400
2	144,000	135,000	3,600
3	192,000	150,000	4,800
4	192,000	150,000	4,800
5	192,000	150,000	4,800

[a] Includes depreciation of equipment costing $350,000 over a five-year life, assuming straight-line depreciation.

Mr. Dobbs is aware of the rapid pace of technological change and anticipates that the current equipment, costing $350,000, will need to be replaced at the end of Year 5 for $500,000. He is not concerned about price inflation for his other operating costs because he believes the increased costs can be recovered by increased charges. However, he is concerned about establishing a current charge for the new service that will generate a fund of sufficient size to meet the Year 5 replacement cost. Mr. Dobbs believes that any invested funds will earn interest at a rate of eight percent compounded annually. Assume all payments and receipts are made at year end.

What rate would you recommend charging for the new health screening service? Assume this rate to be effective for the entire five-year period.

7. Two hospitals are considering merging their laundry departments and constructing a new facility to take care of their future laundry requirements. Some relevant cost data are presented below:

	Hospital A	Hospital B	Merged C
Variable cost/pound	.030	.032	.024
Pounds of laundry	300,000	700,000	1,000,000
Fixed costs/year			
Depreciation (lease)	$ 1,000	$ 5,000	$ 8,000
Maintenance	1,400	2,500	3,000
Administrative salaries	8,000	16,000	20,000
Transportation	0	0	3,000
Total fixed cost	$10,400	$23,500	$34,000

The new laundry facility will cost approximately $40,000 to construct and will be located between the two hospitals in a leased building. Average life of the equipment is assumed to be eight years, which generates a $5,000 yearly depreciation charge. Lease payment is fixed at $3,000/year for the next eight years. Financing for the project will be generated from available funds in each institution: $12,000 from Hospital A, and $28,000 from Hospital B. Expenses will be shared using the same ratios (30 and 70 percent). Both hospitals employ a discount factor of ten percent on their cost reduction investment projects.

Given this information, do you think the merger is beneficial to both individual hospitals? What other information would you like to have to help you evaluate this investment project?

8. In the preceding laundry merger problem, assume that Hospital B would expect to replace its present equipment with new equipment in two years at a cost of $64,000. The equipment would have an eight-year life. Ignoring cost reimbursement considerations, does the merger make economic sense for Hospital B under these conditions?

9. Scioto Valley Convalescent Center is considering buying a $25,000 computer to improve its medical record and accounting functions. It is estimated that, with the computer, operating costs will be reduced by $7,000 per year. The computer has an estimated five-year life with an estimated $5,000 salvage value. What is this investment's profitability index if the discount rate is eight percent? Ignore reimbursement considerations.

10. In Problem 9, assume that capital costs are reimbursed 80 percent and there is no reimbursement based on operating costs. Further assume that Scioto Valley is a tax-paying entity with a marginal tax rate of 40 percent. What is the profitability index for this project now?

SOLUTIONS AND ANSWERS

1. The cash flow of the equipment investment by the health care firm may be calculated as follows:

Cash flow = Annual depreciation × Proportion of capital cost payers
+ (Annual operating savings × [1–Proportion of operating cost payers])
= $200 × .80 + ($400 [1–.10])
= $160 + $360 = $520

2. The investment in a new boiler would have benefits for the hospital in the area of operational continuance. Failure to make the needed investment would mean a discontinued service. In this case, less analysis is needed, but care should still be exercised in identifying alternatives. The lowest-cost alternative to meet the need should be selected.

3. If it does not compare actual with projected results, management may lose some of the benefits that were originally expected to be realized with its investment. If the control loop is not closed, management will not know, and therefore cannot correct for, deviations from forecasted results. It is also possible that some departmental managers will overstate benefits for their favorite capital projects and that such actions will not be perceived as having any adverse consequences since no comparison of forecast with actual results was made.

4. The following calculations show the payback, the net present value, and the profitability index for the laundry service investment:

$$\text{Payback} = \frac{\text{Investment cost}}{\text{Annual cash flow}} = \frac{\$90{,}000}{\$20{,}000} = 4.5 \text{ years}$$

$$\text{Net present value} = \text{Present value of cash inflows} - \text{Investment cost}$$

$$= \$20{,}000 \times P(8\%,6) - \$90{,}000$$

$$= \$20{,}000 \times 4.623 - \$90{,}000 = \$2{,}460$$

$$\text{Profitability index} = \frac{\text{Net present value}}{\text{Investment cost}} = \frac{\$2{,}460}{\$90{,}000} = .0273$$

5. The net present value of Lucas Valley's TV-purchase project is shown in the following data:

Item	Amount	Year	Probability	Expected Value	Present Value Factor	Expected Present Value
Rental income	$12,000	1	.40	$4,800	.909	$4,363.20
Rental income	15,000	1	.60	9,000	.909	8,181.00
Rental income	4,000	2	.16	640	.826	528.64
Rental income	7,000	2	.24	1,680	.826	1,387.68
Rental income	6,000	2	.18	1,080	.826	892.08
Rental income	8,000	2	.42	3,360	.826	2,775.36
TV cost	(18,000)	0	1.00	(18,000)	1.000	(18,000.00)
Expected net present value						$ 127.96

6. The first step in determining the rate that Mr. Dobbs should charge for the new health screening service is to calculate the present value of the cash flow requirements that need to be covered by the charge for the service:

Item	Amount	Year	Present Value Factor (8%)	Present Value
Costs less depreciation	$146,000	1	.926	$ 135,196
Costs less depreciation	209,000	2	.857	179,113
Costs less depreciation	272,000	3	.794	215,968
Costs less depreciation	272,000	4	.735	199,920
Costs less depreciation	272,000	5	.681	185,232
Replacement	500,000	5	.681	340,500
				$1,255,929

The second step is to define the rate that will generate the required present value as calculated above. If we define r as the required rate per screening, the following calculation can be made:

$$\$1,255,929 = (2,400 \times r \times p[8\%,1]) + (3,600 \times r \times p[8\%,2])$$
$$+ (4,800 \times r \times p[8\%,3]) + (4,800 \times r \times p[8\%,4])$$
$$+ (4,800 \times r \times p[8\%,5])$$

$$\$1,255,929 = (2,400r[.926]) + (3,600r[.857]) + (4,800r[.794])$$
$$+ (4,800r[.735]) + (4,800r[.681])$$

$$\$1,255,929 = 15,915.6r$$
$$r = \frac{\$1,255,929}{15,915}$$
$$r = \$78.91$$

7. The relevant data and calculations in the laundry service merger between Hospital A and Hospital B are presented below:

	Hospital A	Hospital B
Cash outflows—unmerged		
Variable costs	$ 9,000	$22,400
Maintenance	1,400	2,500
Salaries	8,000	16,000
Total	$18,400	$40,900
Cash outflow—merged		
Variable costs	$ 7,200	$16,800
Lease	900	2,100
Maintenance	900	2,100
Salaries	6,000	14,000
Transportation	900	2,100
	$15,900	$37,100
Net savings	$ 2,500	$ 3,800

Hospital A:

Present value savings = $2,500 × P (10%,8) = $2,500 × 5.335 = $13,337.50

Profitability index = $\dfrac{\$1,337.50}{\$12,000.00}$ = .111

Hospital B:

Present value of savings = $3,800 × P (10%,8) = $3,800 × 5.335 = $20,273

Profitability index = $\dfrac{-7,727}{28,000}$ = -.276

Thus, given present data, the merger would be beneficial to Hospital A but not to Hospital B. A key piece of additional data that is needed is the replacement cost of the existing equipment. If Hospital B would need to acquire new equipment in the near future, the merger might also be favorable to them. The effects of cost reimbursement should also be considered.

8. The laundry merger project in these new circumstances would require use of the equivalent annual cost method. The merged alternative would have an eight-year life, while the unmerged alternative would have a ten-year life cycle.

Merged:

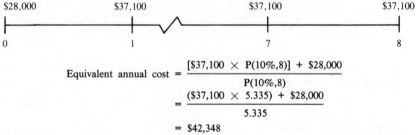

Equivalent annual cost = $\dfrac{[\$37,100 \times P(10\%,8)] + \$28,000}{P(10\%,8)}$

$= \dfrac{(\$37,100 \times 5.335) + \$28,000}{5.335}$

$= \$42,348$

Unmerged:

Equivalent annual cost = $\dfrac{(\$40,900 \times P[10\%,10]) + (\$64,000 \times p[10\%,2])}{P(10\%,10)}$

$= \dfrac{(\$40,900 \times 6.145) + (64,000 \times .826)}{6.145}$

$= \$49,503$

The merger alternative is now more desirable for Hospital B because it has a lower equivalent annual cost compared to the nonmerger alternative.

9. The profitability index for the computer investment by Scioto Valley Convalescent Center is calculated as follows:

Present value of cash inflows = ($7,000 × P[8%,5]) + ($5,000 × p[8%,5])
= ($7,000 × 3.993) + ($5,000 × .681)
= $31,356

$$\text{Profitability index} = \frac{\$31,356 - \$25,000}{\$25,000} = .254$$

10. The calculation of the profitability index for the computer investment in these new circumstances is now:

Calculation of present value of cash inflows:

Operating savings

$7,000 × (1 − .40) × 3.993 = $16,770.60

Reimbursed depreciation

$4,000 × .80 × (1 − .40) × 3.993 =   7,666.56

Depreciation tax shelter effect

$4,000 × .40 × 3.993 =   6,388.80

Salvage value

$5,000 × .681 =   3,405.00

Total present value $34,230.96

$$\text{Profitability index} = \frac{\$34,230.96 - \$25,000}{\$25,000} = .369$$

Chapter 14

Capital Formation

In this last chapter, we shall examine the concepts and principals of capital formation in the health care industry. There are few areas that are more important to the financial well-being of a health care firm. A firm that cannot obtain the amounts of capital specified in its strategic financial plan will not be able to achieve its long-run objectives. Indeed, if the firm finds it difficult to acquire capital in any amount at a reasonable cost, its future survival may be questionable. Successful firms have the capability to provide capital financing when needed, and at a cost that is reasonable.

Three key questions are relevant to our discussion of capital formation in the health care industry. First, how much capital is needed? Ideally, the firm should have defined its capital needs in its strategic financial plan. Capital needs should include working capital requirements and replacement reserves, as well as the funding needs for buildings and equipment.

Second, what sources of capital financing are available? At the time of this writing, the future availability of tax exempt financing is unclear. Tax exempt financing has been the largest source of capital for the hospital industry for the last 20 years. If it were eliminated, a major shift in financing patterns would take place. The exact direction of this shift is unclear at this time, although it would seem that taxable sources of debt would have to be substituted for tax exempt sources.

Third, how are the costs of capital financing provided for in third party payment plans? This area is critical to the discussion of capital financing and selection of capital financing alternatives. At the time of this writing, the majority of third party payment plans provide for the payment of actual capital costs, such as interest expense. It is expected, however, that this situation will change and that cost reimbursement of capital costs will be replaced by some scheme of prospective prices.

Table 14–1 presents a summary of investment and financing patterns in the hospital industry for the period 1980 to 1984. In general, we can classify the sources of financing into the following two categories: (1) equity and (2) debt. In the hospital industry, approximately 50 percent of total assets are financed with equity and 50 percent financed with debt. However, financing patterns may vary somewhat in different sectors of the health care industry. For example, many long-term care facilities have much higher proportions of debt. Debt financing in such facilities may run as high as 90 percent.

EQUITY FINANCING

In general there are only two ways that a firm can generate new equity capital:

1. profit retention
2. contributions

Table 14–1 Percentage Balance Sheet for the Hospital Industry

	Percentages				
	1980	1981	1982	1983	1984
Assets					
Cash and marketable securities	4.2	4.2	4.5	4.5	5.1
Net accounts receivable	15.7	16.2	15.7	15.4	15.4
Inventory	1.7	1.6	1.5	1.4	1.2
Other current assets	2.3	2.2	2.3	2.5	2.7
Total current assets	23.9	24.2	24.0	23.8	24.4
Other investments	9.9	10.1	11.6	12.0	13.2
Net fixed assets	59.7	58.2	55.6	55.1	52.2
Other assets	6.5	7.5	8.8	9.1	10.2
Total assets	100.0	100.0	100.0	100.0	100.0
Liabilities and Fund Balance					
Current liabilities	12.7	13.4	13.6	13.5	12.9
Long-term liabilities	35.7	35.0	37.2	38.7	38.2
Other	1.4	2.2	2.4	1.7	1.8
Fund balance	50.2	49.4	46.8	46.1	47.1
Total liabilities and fund balance	100.0	100.0	100.0	100.0	100.0

Source: Reprinted from *Hospital Industry Analysis Report 1980-1984* by W. Cleverley, p. 113, with permission of Healthcare Financial Management Association, © 1984.

We have already stressed in past chapters the importance of earning adequate levels of profit. Hence, our discussion at this point is focused primarily on contributions. A contribution may be given to a firm for a variety of reasons. Normally, in tax exempt health care firms, a contribution is given with no thought of a future return. The donor may derive some immediate or deferred tax benefit, but there is no expectation of a financial return to be paid by the health care entity. In contrast, contributions are given to a taxable health care entity in the expectation of a future financial return. The contribution may be in the form of a stock purchase or a limited partnership unit. It is important to note that this form of contribution may also be available to tax exempt entities through a corporate restructuring arrangement. We shall discuss this point in more detail shortly.

Philanthropy is definitely not dead in our nation. In 1983, approximately two percent of our nation's Gross National Product, or $64.93 billion, was in the form of philanthropic gifts. Tables 14–2 and 14–3 provide data showing the sources and the distribution of giving for the period 1979 to 1983. These data present an encouraging picture. Total giving was up almost 50 percent over the four-year period 1979 to 1983. That is a promising growth rate in almost anyone's book. Even better, giving in the health and hospital area grew 54 percent over the same four-year period. Individuals were clearly the largest source of giving, representing well over 80 percent of total giving.

To be successful, an equity financing program should have the following key elements:

- *A "case statement."* This document should carefully and persuasively define why you need money.

- *A designated development officer.* This individual may not be full-time, but duties and expectations should be precisely defined. Incentives for development officers should be related to expectations for giving.

- *Trustee and medical staff involvement.* People give to people, not organizations.

- *Prospect lists.* You should know who in the community are prime prospects for giving.

- *Programs for giving.* This is critical. You should have a variety of methods and means to encourage giving. For example, you may have a number of deferred giving plans, such as unitrusts, annuity trusts, or pooled income funds. Your development officer should be familiar with these methods.

- *Goals.* You need to define realistic targets for long-range planning.

Table 14–2 Sources of Giving

	1979		1983	
	Dollars (billions)	Percent	Dollars (billions)	Percent
Individuals	$36.54	84.4	$53.85	82.9
Bequests	2.23	5.1	4.52	7.0
Foundations	2.24	5.2	3.46	5.3
Corporations	2.30	5.3	3.10	4.8
Total	$43.31	100.0	$64.93	100.0

Table 14–3 Distribution of Giving

	1979		1983	
	Dollars (billions)	Percent	Dollars (billions)	Percent
Religion	$20.14	46.5	$31.03	47.8
Health and hospitals	5.95	13.7	9.15	14.1
Education	5.99	13.8	9.04	13.9
Social welfare	4.35	10.0	6.94	10.7
Arts and humanities	2.70	6.2	4.08	6.3
Civic and other	1.24	2.9	1.80	2.8
Other	2.94	6.9	2.89	4.4
Total	$43.31	100.0	$64.93	100.0

Source: Reprinted from Giving U.S.A., with permission of American Association of Fund-Raising Council, Inc.

There are many ways to encourage individuals to give to charitable tax exempt health care firms. Many large firms employ full-time development staff. These individuals can do much to increase charitable giving.

One of the most promising areas of philanthropic giving is deferred gift arrangements. In a deferred giving plan, a tax payer donor may get an immediate tax benefit in return for a later gift to the tax exempt firm. An interesting recent example of deferred giving is the case of a hospital in California that initiated a provocative new fund raising effort, called the Home Value Program (HVP). HVP was designed for senior citizens, age 70 or above, who own mortgage free homes. The homeowners sign a revocable agreement that, upon their death, transfers title to their homes to the hospital. In return, they receive from the hospital a monthly payment that is based on a loan. In concept, HVP is very similar to the reverse annuity mortgages that are being used in some banking circles.

The following case illustrates the mechanics of HVP. Assume Mrs. Jones, age 70, has a mortgage-free home with a market value of $100,000. The hospital, or its foundation, executes a loan of $50,000 at 12 percent interest that will pay Mrs. Jones $717 per month for ten years. Mrs. Jones signs a revocable agreement.

How does the hospital benefit? First, for a $50,000 loan, the hospital receives title to property that is valued at $100,000. Second, the hospital benefits from any appreciation on the property. In ten years, if the annual appreciation rate is 5 percent, Mrs. Jones's $100,000 home will be worth $163,000. Third, the hospital establishes a relationship with Mrs. Jones that may lead to other donations.

How does Mrs. Jones benefit? First, the monthly payment is considered tax-free income. Second, there is no risk to Mrs. Jones since the agreement is revocable and can be rescinded with payment of the loan plus a penalty. Third, HVP provides Mrs. Jones with a tangible way of supporting the hospital. The last factor is the key to the ultimate success of the program.

An HVP, or some adaption of it, can provide a significant return to a hospital. However, some forethought is required. For one thing, working capital obviously is necessary. Payments to homeowners will precede any recovery through sale of the donated homes. Also, a significant amount of legal, accounting, and actuarial consulting is essential. Finally, such a program should not be perceived as a pure donation program. It is intended to be a method of investment diversification, albeit one with unusually high returns. Thus, a program like HVP can provide an excellent vehicle for long-term equity capital growth.

Both taxable and tax exempt health care providers have shown great interest in the issuance of equity to investors. For taxable health care firms, this interest is not new; for most such firms, the issuance of equity has been a major source of financing over the years. Most taxable health care firms began with a small amount of venture capital. They were able to use that original funding to develop a successful track record of operations. Based on that record of success, an initial public offering (IPO) of stock was made. The resulting funds were then used to expand operations, part of which was fueled by leveraging funds acquired in the IPO.

The technique of expanding operations quickly through the issuance of equity and then leveraging that equity has been used extensively in the tax exempt sector. The following data illustrate the growth potential of a taxable entity:

Organizational Type	Historical Net Income	Equity Issue (Stock)	Debt Addition	Possible Total Capital
Tax exempt	$1.0	.0	$ 2.0	$ 3.0
Taxable	$ .5	$10.0	$21.0	$31.5

These data indicate that a taxable entity could raise approximately ten times the amount of total capital that a tax exempt entity could. Let us examine these data and their related assumptions more closely to understand clearly the underlying process behind capital formation. It is assumed that some business unit or firm has generated $1.0 million in before-tax income. If the firm were a taxable entity, it would be required to pay approximately 50 percent of this income as tax. However the taxable firm could issue stock, limited partnership units, or some other type of equity security. Further, it is assumed that a price-to-earnings multiple of 20 is in effect. This means that the taxable firm could raise $10.0 million in equity based upon its net income of $500,000. Both the tax exempt and the taxable firms could issue debt based upon their equity positions. We have assumed that a leverage ratio of two to one exists; that is the firms could borrow $2.00 for every $1.00 of equity. The taxable firm could issue $21.0 million in debt, while the tax exempt firm would be limited to $2.0 million in debt. Total capital, both debt and equity, would be $3.0 million for the tax exempt firm and $31.5 million for the taxable firm.

In the preceding example, some of the assumptions might be changed, but the relative growth potential would remain the same. In this situation, is there any way that a tax exempt firm can take advantage of this growth potential? The answer is yes: A tax exempt firm could change its status to taxable. This is not an easy thing to do, but it is not impossible. Several large HMOs started out as tax exempt firms but changed their ownership status to maximize their growth potential.

An easier alternative method is to restructure the firm. Figure 14–1 presents a generic structure that is used by many tax exempt health care firms to create an equity capital formation alternative. This structure involves the creation of taxable entities that can issue equity securities directly to investors. In the parent holding company model in Figure 14–1, there are several taxable entities that could issue equity to investors and help generate capital for the entire consolidated structure.

An actual case example may help to illustrate the potential for capital formation created by restructuring a tax exempt health care firm. ABC hospital needed to replace its CT scanner with a new one. The estimated cost of the new scanner was $1,160,000. The hospital did not wish to use any of its

Figure 14–1 A Parent Holding Company

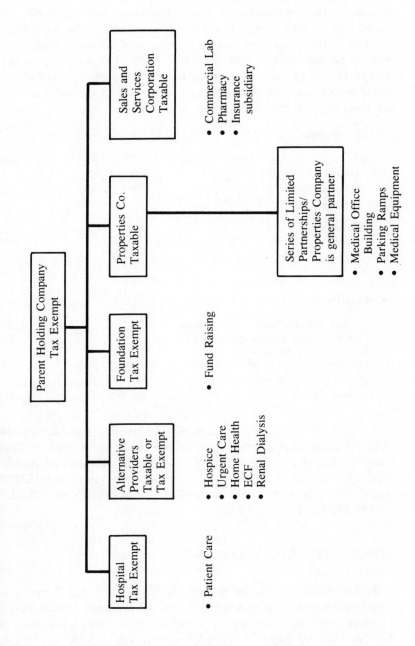

debt capacity in this project. The solution was to create a limited partnership/joint venture with its physicians. A new entity was created, called ABC Scanner, which was a limited partnership. The ABC Properties Company, which was a subsidiary of the hospital's parent holding company, was the general partner. A bank loan of $1,180,000 was obtained; the loan was guaranteed by the limited partners (30 limited partners, all of whom were physicians) and the general partner. The source and use-of-funds statement for the new structure is presented below:

Sources of Funds

Bank loan		$1,180,000
Guaranteed by:		
General partner	$295,000	
Limited partners (@$29,500)	885,000	
General partner's cash contribution		50,000
Limited partner's cash contribution (@$5,000)		150,000
Total sources		$1,380,000

Uses of Funds

Purchase and installation of CT scanner	$1,160,000
Leasehold (suite) improvements	95,000
Loan placement fee	35,400
Legal and other organizational expenses	15,000
Reserve for working capital	74,600
Total uses	$1,380,000

This statement documents the capability of the new structure to enhance ABC hospital's capital position with little funding commitment from the hospital. The general partner, a member of the restructured health care entity, has contributed only $50,000 of cash and guaranteed $295,000 in loans. For this rather modest level of commitment, total funding of $1,380,000 was made available.

LONG-TERM DEBT FINANCING

An examination of the specific sources of long-term debt financing in the health care industry can be a very complex and confusing process. Part of the problem stems from the use of jargon by those involved. Unless one is familiar with this jargon, meaningful communication with financing people may be difficult. Before describing the alternatives for long-term debt financing in the health care industry, we should note five key characteristics of financing that greatly affect the relative desirability of alternative sources of financing. As we describe these characteristics, we shall introduce some new terminology that will facilitate later discussion. The five key characteristics are:

1. cost
2. control
3. risk
4. availability
5. adequacy

Cost

The most important characteristic that affects the cost of alternative debt financing is interest rates. The fixed return of a long-term debt instrument is often called the *coupon rate*. For example, a 9.8 percent hospital revenue bond indicates that the issuer will pay the investor $98 annually for every $1,000 of principal. Sometimes the term *basis point* is used to describe differences in coupon rates. A basis point is one-hundreth of one percent. For example, the difference between a coupon rate of 9.80 percent and 9.65 percent would be 15 basis points.

Although interest is the primary measure of financing cost, it is not the only aspect of cost that should be considered. Issuance costs can be sizable in some types of financing. Issuance costs are simply those expenditures that are essential to consummate the financing. There is a great difference in the amount of issuance costs for *publicly placed* and *privately placed* issues. A privately placed issue is one that is not sold to the general market but is rather purchased directly by only a few major buyers. In a publicly placed issue, there are a number of costs that must be incurred in order legally to sell the securities to the general public. There are printing costs associated with producing the official statements that will be sent to prospective clients. There are costs for attorneys and accountants who must certify various aspects of the issue, such as its financial feasibility and its tax exempt status. Finally, there is the *underwriters spread* that is charged by the investment banking firm that arranges the sale of the securities. When aggregated together, issuance costs can sometimes amount to as much as five percent of the total issue. This means that an issuer must borrow $100 to get $95.

Another large cost of financing is *reserve requirements*. Some types of financing require the creation of fund balances in escrow accounts under the custody of the *bond trustee*. The bond trustee is designated by the issuer to represent the interests of the bondholders. The obligations of the trustee are defined in the Trust Indenture Act of 1939, which is administered by the Securities and Exchange Commission. There are two primary categories of reserve requirements. The first is the *debt service reserve.* This fund represents a cushion for the investors if the issuer gets into some type of fiscal crisis. It is usually set equal to one year's worth of principal and interest payments. The second category of reserve requirement is the *depreciation reserve.* This fund is sometimes set up to equal the cumulative difference between debt principal repayment and depreciation expense on the financed assets. Usually the amount of depreciation expense is greatest in the early years after a major construction program has been completed, when debt principal may be at its lowest level. Since reimbursed depreciation may represent the primary source of debt principal payment, there is a need to accumulate these funds to ensure their availability in later years, when the amount of debt principal payment exceeds depreciation. Figure 14–2 presents a graphic display of this relationship.

Control

Ideally, when issuing debt financing, the issuer would like to have little or no interference by the investors in management. It is usually not possible to avoid such interference, however. The investors will often specify some conditions or restraints that they would like to see included in the bond contract. Such conditions or restrictions are often known as *covenants.* These are spelled out in great detail in the *indenture,* which is the written contract between the investors and the issuing company.

One category of restrictive covenants concerns specific financial performance indicators. For example, most indentures define values for the firm's debt service coverage ratio and its current ratio. If actual values for these indicators are below the defined values, the bond trustee may take certain actions. The trustee may assume a position on the board of trustees, replace current management, or require the entire outstanding principal to be paid immediately.

Another category of covenants concerns future financing. A section in the indenture referred to as *additional parity financing* defines the conditions that must be satisfied before the firm can issue any additional debt. The most important condition is usually prior and projected debt service coverage.

Figure 14–2 Depreciation Reserve Requirement: Relationship Between Depreciation Expense and Debt Principal Payments

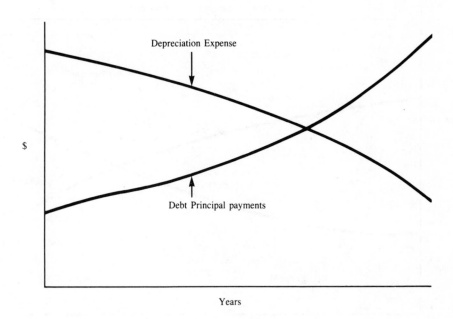

Risk

From the issuer's perspective, flexibility in repayment terms is highly desirable. An issuer with flexible repayment terms can alter payments to meet the issuer's current cash flow. The investor, on the other hand, wants some protection that the principal will be repaid in accordance with some preestablished plan.

One of the most important indenture elements is the *prepayment provision*. This provision specifies the point in time at which the debt can be retired and the penalty that will be imposed for an early retirement. For example, the indenture may prohibit the issuer from prepaying the debt for the first ten years of issue life. Thereafter, the debt may be repaid, but only if there is a *call*

Figure 14–3 Level Debt Service: Relationship Between Interest Payment and Debt Principal

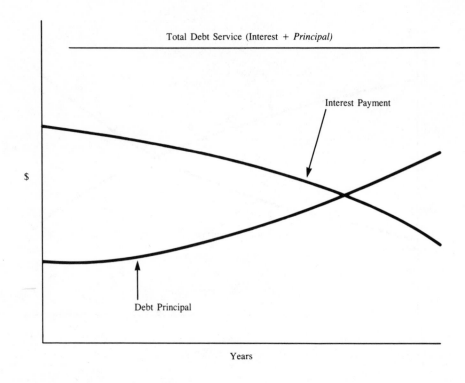

Total Debt Service (Interest + *Principal*)

Interest Payment

$

Debt Principal

Years

---

premium. The call premium is some percentage of the par or face value of the bonds. Thus, a call premium of five percent would mean that a $50 premium would be paid for each $1,000 of bonds. The issuer would like to have the option of retiring outstanding debt at any point with no call premium. However, investors do not usually permit this in debt that has a fixed interest rate.

Another aspect of risk relates to the debt principal amortization pattern. Most debt retirement plans can be categorized as *level debt service* or *level debt principal.* In a level debt service plan, the amount of interest and principal that is repaid each year remains fairly constant. This is the type of repayment that is usually associated with home mortgages. In the early years, the amount of interest is far greater than the debt principal. Over time, this pattern changes and the amount of principal repaid each year begins to

Figure 14–4 Level Debt Principal: Relationship Between Interest
Payment and Total Debt Service

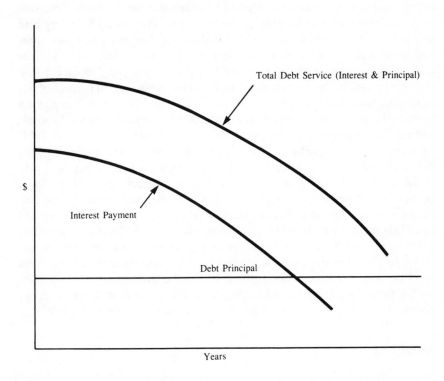

Total Debt Service (Interest & Principal)

$

Interest Payment

Debt Principal

Years

exceed the interest payment. Figure 14–3 presents a graphic view of this
relationship. Level debt principal means that equal amount of debt principal
is repaid each year. In this pattern of debt retirement, the total debt service
payment falls over time. Figure 14–4 shows this relationship.

Many financing plans approximate a level debt service plan. This pattern of
debt amortization extends the debt retirement life and may benefit the issuer.
The benefit is predicated upon three factors:

1. the ability of the issuer to earn a return greater than the interest rate
   on the debt
2. the presence of reimbursement for capital costs
3. the availability of tax exempt financing

To illustrate the desirability of principal repayment delay, we shall examine a simple case. Let us assume that we have two alternative financing plans. One plan will permit us to borrow $10 million for five years with no payment of principal until the fifth year. We will be required to pay 10 percent per year as our interest payment for each of the five years. The second financing plan will permit us to borrow the same $10 million for five years; however, there will be an annual payment of principal equal to $2 million per year. The interest rate on this financing plan will be 8 percent per year, which is below the interest rate in the first plan. Let us further assume that 80 percent of our interest expense will be repaid by our third party payers, who still pay us for the actual costs of capital incurred. Finally, let us assume that any differences in cash flow between the two plans could be invested at 10 percent. Table 14–4 provides a comparison of the net present values for these two financing plans. The table values indicate that the higher interest balloon payment plan is the lower cost source of financing. This is a direct result of the large percentage, 80 percent, of capital cost payment. An 80 percent capital cost payment means that the effective interest rate is $(1 - .80)$ times the interest rate. This means that the effective interest rate for the balloon plan would be 2.0 percent, and the corresponding value for the equal principal plan would be 1.6 percent. The difference in interest rates has decreased from 2.0 percent to .4 percent. An investment yield of 10 percent means that we can make money from delaying principal payment. In short, our cost is less than our return. It is only natural to want to retain money as long as possible.

Availability

Once a health care firm has decided that it needs debt financing, it usually wants to obtain the funds as quickly as possible. A delay can have rather severe consequences. A delay could postpone the start of a construction program. This might increase the cost of the total program because of normal inflation in construction costs. A delay could also result in an unexpected increase in interest rates. Though privately placed issues can usually be arranged more quickly than publicly placed issues, there is usually a higher interest rate associated with privately placed issues. However, the difference in interest rates may more than offset the costs of delay.

Adequacy

A key requirement of any proposed plan of financing is that it cover all the associated costs. One of the key areas of adequacy is that of refinancing costs. In many situations, a new program of construction that requires new

Table 14-4 Cost of Alternative Debt Amortization Plans

Item	Amount Before Reimbursement Effect	Amount After Reimbursement Effect	Years	PV Factor (10%)	PV
	Equal Principal Payment—8%				
Principal	$2,000,000	$2,000,000	1–5	3.791	$7,582,000
Interest	800,000	160,000	1	.909	145,440
Interest	640,000	128,000	2	.826	105,728
Interest	480,000	96,000	3	.751	72,096
Interest	320,000	64,000	4	.683	43,712
Interest	160,000	32,000	5	.621	19,872
Net present value cost					$7,968,848
	Balloon Principal—10%				
Interest	$ 1,000,000	$ 200,000	1–5	3.791	$ 758,200
Principal	10,000,000	10,000,000	5	.621	6,210,000
Net present value cost					$6,968,200

financing may not be possible unless existing financing can be retired or refinanced. Not all types of financing permit the issuer to include the costs of refinancing in the amount borrowed.

Funding during construction is another important area of financing. Some types of financing do not permit the issuer to borrow during the construction period. A loan will be made only after the construction has been completed and the new assets are available for operations. In this situation, the issuer must arrange for a separate source of funding to finance the construction. Permanent financing must then be arranged upon completion of the construction program.

Interest incurred during construction can be rather sizable. For example, a $50 million construction program might incur $10 to $15 million in interest during the construction period. It is thus important to have a source of financing that also permits the issuer to borrow to cover interest costs.

Lastly, it should be noted that the percentage of financing available varies across financing plans. Some plans permit up to 100 percent of the cost, whereas others may limit the amount to 70 or 80 percent. Depending upon the availability of other funds, these limitations may pose real problems in some situations.

ALTERNATIVE DEBT FINANCING SOURCES

Sources

At present time, there are four major alternative sources of long-term debt available to health care facilities:

1. Tax exempt revenue bonds
2. FHA-insured mortgages
3. Public taxable bonds
4. Conventional mortgage financing

Table 14–5 compares these four sources of financing with respect to the factors that affect capital financing desirability.

Tax Exempt Revenue Bonds

Tax exempt revenue bonds permit the interest earned on them to be exempt from federal income taxation. The primary security for such loans is usually a pledge of the revenues of the facility seeking the loan, plus a first mortgage on the assets of the facility. If the tax revenue of a government entity is also pledged, the bonds are referred to as "general obligation bonds." Because of the income tax exemption, the interest rates on a tax exempt bond are usually 1½ to 2 percent lower than other sources of financing.

Most tax exempt revenue bonds are issued by a state or local authority. The health care facility then enters into a lease arrangement with the authority. Title to the assets remains with the authority until the indebtedness is repaid.

FHA-Insured Mortgages

FHA-insured mortgages are sponsored by the Federal Housing Administration, but initial processing begins in the Department of Health and Human Services. Through the FHA program, the government provides mortgage insurance for both proprietary and nonproprietary hospitals. This guarantee reduces the risk of a loan to investors and thus lowers the interest rate that a hospital must pay. However, obtaining the appropriate approvals can often be a time-consuming process.

Table 14–5 Comparative Analysis: Long-Term Debt Alternatives for Hospitals

Program Characteristics	Conventional Mortgage	Taxable Bonds	Tax Exempt Bonds	FHA-Insured Mortgage (GNMA Guarantee)
Security	First mortgage given to lender; pledge of gross revenues (substantially all hospital assets pledged)	First mortgage given to trustee bank for benefit of bondholder; pledge of gross revenue (substantially all assets pledged)	First mortgage given to trustee bank for benefit of bondholders; pledge of gross revenue (substantially all assets pledged)	First mortgage given to FHA-approved mortgagee for benefit of HUD; pledge of gross revenue (substantially all assets pledged)
Timing for alternative financing available	1 to 6 months	4 to 8 months	3 to 6 months	6 to 12 months
Percentage financing available	Usually 70-75% of eligible assets available to be pledged (as determined by appraisal)	Up to 100%, limited by available cash flow and available assets in some cases	Up to 100%, subject to available cash flow	
Construction financing	Normally required	Optional	Not required	Not required
Financing costs	Covers all costs of assets, excluding some movable equipment	Covers all costs	Covers all costs	Covers all costs, including start-up costs
Term of financing	15 to 20 years	15 to 20 years (occasionally with balloon payment based on longer amortization)	30 to 35 years common	25 years subsequent to construction completion.
Front end fees	1% to 2% commitment fee subject to amount financed; other fees $5-$25,000	1% underwriting (private placement) or 2%-4% underwriting (public offering); other expenses approximately ½ of 1% plus feasibility study	1% underwriting (private placement) or 2% to 3.5% underwriting (public offering); other expenses approximate ½ of 1% plus feasibility study	1% placement fee, 0.8% filing fee, 0.5% insurance (FHA) fee, 0.25% GNMA fee
Continuing annual fees	⅛ of 1% servicing if multiple lenders	Trustee fees (nominal)	Trustee fees (nominal)	0.5% FHA insurance fee; 0.25% GNMA fee
Prepayment provisions	Normally 10 year, no prepayment; 5% penalty descending thereafter	Normally 5 year and prepayment; no penalty unless refinancing	10 year, no prepayment; 3% penalty descending thereafter	15% of loan may be prepaid each year; 3% penalty over 15% declining by ⅛ of 1% each year
Required reserves	Usually none. Depreciation reserve optional	None	Debt service reserve equal to one year's P & I; depreciation reserve equal to deficiency amount	Usually none
Restriction on leasing	Yes. Subject to cash flow levels by covenant	None	None	None
Additional parity financing	Yes. Normally subject to lender approval	Yes. Subject to approval of underwriter or to provisions of financing agreement; normally required coverage of 110% to 150%	Yes. Subject to meeting coverage requirement of 110% to 150% on both historical & pro forma basis	Yes. Only with FHA-compatible program
Payment	Monthly	Semiannually	Quarterly/semiannually	Monthly
Reporting	Lender(s) only	Lender(s) or bond trustee and underwriter as appropriate, and rating agencies	Bond trustee, underwriter, and rating agencies as appropriate	HUD and mortgagee

Public Taxable Bonds

Public taxable bonds are issued in much the same way as tax exempt revenue bonds, except that there is no issuing authority and no interest income tax exemption. An investment banking firm usually underwrites the loan and markets the issue to individual investors. Interest rates are thus higher on this type of financing than they are on a tax exempt issue.

Conventional Mortgage Financing

Conventional mortgage financing is usually privately placed with a bank, pension fund, savings and loan institution, life insurance company, or real estate investment trust. This source of financing can be quickly arranged, but, compared with other alternatives, it does not provide as large a percentage of the total financing requirements for large projects. Thus, greater amounts of equity must be contributed.

Parties Involved

Figure 14–5 is a schematic representation of the parties involved and their relationships in issuing a public tax exempt revenue bond. This schematic could also be used to illustrate the process of issuing a public taxable bond. The only change would be the deletion of the issuing authority and addition of a line showing the direct issuance of the bonds by the health care facility. The specific parties in a bond financing include the following:

- issuing authority
- investment banker
- health care facility
- market
- trustee bank
- feasibility consultant
- legal counsel
- bond-rating agency

Issuing Authority

The issuing authority is involved only in tax exempt financing. In most cases, the issuing authority is some state or local governmental authority,

Figure 14–5 Parties Involved in a Public Tax Exempt Revenue Bond Issue

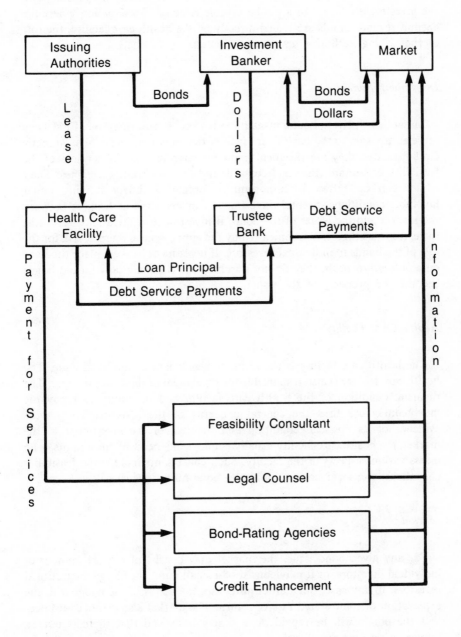

which may be specially created for the sole purpose of issuing revenue bonds. The issuing authority serves as a conduit between the health care facility and the investment banker. In a public taxable issue or in a situation where tax exempt revenue bonds are issued directly by the health care facility, the role of the issuing authority may be eliminated.

Investment Banker

In public or private issues, investment bankers have a dual role. First, they serve as advisors to the health care facility that is issuing the bonds. In many circumstances, they are the focal point for coordinating the services of the feasibility consultant, the legal counsel, and the bond-rating agencies. Their advice can be extremely important in obtaining timely funding under favorable conditions. Second, investment bankers serve as brokers between the market and the issuer of the bond. If investment bankers underwrite the issue, it means that they technically buy the entire issue and are at risk for the sale of the bonds to individual investors. If investment bankers place the issue on a *best efforts basis*, they do not purchase the issue, and any unsold bonds become the property of the issuer.

Health Care Facility

The health care facility is the ultimate beneficiary of the bond issue. The health care facility is also responsible for repayment of the loan principal. The financial condition of the health care facility and its ability to repay the indebtedness are thus the central concerns of the investor. To provide evidence of its financial condition and the risk of the investment to the market, the health care facility usually employs independent consultants, who assess various aspects of the facility. Such consultants include the feasibility consultant, the legal counsel, and the bond-rating agencies.

Market

For any given bond issue, the market may consist of a large number of individual investors, or it may consist of a small number of large institutional investors. In any case, the market purchases the bonds of the issuer with the expectation of some stated rate of return. The market also wants assurances that the bonds will be repaid on a timely basis and that there is not an unreasonable amount of risk.

Trustee Bank

A trustee bank serves as the market's agent once the bonds are sold. Typically, the trustee bank is a commercial bank, in some cases the same bank at which the health care facility has its accounts. The trustee bank may receive the proceeds from the sale of the bond issue and deliver the monies directly to the hospital or to the contractor, as required. The trustee bank also receives the debt service payments from the health care facility and distributes these to the market or investors. It may retire outstanding bonds according to a prearranged schedule of retirement and hold additional reserve requirements deposited by the health care facility. Finally, the trustee bank ensures that the health care facility is adhering to the provisions of the bond contract or indenture, such as those concerning adequate debt service coverage and working capital positions.

Feasibility Consultant

The feasibility consultant is usually an independent CPA who may or may not be the health care facility's outside auditor. The feasibility consultant's primary function is to assess the financial feasibility of the project and the ability of the health care facility to meet the associated indebtedness. Financial projections are usually made for a five-year period. These projections provide a basis for the investor and the bond-rating agency to assess the risk of default.

Legal Counsel

Legal counsel is needed for several reasons. First, in a tax exempt revenue bond issue, the market is concerned with the legality of the tax exemption. If the interest payments are not determined to be tax exempt by the Internal Revenue Service, the investors will suffer a significant loss. Second, legal opinion is necessary to ensure that the security pledged by the health care facility, whether it be revenue or assets, is legal and enforceable.

Bond-Rating Agencies

Moody's and Standard & Poor's are the two primary bond-rating agencies, although other smaller ones exist. Their function is to assess the relative risk associated with a given bond issue. The two agencies have developed detailed coding systems to assess risk (see Table 14–6). The resulting bond rating has important implications. First, there is a definite correlation between the interest rate that an issuer must pay and the bond rating associated with the issue. Generally speaking, the higher the bond rating, the lower the interest rate. Thus, a bond rated AAA by Standard & Poor's would be likely to have a much lower rate of interest than one rated BBB. Second, issues rated below BBB by Standard & Poor's or Baa by Moody's are not classified as investment grade. Many institutional investors are prohibited from investing in bonds that carry a rating lower than investment grade. Thus, the market for such issues is likely to be thin.

Credit Enhancement

Credit enhancement is a term that has only recently come into use in the health care financing field. A credit enhancement device is simply a mechanism by which the risk of default can be shifted from the issuer to a third party. Thus, the FHA-insured mortgage program provides a form of credit enhancement.

Aside from the FHA program, two basic types of credit enhancement are commonly used. The first type is municipal bond insurance. Municipal bond insurance is a surety bond that ensures that the debt service will be repaid. When municipal bond insurance is used, the credit rating for the issue becomes the credit rating of the insurance firm that is writing the insurance. In most cases, this means that the bond rating would be AAA or Aaa. Table 14–7 presents a summary of the major firms that currently provide municipal bond insurance and gives some idea of the relative cost of such insurance.

The second form of credit enhancement is a letter of credit. A letter of credit, usually issued by a commercial bank, provides a formal assurance that

Table 14–6 Bond Ratings

Classification	Moody's	Standard & Poor's
Investment	Aaa	AAA
Grade	Aa	AA
	Al	A+
	A	A
	Baal	BBB+
	Baa	BBB
Not Investment	Ba	BB
Grade	B	B
	Caa	CCC
	Ca	CC
	C	C

Table 14–7 Municipal Bond Insurers

Insurer	Types of Issues	Rating	Premiums	Principal & Interest Insured (all types of issues)	Principal & Interest Insured (health care issues)
AMBAC Indemnity Corp. (1971)	New Issue GOs, tax & revenue anticipation notes, some IDBs	AAA	.5% to 1.25%	$59.1 billion	$2.2 billion
MBIA (1974)	New Issue GOs, utility issues, commercial paper, notes, hospital bonds, unit investment trusts, debt service reserve fund replacement	AAA Aaa	.65% to 1.1%	$39.9 billion	$846 billion
HIBI (1983) (Industrial Indemnity Co.)	Health & Hospital Issues	AAA	.75% to 1.35%	$2.4 billion	$2.4 billion
FGIC (1983)	GOs, revenue bonds, unit investment trusts, industrial pollution control, and lease revenue bonds	AAA	.3% to 1.5%	$4.5 billion	$20 million
Bond Investors Guaranty Insurance Co. (1984)	New Issue GOs, revenue bonds, notes, unit investment trusts, mutual funds, bond portfolios	(Too new to provide detailed information)			

Source: Reprinted from *Hospital Bottom Line*, Vol. 110, November 1984. Published by Hospital Bottom Line, Inc. Columbus, Ohio.

a specified sum of money will be available over some defined time period. Usually the time period matches the maturity of the debt, and the amount provided in the letter of credit corresponds to the amount of indebtedness. As with bond insurance, the credit rating of the bank would be substituted for the credit rating of the issuer. In most situations, this would mean an automatic AAA or Aaa rating. The bank requires a fee for providing the letter of credit, and the issuer must determine if the cost of the letter of credit exceeds any possible savings in reduced interest expense that would result from an improved bond rating.

NEW DEVELOPMENTS

Three recent modifications in the traditional sources of long-term debt should be noted at this juncture:

1. variable rate financing
2. pooled or shared financing
3. zero coupon/original issue discount bonds

Variable Rate Financing

Recently, in the health care sector as well as in other industries, there has been a shift to the use of variable rate financing. In variable rate financing, the outstanding debt principal is fixed, but the interest rate on the principal is variable. This contrasts with the traditional situation in which the interest rate is fixed for the life of the bonds. Variable rate financing requires that the interest rate be adjusted periodically, weekly in some cases, to a current market index.

A feature that is often associated with variable rate financing is the use of a tender option or put. A tender option or put permits investors to redeem their bonds at some predetermined interval, perhaps daily, at the face value. In reality, this type of financing is short-term, not long-term. As a result, the interest rate may be significantly below a comparable long-term rate at the initiation of the financing. Many firms—not just health care firms—have opted to use variable rate financing to achieve a lower cost of financing. Sometimes this strategy is referred to as "moving down the yield curve." Figure 14–6 shows a typical upward-sloping yield curve.

Pooled Financing

In the health care sector, there has been increasing interest in developing financing packages that encompass more than one entity. The major rationale for this interest lies in the relationship between size and cost of debt; larger organizations are better able to obtain debt capital and to realize lower costs of financing.

In general, there are three ways that pooled or shared arrangements have been created in the health care sector. The first is through the use of master

Figure 14-6 The Yield Curve

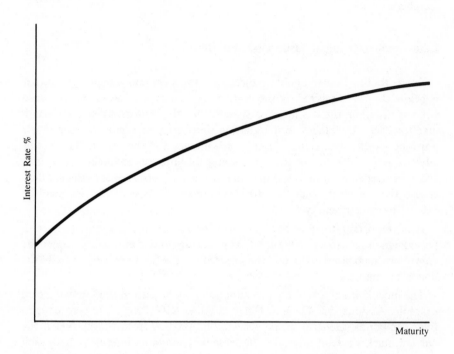

indenture financing by health care systems. In such cases, the master indenture financing means that the debt is guaranteed by all the members who are a part of the master indenture. For example, a system of ten hospitals could finance through some master indenture arrangement in which all ten hospitals, or some subset of the ten hospitals, would be a party to the financing.

A second alternative is the use of pooled equipment financing programs. These programs are often sponsored by the state hospital association or some regional association. Individual hospitals are a party to the financing and can obtain funds from the pool. The interest rate is usually much lower because the risk is spread across several hospitals.

The third alternative is an arrangement similar to the above except that the sponsor is different. Here, the pooled approach is used either for equipment needs or, in some cases, for major building programs. The issuer and sponsor of the pool is not the state or regional association, however, but some voluntary association of health care entities. The Voluntary Hospitals of America (VHA) have created such pooled financings for their members, and other associations are rapidly developing similar financing programs for their members.

Zero Coupon/Original Issue Discount Bonds

Bonds that are issued at a deep discount have a coupon rate of interest that is below the rate required by the market for that type of security. In a zero coupon situation, there is no interest paid, thus the term *zero coupon*. Certain investors see advantages in purchasing zero coupon bonds to meet their portfolio needs. There may also be advantages for the issuer. The major advantage for the issuer is in the delay of interest payments. This can conserve needed cash flow and may match the cash needs of the issuer. There is also the possibility that the after-reimbursement cost of the debt will be below the investment yield.

It is important to note that, in most zero coupon situations, there is a periodic payment to a sinking fund. The sinking fund is an account under the control of the bond trustee, and the proceeds of the fund are used to retire the bonds at maturity.

The mechanics of a zero coupon situation may be seen in the following case example. Assume that General Hospital issues $100,000,000 in zero coupon five-year bonds. General would receive $62,100,000 from the market if the current market rate of interest is 10 percent. Though no interest is paid, each year an amount is recorded for interest expense. This amount is an amortization of the difference between the face value of the bonds ($100,000,000) and the actual cash received ($62,100,000). Thus, during the five-year period, $37,900,000 will be recognized as interest expense. General will also be required to make semi-annual payments of $7,586,793 to a sinking fund. This fund is assumed to earn interest at 12 percent annually or 6 percent semi-annually. Assume also that equal amounts of the total discount will be recognized as interest expense each year. This would amount to $7,580,000. The Table 14–8 calculation shows the net present value cost of this financing, assuming that 50 percent of capital costs are reimbursed and that the appropriate discount rate for the hospital is its investment yield of 12 percent.

The net present value cost of General's financing is $42,175,850, which is significantly less than the $62,100,000 that the hospital will receive. The sinking fund is not recognized as a capital expense item, which explains why the before- and after-reimbursement amounts are the same. The annual amortization of the discount, which is recognized by third party payers as a reimbursable capital item, reduces the cost of the financing significantly. In some cases, this pattern of amortization may not be permitted by the payers.

Table 14–8 Net Present Value of Zero Coupon Financing

Item	Amount Before Reimbursement	Amount After Reimbursement	Years (Periods)	Present Value Factor (12%)	Present Value
Sinking fund	$7,586,793	$7,586,793	1–10[a]	7.360[a]	$55,838,800
Interest expense (amortization)	(7,580,000)	(3,790,000)	1–5	3.605	(13,662,950)
			Net present value cost		$42,175,850

[a] Ten semi-annual payments; the present value factor is for ten periods at 6%.

Instead, the payer may require a type of payment called effective yield. This type of payment requires that the same total amount of interest expense be recorded over the five years ($37,900,000), but the amounts in the earlier years would be less. This would reduce the present value of the benefit somewhat.

EARLY RETIREMENT OF DEBT

In many cases, an issuer would like to retire an existing debt issue prior to its maturity. There are a variety of reasons for wanting to do this. One important reason is that it permits the issuer to take advantage of a reduction in interest rates. An issue may have been marketed several years ago when interest rates were 14 percent, and rates may now have dropped to 9 percent. If the present lower interest rate could be substituted for the original rate, a major improvement in net income could result. Other reasons for wishing to retire an existing indebtedness might be that it would enable the issuer to avoid onerous covenants in the existing indenture or to take advantage of changes in bond ratings or changes in policy regarding tax exempt financing. Whatever the reason, most health care issues in fact do not remain outstanding for their full life cycle; most are retired early.

Two common ways of retiring an issue early are (1) refinancing and (2) refunding. In a refinancing, the issuer buys back the outstanding bonds from the investors. This can be accomplished in either of two ways. In the first way, the issuer may have the option of an early call. If the outstanding bonds are callable, the issuer would notify the present bondholders that the bonds are being called and should be tendered for payment. The principal or face value would then be paid, along with any call premium plus accrued interest. A second way to effect a refinancing would be for the issuer to buy back the bonds in open market transactions or to send a letter to existing bondholders, offering to buy the bonds at some stated price.

Early retirement of existing bonds can also be accomplished through refunding. In a refunding, the outstanding bonds are not acquired by the issuer and the present bondholders continue to maintain their investment. Though the refunding does not actually retire the bonds, they are not shown on the issuer's financial statements, and the covenants present in the indenture are now voided. The process of voiding existing indenture covenants and removing the bonds from the issuer's financial statements is called defeasance. In effect, defeasance in a refunding involves the deposit of a sum of money with the bond trustee, which is then used to buy specially designated securities of the federal government. With these securities, there is a guarantee that all future interest and principal payments can be met from the proceeds controlled by the bond trustee.

Here is a simple example to illustrate the refunding process: On January 1, 1984, $1 million of 15 percent level debt service bonds are issued. The bonds have a five-year life. The earliest call date is January 1, 1986. No call premium is involved. On January 1, 1985, interest rates have dropped to 7 percent, and management advance-refunds the January 1, 1984, issue. In this example, the original January 1, 1984, issue would have the following debt service schedule:

Date	Interest	Principal	Total Debt Service	Ending Debt Principal
Jan. 1, 1985	$150,000	$148,320	$298,320	$851,680
Jan. 1, 1986	127,750	170,570	298,320	681,110
Jan. 1, 1987	102,170	196,150	298,320	484,960
Jan. 1, 1988	72,740	225,580	298,320	259,380
Jan. 1, 1989	38,940	259,380	298,320	0

To retire or advance-refund the issue on January 1, 1985, management must place on deposit with a trustee a sum of money that will guarantee payment of the following amounts on January 1, 1986, (the earliest call date):

Interest due Jan. 1, 1986	$127,750
Debt principal due Jan. 1, 1986	170,570
Ending debt principal on Jan. 1, 1986	681,110
	$979,430

If management borrows all the funds necessary to meet the $979,430 payment on January 1, 1986, how much must it borrow on January 1, 1985? Ignoring placement fees and other debt issuance costs, the hospital would borrow $915,360. Why $915,360? It is assumed that the hospital will be able to invest the proceeds at seven percent, the effective interest rate on January 1, 1985. In tax exempt issues, an arbitrage restriction limits investment yields for all practical purposes to the interest rate of the refunding issue.

Is there any real savings in debt service costs? Yes; the following new issue schedule shows annual savings of $28,080 ($298,320 − $270,240) for the next four years:

Date	Interest	Principal	Total Debt Service	Ending Debt	Savings in Debt Service
Jan. 1, 1986	$64,080	$206,160	$270,240	$709,200	$28,080
Jan. 1, 1987	49,640	220,600	270,240	488,600	28,080
Jan. 1, 1988	34,200	236,040	270,240	252,560	28,080
Jan. 1, 1989	17,680	252,560	270,240	0	28,080

Thus far, the refinancing looks good. However, there is an accounting loss that must be recorded. At the end of the first year (January 1, 1985), the value for the old debt, $851,680, will be removed from the balance sheet. But the defeased debt will be replaced by $915,360 of new debt, and this will reduce income in that year by $63,680 ($915,360 − $851,680). This will be treated as an extraordinary loss in the period in which refunding takes place.

A real world case may make the magnitude of these numbers more apparent. A hospital recently refunded $65 million of two-year-old debt with $79 million of new debt at a lower effective interest rate. Estimated savings in debt service over the life of the issue were $22 million, but there was an accounting loss of approximately $13 million in the initial year. More importantly, this loss reduced the hospital's ratio of equity to assets from 26 percent to 16 percent. This is a rather sizable reduction that could have some impact on future credit availability. Many lenders establish target equity-to-debt ratios beyond which they will not lend funds at reasonable interest rates.

In sum, refunding to take advantage of reduced interest rates usually makes a lot of economic sense. But, the presence of an accounting loss should be considered, especially in light of its potential impact on future credit availability.

SUMMARY

The major sources of capital financing available to health care firms may be categorized as (1) equity and (2) debt. Equity has become an important source of capital, even for traditional tax exempt health care firms. Corporate restructuring can greatly facilitate the process of accessing equity capital. However, long-term debt will probably continue to represent the major source of capital for most health care firms. Evaluation of alternative sources of long-term debt requires more than a simple comparison of interest rates. The impact of other factors should also be carefully reviewed to determine the overall attractiveness of alternative financing packages.

ASSIGNMENTS

1. Explain the term *defeasance.* What does it mean?
2. Assuming a normal or typical yield curve (that is, upward-sloping), discuss the advantages and disadvantages of borrowing money for a major construction program with three-year term financing.
3. When is a master trust indenture used, and what is its value?
4. In what circumstances might your hospital be interested in issuing zero coupon bonds?
5. In an advance refunding of debt, accounting gains or losses usually occur. Under what conditions could there be an accounting gain?
6. United Hospital has received a leasing proposal from Leasing, Inc., for a Siemens cardiac catheterization unit. The terms are:

   • five-year lease
   • annual payments of $200,000 payable one year in advance
   • payment of property tax, estimated to be $23,000 annually
   • renewal at end of Year 5 at fair market value

   Alternatively, United can buy the catheterization unit for $725,000. United must debt-finance this equipment. It anticipates a bank loan with an initial down payment of $125,000 and a three-year term loan at 16 percent with equal principal payments. The residual value of the equipment at Year 5 is estimated to be $225,000. The lease is treated as an operating lease. Depreciation is calculated on a straight-line basis. Assuming a discount rate of 14 percent, what financing option should United select? Assume that there is no reimbursement of capital costs.

7. Nutty Hospital wishes to advance-refund its existing 15 percent long-term debt. The present $30,000,000 is not callable until five years from today. The payout on the issue over the next five years is as follows:

	Interest	Principal	Total
End of Year 1	$4,500,000	$1,000,000	$5,500,000
End of Year 2	4,350,000	1,000,000	5,350,000
End of Year 3	4,200,000	1,000,000	5,200,000
End of Year 4	4,050,000	1,000,000	5,050,000
End of Year 5	3,900,000	1,000,000	4,900,000

   At the end of the fifth year, the debt ($25,000,000 outstanding balance at that time) may be called with a 10 percent penalty. If present interest rates are 10 percent and the investment rate on the funds to be received from the new issue cannot exceed 10 percent, what amount must Nutty Hospital borrow today? Assume that underwriting fees and other issuance costs will be 5 percent of the issue and that all debt service on the old issue must be met from the proceeds of the refunding issue and related investment income.

8. You have the option of leasing an asset for $100,000 per year, with payments to be made at the end of each year of use. This is a noncancelable lease. Alternatively, you may buy the

asset for $248,700. For reimbursement purposes, the lease must be capitalized. If the asset is purchased, it will be debt-financed with $210,000 of three-year serial notes (that is, $70,000 of principal will be repaid each year). The effective interest rate on this loan will be 8 percent. Assume that the asset has an allowable useful life of three years with no estimated salvage value.

Assignment:

- Determine the amount of expense that would be reported in each of the three years under the two financing plans.
- Assuming that 80 percent of all reported capital expenses are reimbursed and that the discount rate is 6 percent, determine the present value of the asset in these two methods of financing.

9. Happy Valley Hospital is considering moving from its present 200-bed facility and constructing a new facility. Estimated construction cost for the new facility is $20 million. The hospital has virtually no internally generated funds available and is considering financing the construction project with a 20-year first mortgage.

Approximately 80 percent or $16 million of the construction cost is in bricks and mortar and fixed equipment. For reimbursement purposes, the average allowed depreciable life is 40 years. The remaining $4 million in cost is for major movable equipment with an average depreciable life of 10 years.

The 20-year first mortgage bonds can be marketed at an expected yield rate of 12 percent, given current money market conditions. The issue is to be repaid over the 20-year life with equal yearly principal payments of $1,000,000. Thus, interest expense for the issue will be decreased each year by $120,000 ($2,400,000 in Year 1, $2,280,000 in Year 2, $2,160,000 in Year 3, and so on.). Assume that the $4 million in equipment will need to be replaced in 10 years at an estimated cost of $10 million and that the $16 million in plant will need replacement in 40 years at an estimated cost of $724 million (inflation factor of 10 percent for both components).

The patient mix at Happy Valley is approximately 90 percent Blue Cross, Medicare, and Medicaid patients, with the remaining 10 percent self-pay. There is no other significant third party payer. Because Happy Valley is located in a rural, economically depressed area, the number of bad debts is extremely high—20 percent of self-pay charges. Blue Cross and Medicaid reimbursement formulas are identical to those of Medicare. Assume for the purposes of this problem that these three payers pay average cost, both operating and capital.

Happy Valley currently operates at a 90 percent occupancy ratio (180 patients per day) and expects this to remain constant for the next 20 years. It is the only provider of hospital services in its area. Average operating costs in the new facility, excluding depreciation and interest, will be $110 per day in the first year of operation. Expectations are that this will increase by $10/patient day per year for the next 10 years, reaching $200/patient day in Year 10. Assume no existing depreciation or interest charges.

Assignment:

- Assuming that Happy Valley intends to break even on a cash flow basis over the coming five-year period, what charge per day must it set for each of the next five years to break even?
- What impact would the provision for an investment fund have on the per diem charge to self-pay patients over the five-year period? Assume Happy Valley can net 8 percent on its investments and wants to establish a fund that will be of sufficient size to meet the replacement costs in Years 10 and 40. Further assume that, after an analysis of the hospital's credit position, it is expected that no more than 50 percent of the 10th year's replacement cost and no more than 80 percent of the 40th year's replacement cost may be

debt-financed. What annual amount must be deposited to meet these expected replacement costs, and what impact will that have on the per diem charge to self-pay patients? (Incorporate the 20 percent bad debt write-off.)

10. Mayberry Hospital is considering a joint-venture relationship with your physicians to acquire a full-body CAT scanner. Projected revenues and expenses for the scanner are presented below:

	Year 1	Year 2	Year 3	Year 4	Year 5
Revenues	$521,000	$531,000	$542,000	$533,000	$564,000
Less bad debts and discounts	52,100	53,100	54,200	53,300	56,400
Net revenues	468,900	477,900	487,800	479,700	507,600
Expenses					
Wages and employee benefits	60,000	63,000	66,150	69,458	72,930
Maintenance	55,000	57,750	60,638	63,669	66,853
Supplies	20,000	21,000	22,050	23,153	24,310
Rent	18,000	18,900	19,845	20,837	21,879
Administrative	10,000	10,500	11,025	11,576	12,155
Utilities	5,000	5,250	5,513	5,788	6,078
Insurance	5,000	5,250	5,513	5,788	6,078
Taxes	10,000	10,000	10,000	10,000	10,000
Depreciation	94,050	137,940	131,670	131,670	131,670
Interest	40,620	33,384	25,271	16,176	5,977
Total expenses	317,670	362,974	357,675	358,115	357,930
Net income before tax or interest	$151,230	$114,926	$130,125	$121,585	$149,670

The scanner is expected to cost $627,000 and have a useful life of five years. Two possible financing plans have been proposed. The first plan would be a limited partnership arrangement. There would be 34 shares; 33 would be sold to physicians for $19,000 apiece. The 34th would be retained by the hospital for its development effort. In the second financing plan, a $380,000 level debt service plan with a five-year maturity and interest at 10 percent would be arranged. The remainder of the funding would be generated through the sale of 33 limited partnership shares at $7,500 per share. Again, a 34th share would be issued to the hospital for its development efforts. Assuming that an investment tax credit of 10 percent would be available to the partners and that a 50 percent marginal tax rate will exist, project cash flow per partnership unit under each financing alternative for each of the five years.

SOLUTIONS AND ANSWERS

1. Defeasance means that, upon final payment of all interest and principal, the rights of the bond trustee cease to exist, that is, they are defeased. The security covenants in an indenture may also be satisfied through the creation of a trust (escrow) in which sufficient monies are held to guarantee payment at some future date. Defeasance means that the issue defeased is no longer an obligation of the issuer and can be removed from the issuer's books.

2. The typical, upward-sloping yield curve implies that a 3-year interest rate will probably be much lower than a 20- to 25-year rate. Therefore, cost will be lower with a 3-year construction loan. At the end of the third year, however, permanent financing must be

sought. And there is no guarantee that interest rates will not have increased during the period or that financing will be available at the end of the third year.

3. A master trust indenture usually pledges the assets and revenues of several firms in a combined financing package. It is often used by health care systems to gain better access to capital and lower interest rates.

4. Zero coupon bonds are especially desirable if the issuer's effective interest rate on the bonds is well below the yield or discount rate of the issuer. In a zero coupon bond issue, the postponement of interest payment maximizes the possibility for additional arbitrage, that is, for investing at a yield greater than the cost of funds.

5. Accounting gains usually take place when the advance-refunding issue has a higher rate of interest than the refunded issue. Accounting losses often occur when the reverse is true.

6. United Hospital's financing options for the cardiac catheterization unit are detailed below:

Item	Amount Before Reimbursement	Amount After Reimbursement	Years	Present Value Factor (14%)	Present Value
Lease					
Rent	$200,000	$200,000	0	1.000	$200,000
Rent	200,000	200,000	1–4	2.914	582,800
Property tax[a]	23,000	23,000	1–5	3.433	78,959
			Net present value cost of lease		$861,759
Purchase					
Down payment	$125,000	$125,000	0	1.000	$125,000
Principal	200,000	200,000	1–3	2.322	464,400
Interest	96,000	96,000	1	.877	84,192
Interest	64,000	64,000	2	.769	49,216
Interest	32,000	32,000	3	.675	21,600
Salvage	(225,000)	(225,000)	5	.519	(116,775)
			Net present value of purchase		$627,633

[a] Property tax would be passed on to the lessee. There is no property tax of purchase because the hospital is a tax exempt firm.

From the above data, it can be seen that purchase of the catheterization unit would produce a lower net present value cost, compared with a lease.

7. Nutty Hospital's present borrowing needs are detailed below:

Item	Amount Required	Years	Present Value Factor (10%)	Present Value
Debt service–Year 1	$ 5,500,000	1	.909	$ 4,999,500
Debt service–Year 2	5,350,000	2	.826	4,419,100
Debt service–Year 3	5,200,000	3	.751	3,905,200
Debt service–Year 4	5,050,000	4	.683	3,449,150
Debt service–Year 5	4,900,000	5	.621	3,042,900
Principal at Year 5	25,000,000	5	.621	15,525,000
Call premium	2,500,000	5	.621	1,552,500
			Net present value	$36,893,350

$$\text{Amount borrowed} = \frac{\$36,893,350}{.95} = \$38,835,105$$

8. The following data show the comparative expense and present values for leasing versus debt-financing the asset over the three-year period:

• Expenses for Lease

Interest rate = 10%

$248,700 = \$100,000 \times P\ (i,3)$

$P\ (i,3) = 2.487$

• Interest expense per year:

Year	Beginning Principal	Interest (at 10%)	Reduction in Principal	Total
1	$248,700	$24,870	$ 75,130	$100,000
2	173,570	17,357	82,643	100,000
3	90,927	9,073[a]	90,927	100,000
		$51,300	$248,700	$300,000

[a] Last year's interest is derived by subtracting the principal payment of $90,927 from the total payment of $100,000.

• Depreciation expense per year: $248,700/3 = \$82,900$

• Expenses for debt financing

Interest expense per year:

Year	Interest
1	$.08 \times 210,000 = \$16,800$
2	$.08 \times 140,000 = 11,200$
3	$.08 \times 70,000 = 5,600$

Depreciation expense per year: $82,900

• Comparison of expenses

	Lease Alternative			Debt Alternative		
Year	Interest	Depreciation	Total	Interest	Depreciation	Total
1	$24,870	$ 82,900	$107,770	$16,800	$ 82,900	$ 99,700
2	17,357	82,900	100,257	11,200	82,900	94,100
3	9,073	82,900	91,973	5,600	82,900	88,500
Totals	$51,300	$248,700	$300,000	$33,600	$248,700	$282,300

- Comparison of cash flows—present value basis

Item	Amount Before Reimbursement	Amount After Reimbursement	Years	Present Value Factor (6%)	Present Value
		Lease Financing			
Rentals	$100,000	$100,000	1–3	2.673	$267,300
Depreciation	(82,900)	(66,320)	1–3	2.673	(177,273)
Interest[a]	(24,870)	(19,896)	1	.943	(18,762)
Interest[a]	(17,357)	(13,886)	2	.890	(12,358)
Interest[a]	(9,073)	(7,258)	3	.840	(6,097)
		Net present value cost of lease			$ 52,810
		Debt Financing			
Down Payment	$38,700	38,700	0	1.000	$ 38,700
Principal payment	70,000	70,000	1–3	2.673	187,110
Depreciation	(82,900)	(66,320)	1–3	2.673	(177,273)
Interest	16,800	3,360	1	.943	3,168
Interest	11,200	2,240	2	.890	1,993
Interest	5,600	1,120	3	.840	941
		Net present value cost of debt			$ 54,639

[a]Interest is shown as a reduction of cost because the lease payment reflects the interest paid to the lessor. The interest deduction recognizes third party payments for interest expense.

9. The following data are relevant to a determination of (1) the charge per day Happy Valley Hospital must charge over the five-year period to break even and (2) the impact of the projected investment fund on annual deposits to meet replacement costs and on per diem charges to self-pay patients:

Year	Principal	Interest	Operating	Total Cash Outflow (Col. 2 + 3 + 4)	Depreciation	Reimbursable Cost (Col.3 + 4 + 6)	Reimbursed Cost (Col. 7×.90)	Net Cash Outflow (Col. 5–8)	Required[a] Charge/Day (Col. 9–5,256)	Additional[b] Refinancing Charge
1	$1,000,000	$2,400,000	$7,227,000	$10,627,000	$800,000	$10,427,000	$9,384,300	$1,242,700	$236.44	$171.91
2	1,000,000	2,280,000	7,884,000	11,164,000	800,000	10,964,000	9,867,600	1,296,400	246.65	171.91
3	1,000,000	2,160,000	8,541,000	11,701,000	800,000	11,501,000	10,350,900	1,350,100	256.87	171.91
4	1,000,000	2,040,000	9,198,000	12,238,000	800,000	12,038,000	10,834,200	1,403,800	267.09	171.91
5	1,000,000	1,920,000	9,855,000	12,775,000	800,000	12,575,000	11,317,500	1,457,500	277.30	171.91

[a] Required charge/day:
Number of paid charge days/year = .10 × .80 × 65,700 = 5,256.

[b] Refinancing charge—
Required annual deposit for equipment at Year 10:
Present value of equipment financing = $10,000,000 × .5 × .463 = $2,315,000.
Required deposit = $2,315,000/6.710 = $345,007.
Required annual deposit for replacement at Year 40:
Present value of plant financing = $724,000,000 × .2 × .046 = $6,660,800.
Required deposit = $6,660,800/11.925 = $558,558.

$$\text{Required additional charge/day} = \frac{(\$558,558 + \$345,007)}{5256} = \$171.91.$$

10. The following data show the project cash flow per partnership unit under the two financing alternatives in acquiring the CAT scanner:

- Alternative 1 — No debt

	Years				
	1	2	3	4	5
Income before tax and interest	$ 151,230	$ 114,926	$ 130,126	$ 121,585	$ 149,670
− Income tax	75,615	57,463	65,063	60,793	74,835
+ Investment tax	62,700				
Income after tax	$ 138,315	$ 57,463	$ 65,063	$ 60,793	$ 74,835
+ Depreciation	94,050	137,940	131,670	131,670	131,670
Cash flow	$ 232,365	$ 195,403	$ 196,733	$ 192,463	$ 206,505
Cash flow per share	$6,834.26	$5,747.15	$5,786.26	$5,660.67	$6,073.68
Percent return	36.0%	30.2%	30.5%	29.8%	32.0%

- Alternative 2 — Debt financing

	Years				
	1	2	3	4	5
Income before tax and interest	$ 151,230	$ 114,926	$ 130,126	$ 121,585	$ 149,670
−Interest	38,000	31,776	24,930	17,400	9,116
Taxable income	113,230	83,150	105,196	104,185	140,554
− Tax	56,615	41.575	52,598	52,093	70,277
+ Investment tax credit	$ 62,700				
Income after tax	$ 119,315	$ 41,575	$ 52,598	$ 52,092	$ 70,277
+ Depreciation	94,050	137,940	131,670	131,670	131,670
− Debt principal	62,237	68,461	75,307	82,837	91,158
Cash flow	$ 151,128	$ 111,054	$ 108,961	$ 100,925	$ 110,789
Cash flow per share	$4,444.94	$3,266.29	$3,204.74	$2,968.38	$3,258.50
Percent return	59.3%	43.6%	42.7%	39.6%	43.4%

Index

D